Immune Mechanisms and Biomarkers in Systemic Lupus Erythematosus

Immune Mechanisms and Biomarkers in Systemic Lupus Erythematosus

Guest Editors

Ioannis Parodis
Christopher Sjöwall

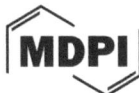

Basel • Beijing • Wuhan • Barcelona • Belgrade • Novi Sad • Cluj • Manchester

Guest Editors

Ioannis Parodis
Department of Medicine Solna
Karolinska Institutet
Stockholm
Sweden

Christopher Sjöwall
Biomedical and Clinical Sciences
Linköping University
Linköping
Sweden

Editorial Office
MDPI AG
Grosspeteranlage 5
4052 Basel, Switzerland

This is a reprint of the Special Issue, published open access by the journal *International Journal of Molecular Sciences* (ISSN 1422-0067), freely accessible at: www.mdpi.com/journal/ijms/special_issues/immune_sle.

For citation purposes, cite each article independently as indicated on the article page online and using the guide below:

Lastname, A.A.; Lastname, B.B. Article Title. *Journal Name* **Year**, *Volume Number*, Page Range.

ISBN 978-3-7258-2594-3 (Hbk)
ISBN 978-3-7258-2593-6 (PDF)
https://doi.org/10.3390/books978-3-7258-2593-6

© 2024 by the authors. Articles in this book are Open Access and distributed under the Creative Commons Attribution (CC BY) license. The book as a whole is distributed by MDPI under the terms and conditions of the Creative Commons Attribution-NonCommercial-NoDerivs (CC BY-NC-ND) license (https://creativecommons.org/licenses/by-nc-nd/4.0/).

Contents

About the Editors . . . . **vii**

Ioannis Parodis and Christopher Sjöwall
Immune Mechanisms and Biomarkers in Systemic Lupus Erythematosus
Reprinted from: *Int. J. Mol. Sci.* **2024**, *25*, 9965, https://doi.org/10.3390/ijms25189965 . . . . . . **1**

Fatima K. Alduraibi and George C. Tsokos
Lupus Nephritis Biomarkers: A Critical Review
Reprinted from: *Int. J. Mol. Sci.* **2024**, *25*, 805, https://doi.org/10.3390/ijms25020805 . . . . **6**

Matthieu Halfon, Aurel T. Tankeu and Camillo Ribi
Mitochondrial Dysfunction in Systemic Lupus Erythematosus with a Focus on Lupus Nephritis
Reprinted from: *Int. J. Mol. Sci.* **2024**, *25*, 6162, https://doi.org/10.3390/ijms25116162 . . . . . . **28**

Susannah von Hofsten, Kristin Andreassen Fenton and Hege Lynum Pedersen
Human and Murine Toll-like Receptor-Driven Disease in Systemic Lupus Erythematosus
Reprinted from: *Int. J. Mol. Sci.* **2024**, *25*, 5351, https://doi.org/10.3390/ijms25105351 . . . . . . **41**

Alessandra Maria Vitale, Letizia Paladino, Celeste Caruso Bavisotto, Rosario Barone, Francesca Rappa and Everly Conway de Macario et al.
Interplay between the Chaperone System and Gut Microbiota Dysbiosis in Systemic Lupus Erythematosus Pathogenesis: Is Molecular Mimicry the Missing Link between Those Two Factors?
Reprinted from: *Int. J. Mol. Sci.* **2024**, *25*, 5608, https://doi.org/10.3390/ijms25115608 . . . . . . **65**

Ioannis Parodis, Alvaro Gomez, Julius Lindblom, Jun Weng Chow, Christopher Sjöwall and Savino Sciascia et al.
B Cell Kinetics upon Therapy Commencement for Active Extrarenal Systemic Lupus Erythematosus in Relation to Development of Renal Flares: Results from Three Phase III Clinical Trials of Belimumab
Reprinted from: *Int. J. Mol. Sci.* **2022**, *23*, 13941, https://doi.org/10.3390/ijms232213941 . . . . . **77**

Bethany Wolf, Calvin R. K. Blaschke, Sandy Mungaray, Bryan T. Weselman, Mariia Stefanenko and Mykhailo Fedoriuk et al.
Metabolic Markers and Association of Biological Sex in Lupus Nephritis
Reprinted from: *Int. J. Mol. Sci.* **2023**, *24*, 16490, https://doi.org/10.3390/ijms242216490 . . . . . **94**

Lina Wirestam, Frida Jönsson, Helena Enocsson, Christina Svensson, Maria Weiner and Jonas Wetterö et al.
Limited Association between Antibodies to Oxidized Low-Density Lipoprotein and Vascular Affection in Patients with Established Systemic Lupus Erythematosus
Reprinted from: *Int. J. Mol. Sci.* **2023**, *24*, 8987, https://doi.org/10.3390/ijms24108987 . . . . . . **115**

Irene Carrión-Barberà, Laura Triginer, Laura Tío, Carolina Pérez-García, Anna Ribes and Victoria Abad et al.
Role of Advanced Glycation End Products as New Biomarkers in Systemic Lupus Erythematosus
Reprinted from: *Int. J. Mol. Sci.* **2024**, *25*, 3022, https://doi.org/10.3390/ijms25053022 . . . . . . **127**

Julia Mercader-Salvans, María García-González, Fuensanta Gómez-Bernal, Juan C. Quevedo-Abeledo, Antonia de Vera-González and Alejandra González-Delgado et al.
Relationship between Disease Characteristics and Circulating Interleukin 6 in a Well-Characterized Cohort of Patients with Systemic Lupus Erythematosus
Reprinted from: *Int. J. Mol. Sci.* **2023**, *24*, 14006, https://doi.org/10.3390/ijms241814006 . . . . . **143**

Agnieszka Winikajtis-Burzyńska, Marek Brzosko and Hanna Przepiera-Bedzak
Elevated Serum Levels of Soluble Transferrin Receptor Are Associated with an Increased Risk of Cardiovascular, Pulmonary, and Hematological Manifestations and a Decreased Risk of Neuropsychiatric Manifestations in Systemic Lupus Erythematosus Patients
Reprinted from: *Int. J. Mol. Sci.* **2023**, *24*, 17340, https://doi.org/10.3390/ijms242417340 . . . . . **157**

About the Editors

Ioannis Parodis

Ioannis Parodis graduated with a medical degree from the National and Kapodistrian University of Athens, Greece, in 2006. His academic and professional focus is in B cell biology and the development of novel treatments for systemic lupus erythematosus (SLE) and lupus nephritis. In February 2017, he completed his doctoral thesis titled "Systemic Lupus Erythematosus: Biomarkers and Biologics" at the Department of Medicine Solna, Karolinska Institutet, Stockholm, Sweden. His research has centered on identifying biomarkers and refining predictive models for diagnostics, therapeutic responses, and long-term prognosis in SLE and lupus nephritis.

Currently, he serves as a senior consultant rheumatologist at Karolinska University Hospital, Stockholm, Sweden, where he also holds leadership roles in medical education as a Director and examiner for clinical courses at Karolinska Institutet. Alongside his clinical and teaching responsibilities, Ioannis Parodis leads clinical and translational research in inflammation and autoimmunity at Karolinska Institutet. Since 2021, he has been affiliated with Örebro University, Sweden, where he continues to advance research efforts in the field of rheumatology.

Christopher Sjöwall

Christopher Sjöwall graduated with a medical degree from Linköping University, Sweden, in 2003. His academic and professional focus is in biomarkers and autoantibodies in systemic lupus erythematosus (SLE). In January 2006, he completed his doctoral thesis titled "C-reactive protein (CRP) and anti-CRP autoantibodies in Systemic Lupus Erythematosus" at the Department of Molecular and Clinical Medicine, Linköping University, Linköping, Sweden. His research has centered on identifying biomarkers and refining predictive models for diagnostics, therapeutic responses, and long-term prognosis in SLE and lupus nephritis.

Currently, he serves as a senior consultant rheumatologist and full professor at Linköping University, Linköping, Sweden.

Editorial

Immune Mechanisms and Biomarkers in Systemic Lupus Erythematosus

Ioannis Parodis [1,2,*] and Christopher Sjöwall [3]

1. Division of Rheumatology, Department of Medicine Solna, Karolinska Institutet and Karolinska University Hospital, SE-171 77 Stockholm, Sweden
2. Department of Rheumatology, Faculty of Medicine and Health, Örebro University, SE-701 82 Örebro, Sweden
3. Division of Inflammation and Infection/Rheumatology, Department of Biomedical and Clinical Sciences, Linköping University, SE-581 85 Linköping, Sweden; christopher.sjowall@liu.se
* Correspondence: ioannis.parodis@ki.se; Tel.: +46-722321322

The immense heterogeneity of the chronic, inflammatory, autoimmune disease systemic lupus erythematosus (SLE), both with regard to immunological aberrancies and clinical manifestations, poses diagnostic difficulties and challenges in the management of patients [1–3]. This is underlined by the lack of generally accepted diagnostic criteria and the numerous clinical trial failures. However, the treatment landscape has witnessed substantial changes during the last decade, facilitated by advances in biotechnology and hence new knowledge on the pathophysiology of SLE.

SLE predominantly affects women, with the onset of the disease typically occurring during their reproductive years. Early diagnosis and treatment initiation are important for the prevention of organ damage accrual [4]. The chronic nature of the disease and its varying course necessitate regular monitoring. The treatment of SLE mainly consists of antimalarial agents, glucocorticoids, non-biological immunosuppressants, and, more recently, biological agents, including B-cell-targeting therapies and a monoclonal antibody against the type I interferon receptor [5]. The recent approvals of new targeted therapies for SLE and lupus nephritis (LN), one of the most severe clinical manifestations of SLE [6], and the increasing awareness of the long-term adverse effects of glucocorticoids changed the focus of research towards the optimisation of therapeutic decision making, surveillance, and treatment evaluations, and technological advances paved the way for a cellular and molecular characterisation of SLE to serve as a basis for disease management [7,8]. In this context, identifying reliable biomarkers is imperative [9], and significant progress has been made in this area over the past few decades [10–12].

Historically, biomarker studies in SLE have focused on serum biomarkers [9,10,13,14]. Nevertheless, urinary, cerebrospinal fluid, and tissue biomarkers for organ-specific monitoring and prognostication are gaining increasing interest [12,15]. In this Special Issue titled "Immune Mechanisms and Biomarkers in Systemic Lupus Erythematosus", we welcomed original works and review articles focusing on the cellular and molecular mechanisms underlying SLE in its different phases, with the goal of contributing novel knowledge of the pathogenesis of SLE and improved diagnostics, surveillance, prevention of long-term damage, and overall patient management. We also welcomed original works or review articles that evaluated immune components that could serve as diagnostic biomarkers, biomarkers of disease activity, or biomarkers of long-term outcomes. We received several contributions, and we hereby summarise the final content of the Special Issue, which is also visually represented in Figure 1.

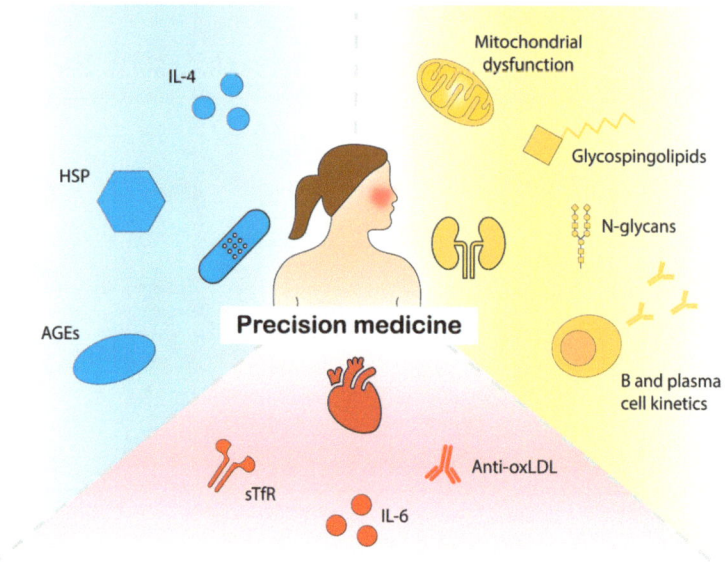

Figure 1. Visual representation of the content of the Special Issue. AGEs: advanced glycation end-products; anti-oxLDL: anti-oxidised low-density lipoprotein; HSP: heat shock protein; IL: interleukin; sTfR: soluble transferrin.

In a cross-sectional study by Irene Carrión-Barberà et al., levels of advanced glycation end-products (AGEs) were found to be significantly higher in SLE patients compared to healthy controls. AGEs showed positive associations with the degree of SLE activity using the SLE disease activity index (SLEDAI) and the degree of organ damage using the Systemic Lupus International Collaborating Clinics (SLICC)/American College of Rheumatology (ACR) damage index (SDI), as well as various clinical features, indicating some potential of AGEs as biomarkers of monitoring and prognosis in SLE [16]. In a study by Bethany Wolf et al., significant differences in urine glycosphingolipids and N-glycans were observed between LN patients and healthy controls, with men showing more pronounced differences [17].

In a cohort study by Agnieszka Winikajtis-Burzyńska et al., elevated serum levels of soluble transferrin receptor (sTfR) were linked to an increased risk of cardiovascular, pulmonary, and haematological manifestations of SLE, while elevated interleukin (IL)-4 levels were associated with a decreased risk of mucocutaneous manifestations, collectively suggesting that sTfR and IL-4 could be useful for differentiating the risk of affliction across organ systems in SLE [18]. In an observational study of 284 SLE patients, Julia Mercader-Salvans et al. found that circulating levels of IL-6 were associated with a higher cardiovascular risk and disruption of the complement system, but not with SLE disease activity or organ damage [19]. Contrary to some prior observations [20,21], a study by Lina Wirestam et al. found no strong association between anti-oxidised low-density lipoprotein (anti-oxLDL) antibodies and vascular affliction in SLE patients [22]. Although a significant correlation was observed with intima media thickness in the common femoral artery, the overall findings do not support anti-oxLDL antibodies as reliable biomarkers for vascular involvement in SLE.

Using data from multiple phase III clinical trials of belimumab, Ioannis Parodis et al. investigated the role of early alterations in circulating B cell and plasma cell subsets in relation to renal flares in SLE patients treated for active extra-renal disease with non-biological standard therapy plus belimumab or placebo. A rapid decrease in short-lived plasma cells or plasmablasts with a subsequent return was associated with renal flares.

Rapid decreases in transitional B cells and long-lived plasma cells upon belimumab therapy indicated greater protection against renal flares, which was not the case for the placebo-treated group of patients [23]. Collectively, B cell and plasma cell kinetics during the early phases of treatment with belimumab for active SLE might be useful early indicators of the need for therapeutic adjustments [24].

In a review by Matthieu Halfon et al., mitochondrial dysfunction was detailed as a significant factor in SLE pathogenesis, particularly in LN. Altered mitochondrial homeostasis and defective mitophagy appears to contribute to immune dysregulation, suggesting mitochondria as potential biomarkers and therapeutic targets in SLE and LN [25]. Based on the current literature, Alessandra Maria Vitale et al. proposed that molecular mimicry between human heat shock proteins (HSPs) belonging to the chaperone system and proteins and metabolites of gut commensal bacteria could link gut microbiota dysbiosis with SLE pathogenesis. The production of autoantibodies against HSPs, which are known to associate with SLE onset and progression, due to shared epitopes between human HSPs and those of gut commensal bacteria, may contribute to disease pathogenesis, warranting a coordinated study of these factors in SLE [26].

In a comprehensive review by Susannah von Hofsten et al., the roles of Toll-like receptors (TLRs) in SLE pathogenesis were discussed, particularly TLR7, TLR8, and TLR9. In brief, the authors detailed the link between the overexpression of TLR7 and SLE severity and further stated that TLR8 and TLR9 may regulate TLR7 activity, offering insights into potential therapeutic strategies targeting these receptors [27]. Last but not least, Fatima K. Alduraibi and George C. Tsokos provided a critical evaluation of biomarkers for LN. Despite improvements in kidney and patient survival, complete clinical and histological remission rates remain limited in LN, highlighting the need for the timely detection of kidney affliction due to SLE and the prompt initiation of therapy, as well as understanding of the specific attributes of proposed LN biomarkers, to further improve patient outcomes and guide disease management [28]. Importantly, despite advancements in biomarker research, kidney biopsy remains the gold standard for the determination of LN activity and the identification of histological features that dictate the pharmacotherapeutic need and guide management.

In summary, our Special Issue provides valuable insights into immune mechanisms and biomarkers relevant to SLE and LN, highlighting recent advancements in understanding the pathogenesis and improving diagnostics and patient management. The collected original works and reviews offer a comprehensive view of the potential biomarkers and therapeutic targets, paving the way for enhanced surveillance, the prevention of long-term organ damage, and optimised therapeutic decision making in SLE.

Author Contributions: I.P. and C.S. have contributed equally to this manuscript. All authors have read and agreed to the published version of the manuscript.

Funding: I.P. has received grants from the Swedish Rheumatism Association (R-995882), King Gustaf V's 80-year Anniversary Foundation (FAI-2023-1055), Swedish Society of Medicine (SLS-974449), Nyckelfonden (OLL-1000881), Professor Nanna Svartz Foundation (2021-00436), Ulla and Roland Gustafsson Foundation (2024-43), Region Stockholm (FoUI-1004114), and Karolinska Institutet. C.S. has received grants from the Swedish Rheumatism Association (R-993724), Region Östergötland (RÖ-960604), Njurfonden (F2023-0030), Ulla and Roland Gustafsson Foundation (2023-36), the King Gustaf V's 80-year Anniversary Foundation (FAI-2020-0663), and the King Gustaf V and Queen Victoria's Freemasons Foundation (2021).

Acknowledgments: The authors express gratitude to Lina Wirestam, Linköping University, for her help with the graphical illustration.

Conflicts of Interest: I.P. has received research funding and/or honoraria from Amgen, AstraZeneca, Aurinia, Bristol Myers Squibb, Eli Lilly, Gilead, GSK, Janssen, Novartis, Otsuka, and Roche. C.S. discloses speaker's bureau from Bristol Myers Squibb, Fresenius Kabi, Novartis, and AstraZeneca. Since April 2024, C.S. has been an employee of Bristol Myers Squibb. The funders had no role in the writing of the manuscript or in the decision to publish.

References

1. Kaul, A.; Gordon, C.; Crow, M.K.; Touma, Z.; Urowitz, M.B.; van Vollenhoven, R.; Ruiz-Irastorza, G.; Hughes, G. Systemic lupus erythematosus. *Nat. Rev. Dis. Primers* **2016**, *2*, 16039. [CrossRef] [PubMed]
2. Hoi, A.; Igel, T.; Mok, C.C.; Arnaud, L. Systemic lupus erythematosus. *Lancet* **2024**, *403*, 2326–2338. [CrossRef] [PubMed]
3. Siegel, C.H.; Sammaritano, L.R. Systemic Lupus Erythematosus: A Review. *JAMA* **2024**, *331*, 1480–1491. [CrossRef] [PubMed]
4. Frodlund, M.; Reid, S.; Wetterö, J.; Dahlström, Ö.; Sjöwall, C.; Leonard, D. The majority of Swedish systemic lupus erythematosus patients are still affected by irreversible organ impairment: Factors related to damage accrual in two regional cohorts. *Lupus* **2019**, *28*, 1261–1272. [CrossRef] [PubMed]
5. Fanouriakis, A.; Kostopoulou, M.; Andersen, J.; Aringer, M.; Arnaud, L.; Bae, S.C.; Boletis, J.; Bruce, I.N.; Cervera, R.; Doria, A.; et al. EULAR recommendations for the management of systemic lupus erythematosus: 2023 update. *Ann. Rheum. Dis.* **2024**, *83*, 15–29. [CrossRef]
6. Anders, H.J.; Saxena, R.; Zhao, M.H.; Parodis, I.; Salmon, J.E.; Mohan, C. Lupus nephritis. *Nat. Rev. Dis. Primers* **2020**, *6*, 7. [CrossRef]
7. Lindblom, J.; Toro-Dominguez, D.; Carnero-Montoro, E.; Beretta, L.; Borghi, M.O.; Castillo, J.; Enman, Y.; Consortium, P.C.; Mohan, C.; Alarcon-Riquelme, M.E.; et al. Distinct gene dysregulation patterns herald precision medicine potentiality in systemic lupus erythematosus. *J. Autoimmun.* **2023**, *136*, 103025. [CrossRef]
8. Parodis, I.; Lindblom, J.; Toro-Domínguez, D.; Beretta, L.; Borghi, M.O.; Castillo, J.; Carnero-Montoro, E.; Enman, Y.; Mohan, C.; Alarcón-Riquelme, M.E.; et al. Interferon and B-cell Signatures Inform Precision Medicine in Lupus Nephritis. *Kidney Int. Rep.* **2024**, *9*, 1817–1835. [CrossRef]
9. Lindblom, J.; Mohan, C.; Parodis, I. Diagnostic, predictive and prognostic biomarkers in systemic lupus erythematosus: Current insights. *Curr. Opin. Rheumatol.* **2022**, *34*, 139–149. [CrossRef]
10. Enocsson, H.; Wirestam, L.; Dahle, C.; Padyukov, L.; Jönsen, A.; Urowitz, M.B.; Gladman, D.D.; Romero-Diaz, J.; Bae, S.C.; Fortin, P.R.; et al. Soluble urokinase plasminogen activator receptor (suPAR) levels predict damage accrual in patients with recent-onset systemic lupus erythematosus. *J. Autoimmun.* **2020**, *106*, 102340. [CrossRef]
11. Chalmers, S.A.; Ayilam Ramachandran, R.; Garcia, S.J.; Der, E.; Herlitz, L.; Ampudia, J.; Chu, D.; Jordan, N.; Zhang, T.; Parodis, I.; et al. The CD6/ALCAM pathway promotes lupus nephritis via T cell-mediated responses. *J. Clin. Investig.* **2022**, *132*. [CrossRef] [PubMed]
12. Fava, A.; Buyon, J.; Magder, L.; Hodgin, J.; Rosenberg, A.; Demeke, D.S.; Rao, D.A.; Arazi, A.; Celia, A.I.; Putterman, C.; et al. Urine proteomic signatures of histological class, activity, chronicity, and treatment response in lupus nephritis. *JCI Insight* **2024**, *9*. [CrossRef] [PubMed]
13. Palazzo, L.; Lindblom, J.; Mohan, C.; Parodis, I. Current Insights on Biomarkers in Lupus Nephritis: A Systematic Review of the Literature. *J. Clin. Med.* **2022**, *11*, 5759. [CrossRef]
14. Lindblom, J.; Mohan, C.; Parodis, I. Biomarkers in Neuropsychiatric Systemic Lupus Erythematosus: A Systematic Literature Review of the Last Decade. *Brain Sci.* **2022**, *12*, 192. [CrossRef]
15. Parodis, I.; Tamirou, F.; Houssiau, F.A. Prediction of prognosis and renal outcome in lupus nephritis. *Lupus Sci. Med.* **2020**, *7*, e000389. [CrossRef]
16. Carrión-Barberà, I.; Triginer, L.; Tío, L.; Pérez-García, C.; Ribes, A.; Abad, V.; Pros, A.; Bermúdez-López, M.; Castro-Boqué, E.; Lecube, A.; et al. Role of Advanced Glycation End Products as New Biomarkers in Systemic Lupus Erythematosus. *Int. J. Mol. Sci.* **2024**, *25*, 3022. [CrossRef]
17. Wolf, B.; Blaschke, C.R.K.; Mungaray, S.; Weselman, B.T.; Stefanenko, M.; Fedoriuk, M.; Bai, H.; Rodgers, J.; Palygin, O.; Drake, R.R.; et al. Metabolic Markers and Association of Biological Sex in Lupus Nephritis. *Int. J. Mol. Sci.* **2023**, *24*, 16490. [CrossRef]
18. Winikajtis-Burzyńska, A.; Brzosko, M.; Przepiera-Będzak, H. Elevated Serum Levels of Soluble Transferrin Receptor Are Associated with an Increased Risk of Cardiovascular, Pulmonary, and Hematological Manifestations and a Decreased Risk of Neuropsychiatric Manifestations in Systemic Lupus Erythematosus Patients. *Int. J. Mol. Sci.* **2023**, *24*, 17340. [CrossRef]
19. Mercader-Salvans, J.; García-González, M.; Gómez-Bernal, F.; Quevedo-Abeledo, J.C.; de Vera-González, A.; González-Delgado, A.; López-Mejías, R.; Martín-González, C.; González-Gay, M.Á.; Ferraz-Amaro, I. Relationship between Disease Characteristics and Circulating Interleukin 6 in a Well-Characterized Cohort of Patients with Systemic Lupus Erythematosus. *Int. J. Mol. Sci.* **2023**, *24*, 14006. [CrossRef]
20. Iseme, R.A.; McEvoy, M.; Kelly, B.; Agnew, L.; Walker, F.R.; Handley, T.; Oldmeadow, C.; Attia, J.; Boyle, M. A role for autoantibodies in atherogenesis. *Cardiovasc. Res.* **2017**, *113*, 1102–1112. [CrossRef]
21. van den Berg, V.J.; Vroegindewey, M.M.; Kardys, I.; Boersma, E.; Haskard, D.; Hartley, A.; Khamis, R. Anti-Oxidized LDL Antibodies and Coronary Artery Disease: A Systematic Review. *Antioxidants* **2019**, *8*, 484. [CrossRef]
22. Wirestam, L.; Jönsson, F.; Enocsson, H.; Svensson, C.; Weiner, M.; Wetterö, J.; Zachrisson, H.; Eriksson, P.; Sjöwall, C. Limited Association between Antibodies to Oxidized Low-Density Lipoprotein and Vascular Affection in Patients with Established Systemic Lupus Erythematosus. *Int. J. Mol. Sci.* **2023**, *24*, 8987. [CrossRef] [PubMed]
23. Parodis, I.; Gomez, A.; Lindblom, J.; Chow, J.W.; Sjöwall, C.; Sciascia, S.; Gatto, M. B Cell Kinetics upon Therapy Commencement for Active Extrarenal Systemic Lupus Erythematosus in Relation to Development of Renal Flares: Results from Three Phase III Clinical Trials of Belimumab. *Int. J. Mol. Sci.* **2022**, *23*, 13941. [CrossRef] [PubMed]

24. Parodis, I.; Gatto, M.; Sjöwall, C. B cells in systemic lupus erythematosus: Targets of new therapies and surveillance tools. *Front. Med.* **2022**, *9*, 952304. [CrossRef] [PubMed]
25. Halfon, M.; Tankeu, A.T.; Ribi, C. Mitochondrial Dysfunction in Systemic Lupus Erythematosus with a Focus on Lupus Nephritis. *Int. J. Mol. Sci.* **2024**, *25*, 6162. [CrossRef] [PubMed]
26. Vitale, A.M.; Paladino, L.; Caruso Bavisotto, C.; Barone, R.; Rappa, F.; Conway de Macario, E.; Cappello, F.; Macario, A.J.L.; Marino Gammazza, A. Interplay between the Chaperone System and Gut Microbiota Dysbiosis in Systemic Lupus Erythematosus Pathogenesis: Is Molecular Mimicry the Missing Link between Those Two Factors? *Int. J. Mol. Sci.* **2024**, *25*, 5608. [CrossRef]
27. von Hofsten, S.; Fenton, K.A.; Pedersen, H.L. Human and Murine Toll-like Receptor-Driven Disease in Systemic Lupus Erythematosus. *Int. J. Mol. Sci.* **2024**, *25*, 5351. [CrossRef]
28. Alduraibi, F.K.; Tsokos, G.C. Lupus Nephritis Biomarkers: A Critical Review. *Int. J. Mol. Sci.* **2024**, *25*, 805. [CrossRef]

Disclaimer/Publisher's Note: The statements, opinions and data contained in all publications are solely those of the individual author(s) and contributor(s) and not of MDPI and/or the editor(s). MDPI and/or the editor(s) disclaim responsibility for any injury to people or property resulting from any ideas, methods, instructions or products referred to in the content.

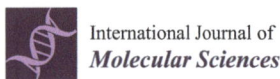

Review

Lupus Nephritis Biomarkers: A Critical Review

Fatima K. Alduraibi [1,2,3,*] and George C. Tsokos [1]

1. Department of Medicine, Division of Clinical Immunology and Rheumatology, Beth Israel Deaconess Medical Center, Harvard Teaching Hospital, Boston, MA 02215, USA
2. Department of Medicine, Division of Clinical Immunology and Rheumatology, University of Alabama at Birmingham, Birmingham, AL 35294, USA
3. Department of Medicine, Division of Clinical Immunology and Rheumatology, King Faisal Specialist Hospital and Research Center, Riyadh 11564, Saudi Arabia
* Correspondence: faldurai@bidmc.harvard.edu; Tel.: +1-617-735-4160

Abstract: Lupus nephritis (LN), a major complication in individuals diagnosed with systemic lupus erythematosus, substantially increases morbidity and mortality. Despite marked improvements in the survival of patients with severe LN over the past 50 years, complete clinical remission after immunosuppressive therapy is achieved in only half of the patients. Therefore, timely detection of LN is vital for initiating prompt therapeutic interventions and improving patient outcomes. Biomarkers have emerged as valuable tools for LN detection and monitoring; however, the complex role of these biomarkers in LN pathogenesis remains unclear. Renal biopsy remains the gold standard for the identification of the histological phenotypes of LN and guides disease management. However, the molecular pathophysiology of specific renal lesions remains poorly understood. In this review, we provide a critical, up-to-date overview of the latest developments in the field of LN biomarkers.

Keywords: biomarker; systemic lupus erythematosus; lupus nephritis

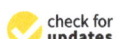

Citation: Alduraibi, F.K.; Tsokos, G.C. Lupus Nephritis Biomarkers: A Critical Review. *Int. J. Mol. Sci.* **2024**, *25*, 805. https://doi.org/10.3390/ijms25020805

Academic Editors: Christopher Sjöwall and Ioannis Parodis

Received: 6 December 2023
Revised: 2 January 2024
Accepted: 5 January 2024
Published: 9 January 2024

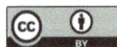

Copyright: © 2024 by the authors. Licensee MDPI, Basel, Switzerland. This article is an open access article distributed under the terms and conditions of the Creative Commons Attribution (CC BY) license (https://creativecommons.org/licenses/by/4.0/).

1. Introduction

Systemic lupus erythematosus (SLE) is a chronic systemic autoimmune disease characterized by the presence of autoantibodies (autoAbs), autoreactive B and T cells, and the dysregulation of cytokines, which lead to inflammation and cause damage to multiple organs [1–4]. The prevalence of SLE in the United States ranges from 20 to 150 cases per 100,000 people [5–8]. The etiology and pathogenesis of SLE are not well understood; the factors that lead to disease onset are highly variable, and the disease manifests systemically with manifestations resulting from the injury of multiple tissues. The kidney is the most commonly involved organ in this disease and contributes extensively to morbidity and mortality [9–11].

Lupus nephritis (LN) has been classified histologically into six types, which are determined by the location and the type of histological changes. There is variability among the six classes in terms of response to treatment and preservation of the kidney function and the development of end-stage disease [12]. LN is characterized by inflammation of the kidney arising from complex interactions between the innate and adaptive immune responses and the kidney parenchyma [13,14]. Extensive research has recognized the contributions of genetic, epigenetic, and environmental factors to LN; however, the precise etiology and pathogenesis of LN remain unclear. The onset and progression of LN, as well as the response to treatment, are highly variable among patients, highlighting the need to develop biomarkers to assess these diverse aspects of this disease [15]. The pathogenesis involves several genetic variants, including those that hinder the efficient elimination of dying cells, resulting in the persistence of nuclear antigens in the extracellular space. The released autoantigens act as triggers for innate and adaptive immune responses, while other genetic variants influence the magnitude of these immune reactions and the proper function of immune tolerance checkpoints, ultimately promoting the expansion of autoreactive T and B lymphocytes [15,16]. Consequently, circulating antinuclear antibodies, along with other autoAbs, lead to the formation of ICs that propagate systemic inflammation, leading to organ damage. The deposition of ICs in the renal microvasculature triggers inflammation and organ injury, accounting for the extensive morbidity and mortality associated with the disease [17]. The persistence of autoAbs amplifies systemic autoimmunity and exacerbates LN by facilitating an inflammatory response. These events may accentuate autoantigen presentation and induce immune responses specific to kidney-specific autoantigens [18]. Furthermore, ICs, local complement system activation, and the recruitment of immune cells cumulatively contribute to kidney damage. In response to autoantigens, immune cell memory may introduce further complications in the context of SLE, LN disease progression, and flares. The persistence of memory T cells and plasma cells in the bone marrow and other lymphoid organs makes them less susceptible to traditional therapeutic interventions [19–23].

In recent years, remarkable progress has been made in understanding the pathophysiology of LN, leading to the identification of novel biomarkers related to cellular and inflammatory mechanisms. For instance, advanced techniques, such as single-cell (sc) RNA sequencing, have offered valuable insights into the intricate composition of immune cell populations in the kidney tissues of patients with LN [13]. As LN can be categorized into different types, there is the possibility that certain biomarkers correlate with specific types of LN. For instance, the signature of type I interferon (IFN) is predominantly observed in the kidneys and skin of individuals diagnosed with proliferative LN [3,24], whereas patients with membranous LN exhibit different transcriptomic patterns [24], and transcriptome-based investigations using animal models have provided insights into the progression and phases of LN development [25].

Recently, there has been increasing interest in the development of early prediction and detection methods to prevent the onset, manage relapses, and mitigate the complications associated with chronic kidney disease (CKD) as alternatives to renal biopsy. Although invasive, the current diagnostic approach for LN typically involves renal biopsy, which is considered the gold standard for establishing an initial diagnosis. However, it poses challenges regarding the frequent monitoring of disease progression and treatment response.

Currently, the scientific community is building momentum to incorporate more comprehensive approaches, including proteomics and metabolomics, to develop reliable diagnostic and prognostic markers. Here, we review various published approaches regarding the development of biomarkers for LN.

2. LN Biomarkers
2.1. Serum AutoAbs

AutoAbs have emerged as invaluable biomarkers that provide insights into disease activity and progression. Several autoAbs have been found to be associated with LN [13]. Associations between specific autoAbs, including antibodies against ds DNA (dsDNA) and -C1q, and distinct histological classifications of LN have been reported [26–28]. Anti-phospholipid antibodies are also associated with renal thrombotic microangiopathy [29,30]. Crescent formation in the kidney often indicates the presence of antibodies that damage the renal capillaries [30–32].

Anti-dsDNA antibodies and C1q are frequently used as LN biomarkers and have been endorsed by guidelines for disease monitoring [33]. The presence of antibodies against C1q is associated with LN [34], with high specificity (92%) and sensitivity (56%) [35]. This suggests that the level of antibodies against C1q can serve as a valuable diagnostic tool and help distinguish LN cases from those of other nephritides [35]. Additionally, antibodies against C-reactive protein (CRP) have been detected in patients with active LN, and their levels were found to be correlated with the Systemic Lupus Erythematosus Disease Activity Index (SLEDAI) score ($p = 0.002$) [36]. Moreover, high baseline levels of antibodies against CRP significantly predict an unfavorable outcome ($p = 0.021$) during the second year of therapy [36]. This finding highlights the potential of using antibodies against CRP as valuable biomarkers of disease activity in LN.

Antibodies against α-enolase (anti-ENO-1) are formed when α-enolase externalizes during NETosis [37]. Their presence has demonstrated significant potential in predicting LN in patients with SLE, with an area under the curve (AUC) of 0.81 and a p-value of 0.001 [38]. Furthermore, an increased prevalence of the anti-ENO-1 IgG2 isotype discriminates patients with LN from those with other nephritides and non-renal SLE, with an AUC of 0.82 and a p-value of 0.02 [39,40].

Antibodies against alpha-actinin (AaA) have shown promise as diagnostic markers for LN. In a previous study that compared patients with LN and those with SLE without nephritis, the serum AaA levels were considerably lower in those with LN, with a sensitivity of 60%, a specificity of 90%, and a positive predictive value (PPV) of 85.7% [41]. These findings indicate that serum AaA levels may serve as a marker for distinguishing patients with LN from those with SLE without nephritis [41].

Histones are a primary component of the nucleosome, and studies have indicated a strong correlation between antibodies against chromatin/nucleosomes and LN as well as an increased risk of developing proliferative LN [42,43]. Histone 1 forms part of the apoptotic chromatin constituents in the dense electron deposits of the glomerular basement; these are recognized targets of nephritogenic dsDNA antibodies [44–47]. Antibodies to chromatin are present in patients with LN, but they are not particularly useful in monitoring disease activity or response to treatment [48].

Interestingly, numerous studies have reported that patients with LN and antineutrophil cytoplasmic antibodies (ANCA), specifically those who are anti-myeloperoxidase (MPO)/proteinase 3 (PR3)-positive or double positive for anti-MPO and anti-PR3 antibodies, exhibit serologically active SLE (higher dsDNA antibody titers and lower serum C4 concentrations) compared with ANCA-negative LN patients. Additionally, patients in the subgroup with proliferative LN display more necrosis in renal biopsy specimens than ANCA-negative patients. However, it is noteworthy that no significant difference was reported between the outcomes of these groups [32,49,50]. Yet, given the poor prognosis of ANCA-positive cases, it is suggested that all patients with LN be screened for ANCA. The measurement of autoAb levels could potentially enhance the early detection, monitoring, and management of LN. Nevertheless, rigorous prospective studies are required to establish their utility as biomarkers.

2.2. Cytokines/Chemokines

In addition to autoAbs, various serum proteins have emerged as potential LN biomarkers. These include cytokines, chemokines, and adhesion molecules. Cytokines regulate the immune response and are crucial in the pathogenesis of LN, particularly in attracting leukocytes and in the development of the inflammatory response [51,52]. The deposition of ICs on glomeruli initiates and activates the complement pathway, attracting immune cells and triggering the release of inflammatory cytokines, thereby exacerbating glomerular damage. For instance, B-cell activating factor (BAFF or BLyS), produced by glomerular macrophages and mesangial cells, stimulates B-cell activation both directly and by inducing the production of pro-inflammatory molecules, such as IFN-α, perpetuating a detrimental cycle in the renal microenvironment. Moreover, cytokines, such as urinary monocyte chemoattractant protein-1 (MCP-1/CCL2), BAFF, and TNF-related weak inducer of apoptosis (TWEAK), are pertinent in predicting active LN, assessing therapeutic responses, and forecasting disease flares [53,54].

Furthermore, distinct cytokines predominate in different types of LN. For example, in proliferative LN (class III/IV), the deposition of ICs beneath the endothelium leads to mesangial cell proliferation, an increase in extracellular matrix production, and the release of a remarkable array of pro-inflammatory cytokines, such as type I IFN, interleukin (IL)-1β, IL6, IL8, IL-37, and IL-17A [55]. Conversely, membranous LN (class V) is characterized by the subepithelial localization of ICs, resulting in increased complement activation and reduced inflammatory responses [55]. Levels of cytokines may prove useful in distinguishing between proliferative and non-proliferative forms of LN, and this information may be useful in guiding precise treatment and management strategies and may eliminate the need for invasive LN biopsy [55]. Several cytokines have been examined as potential biomarkers to assess the activity, severity, and renal involvement of SLE.

Chemokines are small chemotactic cytokines that typically range in size from 8 to 10 kDa and play crucial roles in regulating the migration and localization of immune cells [56]. Chemokines and their receptors have been implicated in the pathogenesis of LN in both patients with SLE and lupus-prone mice. Several chemokines have shown promising results as biomarkers for the diagnosis and prognosis of LN.

2.2.1. Serum

BAFF and a proliferation-inducing ligand (APRIL) are cytokines belonging to the tumor necrosis factor (TNF) family; they act on B cells and drive the activation of these cells, thereby contributing to the pathogenesis of LN [57,58]. Reduced baseline serum levels of BAFF are predictive of clinical and pathological responses, demonstrating a 92% PPV for clinical responders in cases of proliferative LN [59]. Furthermore, the inhibition of BAFF activity with belimumab, which has been approved for treating patients with active LN, has shown promising results [60]. Serum levels of APRIL (sAPRIL) are associated with its presence in the urine and its histological activity and can help predict the likelihood of treatment failure [61]. A previous study showed that the urine levels of BAFF and APRIL were notably higher in patients with active proliferative LN than in those with SLE with no renal involvement [53]. Moreover, the AUC values of 0.825 for urine BAFF and 0.781 for urine APRIL helped in differentiating between active LN and active SLE without renal involvement [53].

IFN inducible protein-10 (IP-10 or CXCL10) is a chemokine belonging to the ELR CXC family which is secreted by immune and non-immune cells [62]. It is produced in response to IFN activation and guides lymphocytes to the affected organs in lupus-prone mice and patients with SLE [63]. The urine and serum levels of IP-10 are promising potential biomarkers of lupus activity, as they can be used to distinguish between active and inactive lupus cases [54,64].

The serum IL-6 levels are higher in patients with SLE than in healthy individuals and correlate with the SLEDAI ($p = 0.018$) [65]. In a previous study, despite the association of serum and urine IL-6 levels with clinical manifestations of LN, the inhibition of IL-6 activity failed to show therapeutic benefits in clinical tests [66].

Serum IL-10 levels display high accuracy in distinguishing active LN from inactive LN, as evidenced by an AUC of 0.87 ($p = 0.003$), 70.6% sensitivity, 100% specificity, and a notable correlation with the SLEDAI ($p = 0.004$) [65,67].

IL-16, produced by immune and non-immune cells [68,69], exhibits markedly increased levels in the urine of patients with active LN, particularly in proliferative cases. The observed decrease in urine IL-16 levels during therapeutic intervention may serve as a useful marker for assessing therapeutic responses in LN [70].

The serum angiopoietin-2 (Ang2) levels are higher in patients with SLE and those with LN than in healthy individuals [71]. Ang2 levels correlate with the SLEDAI, 24 h proteinuria, and histological activity, which suggests their usefulness as a biomarker for LN [71]. Nevertheless, Ang2 cannot distinguish between the types of LN lesions, particularly the proliferative and non-proliferative forms [71]. Serum angiopoietin-like protein 4 (Angptl4) and angiostatin are gaining attention as potential biomarkers for LN [51,72,73]. The serum Angptl4 levels effectively differentiated patients with active LN from those with active SLE without renal involvement and displayed a strong link with the renal SLEDAI (rSLEDAI), with an AUC of 0.96 [73]. Angiostatin has a strong association with LN, as reported by several studies (AUC = 0.95–0.99; $p < 0.001$) [51,74,75]. Its correlation with the rSLEDAI, SLEDAI, and National Institutes of Health LN index underscores its value as a primary marker for LN monitoring [74,75]. Furthermore, comprehensive proteomic analyses have focused on Angptl4 and angiostatin as valuable urine indicators for monitoring LN progression and renal histology in patients with SLE [51,72,73]. Likewise, in another study, urine angiostatin levels could not be used to discriminate between patients with LN and those with CKD, with an AUC of 0.56 [76].

Serum TNF receptor-associated factor 6 is a cytokine associated with LN activity and has shown promise as a diagnostic marker for LN [77]. Serum human epididymis protein 4 levels are high in SLE, especially in patients with LN, particularly in those with increased anti-dsDNA antibody levels and decreased C3 levels. Moreover, these levels have been shown to have a predictive value for the diagnosis of LN [78].

2.2.2. Urine

MCP-1/CCL2 is a chemokine belonging to the C-C family, and its function is to recruit leukocytes. In a meta-analysis, the urine MCP-1 (uMCP-1) levels were found to have a sensitivity of 89% and a specificity of 63% in differentiating active LN from inactive disease [79]. Furthermore, its levels correlated with kidney disease activity and ongoing kidney impairment and were increased in cases of proliferative glomerulonephritis [80–83]. Interestingly, uMCP-1 has the potential to predict upcoming kidney disease flares 2–4 months in advance and to reflect the effectiveness of treatment [81,82].

Urine IL (uIL)-17 and urine transforming growth factor beta 1 (uTGF-β1) have shown promise as potential LN biomarker candidates [84,85]. A previous study reported significantly elevated levels of uTGF-β1 and uIL-17 in patients with severe LN compared to those in healthy participants ($p < 0.05$) [84]; the AUCs for uTGF-β1 and uIL-17 were 66.50% and 71.70%, respectively [84]. These findings suggest that uTGF-β1 and uIL-17 are potential indicators of disease severity and that they can be valuable in distinguishing severe LN cases from mild ones [84].

Several urine proteins have emerged as promising tools for the diagnosis and ongoing monitoring of LN [51,86]. Notably, a study showed that TWEAK had an AUC of 0.82, demonstrating its predictive efficacy in LN [54]. Furthermore, when combined with UMCP-1, TWEAK effectively distinguishes between active and inactive LN (AUC = 0.89) and predicts the progression of end-stage kidney disease (ESRD) (AUC = 0.78) [54,87,88]. Additionally, urine levels of IL-12p40, IL-15, and thymus- and activation-regulated chemokine have been reported to be higher in patients with active LN than in those with inactive SLE and healthy individuals and to be correlated with the rSLEDAI [89]. Furthermore, urine clusterin has shown promise as a marker for tubulointerstitial lesions in LN [90]. Urine osteoprotegerin levels are notably elevated in patients with active LN; they correlate with disease activity, and it has been suggested that they predict poor treatment response and LN relapse [91]. Finally, urine levels of transferrin and ceruloplasmin are elevated in patients with LN compared to those in individuals without LN [92].

2.3. Cell Adhesion Molecules (CAMs)

CAMs are essential for guiding leukocyte movement across the endothelium toward the sites of inflammation [93]. Existing studies have investigated the use of specific CAMs, including the activated leukocyte cell adhesion molecule (ALCAM), intercellular adhesion molecule 1 (ICAM-1), vascular cell adhesion molecule 1 (VCAM-1), neural cell adhesion molecule 1 (NCAM-1), and L-selectin, as biomarkers in LN [51,72,73,75,80,94–99].

Urine CAMs (uCAMs) have demonstrated remarkable precision in distinguishing between active and inactive LN as well as SLE without LN [95]. The discriminative power of these molecules is reflected in an AUC that consistently surpasses the 0.8 threshold, except for neutrophil gelatinase-associated lipocalin (NGAL) [100–102]. Moreover, a combination of urine markers (uVCAM-1, uCystatinC, and uKIM-1) yielded a promising AUC of 0.80 (95% CI: 0.69–0.90), highlighting the potential to differentiate between the proliferative and membranous forms of LN [54]. Levels of uCAMs collectively serve as robust tools in evaluating LN activity and informing clinical decisions [103]. It has been suggested that urine ALCAM (uALCAM) levels are more efficient in distinguishing proliferative LN from membranous LN [95]. Moreover, uALCAM and urine VCAM-1 (uVCAM-1) levels exhibit a strong correlation with renal histological activity, underscoring their potential value as LN activity markers [75,80,95,99]. Elevated initial levels of uALCAM and uVCAM-1 might signal the waning of renal function [94]. The incremental benefit of integrating these markers is yet to be conclusively assessed. A longitudinal study revealed an elevation in serum VCAM-1 levels approximately 4.5 months before a recorded renal flare, which decreased after treatment [103]. The urine-soluble VCAM-1 and VCAM-1 levels are higher in patients with LN than in healthy individuals [76]. Furthermore, VCAM-1 has outstanding potential as a biomarker for predicting a renal biopsy activity index score greater than 7, which is associated with a poor long-term prognosis [75]. Serum NGAL levels have also been shown to be a potential biomarker for differentiating patients with LN from those without nephritis [76]. Specifically, at onset, NGAL levels serve as the best predictor, outperforming VCAM and KIM1 levels in identifying treatment responders versus non-responders 6 months after the induction phase, registering an AUC of 0.78 [80]. Furthermore, serum NGAL levels are elevated in patients with active SLE and could be used to gauge the response to treatment [80,104,105]. Additionally, serum NGAL levels are elevated in patients with active SLE, and urine NGAL levels can serve as a predictor of the response to treatment. Serum levels of Axl can distinguish active LN from non-renal SLE and provide insights into long-term renal outcomes [106–108]. Finally, L-selectin levels are closely associated with LN activity and related organ damage metrics [73,75,98].

2.4. Other Protein/Lipid Molecules

Urine-soluble CD163 (uCD163), a transmembrane scavenger receptor, is expressed by macrophages and monocytes and is a useful biomarker with an AUC of 0.998 for differentiating between active and inactive LN [109]. In addition, uCD163 levels are indicative of clinical and histological renal activities in LN [110,111]. Furthermore, uCD163 levels measured 6 months after therapy initiation have been shown to predict kidney recovery in LN, with more than 87% accuracy [109].

Epidermal growth factor (EGF) concentrations are reduced in the urine of patients with active nephritis and are associated with severe renal outcomes, such as elevated serum creatinine levels and ESRD [112].

Ceramides, characterized by modifications of the sphingosine backbone, are emerging as potential biomarkers of LN [113,114]. These diverse lipids play crucial roles in cellular signaling. The serum levels of ceramides, such as C16cer, C18Cer, C20Cer, and C24:1Cer, are higher in patients with LN with kidney impairment than in healthy individuals and patients with SLE without kidney impairment [113]. C24:1dhCer is being recognized as a remarkable indicator of kidney impairment in patients with SLE [113].

2.5. Complement

The complement system plays a crucial role in the pathogenesis of SLE, and the serum levels of certain components have been used to monitor disease activity [115–118]. In a study of patients with LN who underwent a repeat renal biopsy two years later, the prolonged depression of serum C3 levels was associated with a trend toward a worsening chronicity index, whereas normalization of C3 was associated with a reduction in the activity index in the repeat biopsy [118]. Hypocomplementemia, particularly low levels of C3 and C4 alone, may not adequately reflect disease activity, as the sensitivity and specificity of C3 for SLE are 80% and 14%, respectively [117]. The levels of the C4 component breakdown product C4d have been found to be considerably increased during disease flares in patients with SLE, with a 68% PPV. C4d levels also correlate with LN, with a 79% sensitivity [119]. Additionally, the C4d/C4 ratio has been found to be more specific, sensitive, and effective in distinguishing LN from non-LN cases [120]. Complement factor H-related proteins (CFHRs), which encompass CFHR1 through CFHR5, are part of the broader factor H/CFHR family. The levels of CFHR3 and CFHR5 are associated with disease activity in LN [121].

2.6. MicroRNAs (miRNAs)

miRNAs have been reported to play important roles in the development of LN and kidney fibrosis [122,123]. The stability of miRNAs in body fluids makes them attractive diagnostic and prognostic biomarker candidates for human diseases [124]. Several miRNAs serve as potential disease biomarkers for LN. Epigenetic studies regarding SLE have highlighted a set of urinary miRNAs, including miR-146a, miR-204, miR-30c, miR-3201, and miR-1273e, that are associated with LN [125]. These miRNAs play roles in LN-specific pathways, such as nucleic acid processes and inflammation, as well as in kidney function regulation through WNT and TGF-β signaling. The levels of miR-146a are reduced in the sera of patients with LN and are associated with disease activity [77]. Notably, baseline miR-146a levels are associated with renal flares and ESRD progression [126]. The urine levels of miRNA-135b, which originates from tubular cells, vary between treatment responders and non-responders [127]. Circulating miR-21 levels have been reported to be markedly increased in patients with LN compared to those in healthy controls; thus, they can be used to discriminate between patients with LN and controls [128]. A combined calculated value of circulating miRNAs in plasma, including miR-125a, miR-142-3p, miR-146, and miR-155, has shown promise in distinguishing patients with LN from healthy individuals [129]. Additionally, urine exosomal miR-29c levels negatively correlate with the histological chronicity index and glomerular sclerosis. Its expression levels have a remarkable predictive value for chronicity in patients with LN [130]. In addition to miRNAs, long non-coding RNAs (lncRNAs) are also involved in LN development. The levels of lncRNA RP11-2B6.2 are usually elevated following the kidney biopsies of patients with LN and positively correlate with IFNa signature scores and disease activity [131]. Additionally, the lnc3643 levels are considerably reduced only in patients with SLE and proteinuria; accordingly, these levels can distinguish LN from SLE without nephritis [131].

2.7. Genetics

Genetic susceptibility contributes to the complex etiology of LN. Variants in certain genes have been linked to worse outcomes in patients with LN. Owing to the widespread availability of whole-genome sequencing, these variants can be identified and used to predict disease outcomes. One to three percent of patients with SLE may have a single-gene (monogenic) defect, and these patients experience a high incidence of LN [132–134]. Such cases often involve DNA/RNA clearance (e.g., DNASE1L3), complement pathways (e.g., C1q or C4), and DNA/RNA detection, which lead to type I IFN activation (e.g., TLR7), and some LN cases were reported to harbor variants of these genes. In-depth genomic studies spanning the sporadic to polygenic manifestations of SLE have identified more than 100 susceptibility genes. These variants include the genes involved in cell death (e.g., FAS), effective IC management (e.g., FcGR), and the amplified immune responses of T and B cells [10,135]. For example, recent advances in whole-exome sequencing have revealed that novel mutations in the TNF alpha-induced protein 3 (TNFAIP3) gene are linked to LN. These mutations lead to increased activity in nuclear factor kappa B and type I IFN pathways, along with a rise in pro-inflammatory cytokines [136]. Specifically, this study linked three novel mutations with LN: c.634+2T>C, exon 7–8 deletion, and c.1300_1301delinsTA (p. A434*) [136]. Additionally, various databases have reported TNFAIP3 mutations associated with kidney involvement, such as the p.Q187* mutation in a patient with proliferative LN and the p.F224Sfs*4 mutation in a patient with membranous LN [136–138]. Moreover, a genome-wide association study focusing on female SLE patients of European ancestry with LN has identified genes, such as FCGR, STAT4, and BANK1. These genes have been shown to correlate with both the occurrence and severity of LN; this has been confirmed across various cohorts [139–143]. Wang et al. used weighted gene co-expression network analysis to identify four hub genes, namely CD53 (AUC = 0.995), TGFBI (AUC = 0.997), MS4A6A (AUC = 0.994), and HERC6 (AUC = 0.999), which are involved in the development of the inflammatory response and immune activation in LN ($p < 0.0001$) [144]. Yavuz et al. discovered that MERTK, a novel genetic region, contributes to the risk of developing LN and ESRD in patients with SLE, a finding that has been replicated across various ethnicities [145]. MERTK, a member of the Tyro3/Axl/Mer receptor kinase family, is the primary receptor on macrophages for apoptotic cells [146,147]. It plays a key role in the regulation of the innate immune response through efferocytosis and notably influences the production of cytokines, such as IL-10, TGF-β, IL-6, and IL-12 [148,149]. Furthermore, *MERTK* is critical in suppressing TLR-mediated innate immune responses by activating STAT1, which leads to an anti-inflammatory feedback through the production of the cytokine signaling suppressors *SOCS1* and *SOCS3* [150]. Other genes, such as *PRDM1*, are associated with proliferative LN [145] and play a vital role as modulators of dendritic cell function and repressors of the IFN-β gene [151].

Moreover, an *APOL1* gene variant has been identified as an independent risk factor for faster progression to ESRD in patients with LN [152–154]. Although the precise mechanisms by which *APOL1* facilitates kidney disease progression have not been fully elucidated, it is believed that these variants directly affect the function and structure of kidney parenchymal cells and may exacerbate tissue inflammation, thereby influencing the severity of LN. Additionally, human leukocyte antigen (HLA) variants have long been found to be linked to the development of LN, with HLA-DR3 and HLA-DR15 increasing the risk significantly [155].

In terms of classifying patients based on their risk of nephritis, Chen et al. observed that a high polygenic risk score for SLE correlates with poorer prognostic factors like earlier age of onset and LN [156]. Kwon et al. reported in a Korean cohort that an individual's highest weighted genetic risk score (wGRS), calculated from 112 well-validated non-HLA single nucleotide polymorphisms and HLA haplotypes of SLE risk loci, was independently associated with the development of LN and the production of the anti-Sm antibody, compared to those in the lowest wGRS quartile [157]. This association was observed regardless of the age of onset [157]. Webber et al. observed that both HLA and non-HLA SLE risk-weighted genetic risk scores were significantly associated with the risk of proliferative LN in two large, multi-ethnic cohorts of 1251 SLE patients [158]. This may indicate that SLE risk loci are of greater importance in the development of proliferative LN, as opposed to non-proliferative LN [158]. Despite these developments, the full spectrum of genetic risk factors for LN and its progression to ESRD still needs to be better understood and further developed. Taken together, a gene expression score, including all variants known to contribute to the development of LN (class, severity, and risk of ESRD), can be used to screen all patients with SLE, identify patients at high risk of LN, and predict various clinical outcomes in SLE patients.

2.8. Epigenetics

Epigenetic processes, particularly those involving DNA methylation and histone modifications, are crucial for LN development [159]. Irregularities in DNA methylation patterns have been observed in genes linked to immune responses and inflammatory processes in patients with LN, which indicates their potential contribution to disease development [159]. For example, alterations in the DNA methylation of the *MERTK* gene may modify its activity and increase the risk of SLE-ESRD [145]. Similarly, histone modifications can influence gene expression profiles in immune cells, potentially contributing to the dysregulation of immune responses observed in LN [160]. New technologies that are used to assess the epigenome of immune cells may evolve into useful diagnostic and disease-monitoring tools.

3. Conclusions and Future Directions

The complexity of LN pathogenesis poses challenges for the development of biomarkers for monitoring disease activity in response to treatment. The biomarkers discussed in this review represent elements that reflect multiple aspects of the immune response as well as aspects of vascular and parenchymal cell injury (Table 1) [161–208]. It is obvious that with each biomarker in patients with LN, variable pathogenetic pathways are involved, bespeaking the heterogeneity of the disease. Although tools that integrate multiple proteins, or other molecules, may have a greater value as biomarkers, the same limitations may apply. Although in some patients the diagnosis of SLE coincides with that of LN, LN may develop at various times after the diagnosis of SLE. It has been documented that the appearance of serum autoAbs [209] and pro-inflammatory cytokines [210] precedes the diagnosis of SLE by months to several years. Therefore, it is plausible to assume that certain biological processes that result in the production of proteins or other molecules occur in the serum or urine prior to the clinical diagnosis of LN. Studies identifying biomarkers for predicting an upcoming renal involvement in LN are lacking. Although our group has shown that IgG from patients with LN, but not from patients with SLE without LN, can injure cultured podocytes [211], it is still unclear when "podocytopathic" IgG first appears in the sera of patients with SLE prior to the development of LN. When injured, podocytes and other parenchymal cells are released into the urine. A more careful study of urine cells for the identification of molecules involved in kidney cell injury [211] can prove useful in monitoring the response to treatment, as the shed cells may provide a window into the events in the kidney tissue itself.

Table 1. Summary of biomarkers for lupus nephritis (LN).

Sample	Biomarker	Association	Reference
\multicolumn{4}{c}{1. Antibodies/immunoglobulins}			
Serum/plasma	Anti-dsDNA	Diagnosis, clinical disease activity, damage, and responses to therapy in LN	[40,106,109]
	Anti-C1q	Diagnosis, clinical disease activity, histological disease activity, and prognosis	[36,162–166]
	Anti-CRP	Clinical disease activity and responses to therapy in LN	[34,35]
	Anti-ENO-1 (+)	Diagnosis and prediction of LN	[37,38,40]
	AaA (Low)	Diagnosis	[41]
	Anti-chromatin	Diagnostic/predictive capacity in LN	[48]
	PTEC-binding IgG (+)	Clinical disease activity	[167]
	PHACTR4 icx (+)	Diagnosis	[168]
	P3H1 icx (+)	Diagnosis	[168]
	RGS12 icx (+)	Diagnosis	[168]
	PTEC-binding IgG (+)	Clinical disease activity	[167]
	IgM ($\uparrow$)	Responses to therapy in LN	[169]
	ANCAs (+)	Prognosis	[32,49,50]
2. Kidney disease-related			
Serum	Hyperuricemia	Diagnosis	[78,170,171]
	Creatinine ($\uparrow$)	Diagnosis and prognostic biomarkers	[78,166,172]
	Urea ($\uparrow$)	Diagnosis and damage (>10.25 mmol/L)	[78]
Urine	Albumin to globulin ratio (low)	Diagnosis	[173]
	Proteinuria ($\uparrow$) (>500 mg/24 h)	Diagnosis, clinical disease activity, histological disease activity, and prognosis	[67,95,109,174]
	Proteinuria ($\downarrow$)	Responses to therapy in LN	[169]
	uPCR ($\downarrow$) (<1.5 g/g at month 6)	Responses to therapy in LN	[109]
	WBC ($\uparrow$)	Clinical disease activity	[67]
	RBC ($\uparrow$)	Clinical disease activity	[67]

Table 1. *Cont.*

	Granular casts (+)	Clinical disease activity	[67]
		3. Complement/Lymphocytes	
Serum	C3 (low)	Diagnosis, clinical disease activity, histological disease activity, responses to therapy in LN, and prognosis	[67,95,109,174]
	C4 (low)	Diagnosis and clinical disease activity	[175]
	C1q (low)	Histological disease activity	[165]
	Lymphocyte count (↑)	Responses to therapy in LN	[169]
		4. Cytokines	
Serum	TWEAK	Diagnosis	[87,105,176–178]
	IL-2R (↓)	Responses to therapy in LN	[179]
	IL-8 (↓)	Responses to therapy in LN	[179]
	IL-10 (↑)	Clinical disease activity	[67,175]
	IL-17	Clinical disease activity and histological disease activity	[85,180]
	IL-23 (↓)	Responses to therapy in LN	[85]
Urine	TWEAK	Diagnosis and clinical disease activity	[87,176,177]
	TGF-β1 (↑)	Clinical disease activity and histological disease activity	[70,73]
	IL-17 (↑)	Diagnostic potential and clinical disease activity	[89]
	IL-12p40 (↑)	Diagnostic potential and clinical disease activity	[89]
	IL-15	Diagnostic potential and clinical disease activity	[89]
	IL-16 (↑)	Histological disease activity	[70]
	TARC (↑)	Diagnostic potential and clinical disease activity	[89]
	PF-4 (↑)	Clinical disease activity	[72]
		5. Chemokines/Cell adhesion molecules	
Serum	APRIL (↑)	Predictive of treatment failure at 6 months	[61]
	BAFF (↓)	Predictive of clinical and histological responses to therapy in LN	[59]
	VCAM-1 (↑)	Clinical disease activity	[103]
	OPG (↓)	Responses to therapy in LN	[179]
Urine	APRIL (↑)	Diagnosis	[53,181]
	BAFF (↑)	Diagnosis	[53,181]
	CXCL4 (↑)	Diagnosis	[98]
	MCP-1 (↑)	Diagnosis, clinical disease activity, histological disease activity (proliferative vs. membranous), and responses to therapy in LN	[79,80,83,99,177,182,183]
	ALCAM (↑)	Diagnosis, clinical disease activity, histological disease activity, and prognosis	[94,95,184]
	VCAM-1 (↑)	Diagnosis, clinical disease activity, histological disease activity (proliferative vs. membranous), damage, and prognostic biomarkers	[72,75,94,98,99]
	ICAM-1 (↑)	Clinical disease activity	[97]
	NCAM-1 (↑)	Clinical disease activity	[97]
	IP-10/CXCL10 (↑)	Diagnostic potential and clinical disease activity (renal)	[67,89]

Table 1. *Cont.*

		6. Other proteins	
Serum	Axl (↑)	Diagnosis, clinical disease activity, responses to therapy in LN, and prognostic biomarkers	[106–108]
	HE4 (↑)	Diagnosis	[78,185]
	IGFBP-2 (↑)	Diagnosis, clinical disease activity, and damage	[186]
	IGFBP-4	Damage	[187]
	sTNFRII (↑)	Diagnosis, clinical disease activity, histological disease activity, damage, responses to therapy in LN, and prognosis	[106,188,189]
	Angiostatin (↑)	Clinical disease activity	[108]
	Ferritin (↑)	Clinical disease activity	[108]
	Progranulin (↑)	Clinical disease activity	[108]
	SDC-1 (↑)	Clinical disease activity and histological disease activity	[103]
	Resistin (↑)	Damage	[190]
	CSF-1 (↓)	Responses to therapy in LN	[191]
	HNP1-3 (↓)	Responses to therapy in LN	[192]
	S100A8/A9 (↑)	Responses to therapy in LN	[193]
	S100A12 (↑)	Responses to therapy in LN	[193]
Urine	Angiostatin	Diagnosis, clinical disease activity, histological disease activity, and damage	[51,74,75,98]
	NGAL (↑)	Diagnosis, clinical disease activity, and (↓) responses to therapy in LN	[80,104,162,194–199]
	TF (↑)	Diagnosis, clinical disease activity and responses to therapy in LN	[92,183,200]
	β2-MG (↑)	Diagnosis	[22,201]
	Angptl4 (↑)	Clinical disease activity	[51,73]
	Calpastatin (↑)	Clinical disease activity	[72]
	CD163 (↑)	Clinical disease activity, histological disease activity (predictor, proliferative vs. non-proliferative), (↓) responses to therapy in LN and prognosis	[70,109,110,182]
	FOLR2 (↑)	Clinical disease activity	[73]
	Hemopexin (↑)	Clinical disease activity	[72]
	L-selectin (↓)	Clinical disease activity	[73]
	PDGFRβ (↑)	Clinical disease activity	[73]
	Peroxiredoxin 6 (↑)	Clinical disease activity	[72]
	Progranulin (↑)	Clinical disease activity	[108]
	Properdin (↑)	Clinical disease activity	[72]
	RBP4 (↑)	Clinical disease activity and (↓) responses to therapy in LN	[202]
	TSP1 (↑)	Clinical disease activity	[73]
	TTP1 (↑)	Clinical disease activity	[73]
	NRP-1 (↑)	Responses to therapy in LN	[203]
	Plasmin (↑)	Clinical disease activity	[200]
	TFPI (↑)	Clinical disease activity	[200]

Table 1. Cont.

	EGF (↓)	Prognosis	[112]
	7. MicroRNAs (miRNAs)		
Serum/plasma	miRNA-21	Diagnosis	[128,204]
Urine	miRNA-31-5p (↑)	Responses to therapy in LN	[127]
	miRNA-107 (↑)	Responses to therapy in LN	[127]
	miRNA-135b-5p (↑)	Responses to therapy in LN	[127]
	8. Microparticles (MP)		
Urine	MP-CX3CR1+ (↑)	Diagnosis	[172]
	MP-HLADR+ (↑)	Diagnosis	[172]
	MP-HMGB1+ (↑)	Diagnosis and clinical disease activity (active vs. non-active)	[172]
	9. Renal tissue		
Kidney biopsy	Mannose-enriched N-glycan expression	Diagnosis and prognosis	[205]
	CSF-1 (↑)	Histological disease activity	[191]
	Periostin (↑)	Damage	[206]
	C9 (+)	Prognosis	[207]
	Podocyte foot process width (↓)	Prognosis	[169]
	Arteriolar C4d deposition (+)	Prognosis	[208]
	Cellular crescents (+)	Prognosis	[172]
	Fibrous crescents (+)	Prognosis	[172]
	Glomerular C3 deposition (+)	Prognosis	[212]
	IFTA (+) (≥25% of the surface cortical area)	Prognosis	[213]
	Vascular injury (+) (≥25% subintimal narrowing of the lumen)	Prognosis	[213]

AaA: Anti-actin antibody; ANCA: Anti-neutrophil cytoplasmic antibody; Ang2: Angiopoietin 2; Angptl4: Angiopoietin-like 4; Anti-C1q: Anti-complement component 1q; Anti-CRP: Anti-C-reactive protein; Anti-dsDNA: Anti-double-stranded deoxyribonucleic acid; Anti-ENO-1: Anti-Enolase 1; APRIL: A proliferation-inducing ligand; BAFF: B-cell activating factor; β2-MG: Beta-2 microglobulin; C1q: Complement component 1q; C3: Complement component 3; C4: Complement component 4; C4d: Complement component 4d; C9: Complement component 9; Cer: Ceramide; CSF-1: Colony stimulating factor 1; CXCL4: C-X-C motif chemokine ligand 4; EGF: Epidermal growth factor; FOLR2: Folate receptor beta; HNP1-3: Human neutrophil peptide 1-3; ICAM-1: Intercellular adhesion molecule 1; IFTA: Interstitial fibrosis and tubular atrophy; IGFBP: Insulin-like growth factor-binding protein; IL: Interleukin; IL-2R: Interleukin 2 receptor; IL-12p40: Interleukin 12 subunit p40; IP-10: Interferon gamma-induced protein 10, also known as CXCL10; MCP-1: Monocyte chemoattractant protein 1; MicroRNAs (miRNAs): Micro-ribonucleic acids, with miRNA-21 being Micro-ribonucleic acid 21; MP-CX3CR1+: Microparticles with CX3CR1 expression; MP-HLADR+: Microparticles with HLA-DR expression; MP-HMGB1+: Microparticles with high mobility group box 1 protein expression; NRP-1: Neuropilin 1; NCAM-1: Neural cell adhesion molecule 1; NGAL: Neutrophil gelatinase-associated lipocalin; OPG: Osteoprotegerin; PDGFRβ: Platelet-derived growth factor receptor beta; PF-4: Platelet factor 4; PHACTR4: Phosphatase and actin regulator 4, with PHACTR4 icx being Phosphatase and actin regulator 4 immune complexes; P3H1: Prolyl 3-hydroxylase 1, with P3H1 icx as Prolyl 3-hydroxylase 1 immune complexes; PTEC-binding IgG: Proximal tubular epithelial cell-binding immunoglobulin G; RBC: Red blood cells; RGS12: Regulator of G-protein signalling 12, with RGS12 icx as Regulator of G-protein signalling 12 immune complexes; SDC-1: Syndecan-1; sTNFRII: Soluble tumor necrosis factor receptor II; TARC: Thymus and activation-regulated chemokine, also known as CCL17; TFPI: Tissue factor pathway inhibitor; TGF-β1: Transforming growth factor-beta 1; TSP1: Thrombospondin 1; TTP1: Tripeptidyl peptidase 1; Type I IFN: Type I Interferon; TWEAK: Tumor necrosis factor-like weak inducer of apoptosis; uPCR: Urine protein to creatinine ratio; VCAM-1: Vascular cell adhesion molecule 1; WBC: White blood cells; (+): Positivity; ↓: Decreased; ↑: Increased.

Several reasons may account for the fact that none of the discussed biomarkers has reached the bedside. There are challenges in both the discovery and clinical phase of biomarker validation [161]. During the discovery phases a major weight is placed on the formulation of clinically relevant questions and the identification of markers closely linked to the pathogenesis of LN, while less effort is made to consider the clinical and pathogenetic heterogeneity of LN in long prospective studies. In the efforts to validate the reported putative biomarkers, problems arise from the geographical and ethnic heterogeneity of the disease, the lack of standardized treatment protocols, sample collection and processing, and the methods used to measure various biomarkers.

Author Contributions: Conceptualization, F.K.A. and G.C.T.; writing—review and editing, F.K.A. and G.C.T.; writing—original draft preparation, F.K.A. Both authors have read and approved the final manuscript. All authors have read and agreed to the published version of the manuscript.

Funding: This research received no external funding.

Institutional Review Board Statement: Not applicable.

Informed Consent Statement: Not applicable.

Data Availability Statement: Not applicable.

Conflicts of Interest: The authors declare that they have no conflicts of interest.

References

1. Mason, L.J.; Isenberg, D.A. Immunopathogenesis of SLE. *Baillieres Clin. Rheumatol.* **1998**, *12*, 385–403. [CrossRef]
2. Hahn, B.H.; Ebling, F.; Singh, R.R.; Singh, R.P.; Karpouzas, G.; La Cava, A. Cellular and molecular mechanisms of regulation of autoantibody production in lupus. *Ann. N. Y. Acad. Sci.* **2005**, *1051*, 433–441. [CrossRef]
3. Alduraibi, F.; Fatima, H.; Hamilton, J.A.; Chatham, W.W.; Hsu, H.C.; Mountz, J.D. Lupus nephritis correlates with B cell interferon-β, anti-Smith, and anti-DNA: A retrospective study. *Arthritis Res. Ther.* **2022**, *24*, 87. [CrossRef] [PubMed]
4. Alduraibi, F.K.; Sullivan, K.A.; Chatham, W.W.; Hsu, H.C.; Mountz, J.D. Interrelation of T cell cytokines and autoantibodies in systemic lupus erythematosus: A cross-sectional study. *Clin. Immunol.* **2023**, *247*, 109239. [CrossRef] [PubMed]
5. Stojan, G.; Petri, M. Epidemiology of systemic lupus erythematosus: An update. *Curr. Opin. Rheumatol.* **2018**, *30*, 144–150. [CrossRef]
6. Chakravarty, E.F.; Bush, T.M.; Manzi, S.; Clarke, A.E.; Ward, M.M. Prevalence of adult systemic lupus erythematosus in California and Pennsylvania in 2000: Estimates obtained using hospitalization data. *Arthritis Rheum.* **2007**, *56*, 2092–2094. [CrossRef] [PubMed]
7. Pons-Estel, G.J.; Alarcón, G.S.; Scofield, L.; Reinlib, L.; Cooper, G.S. Understanding the epidemiology and progression of systemic lupus erythematosus. *Semin. Arthritis Rheum.* **2010**, *39*, 257–268. [CrossRef] [PubMed]
8. Tian, J.; Zhang, D.; Yao, X.; Huang, Y.; Lu, Q. Global epidemiology of systemic lupus erythematosus: A comprehensive systematic analysis and modelling study. *Ann. Rheum. Dis.* **2023**, *82*, 351–356. [CrossRef]
9. Lerang, K.; Gilboe, I.M.; Steinar Thelle, D.; Gran, J.T. Mortality and years of potential life loss in systemic lupus erythematosus: A population-based cohort study. *Lupus* **2014**, *23*, 1546–1552. [CrossRef]
10. Danila, M.I.; Pons-Estel, G.J.; Zhang, J.; Vila, L.M.; Reveille, J.D.; Alarcon, G.S. Renal damage is the most important predictor of mortality within the damage index: Data from LUMINA LXIV, a multiethnic US cohort. *Rheumatology* **2009**, *48*, 542–545. [CrossRef]
11. Mok, C.C.; Kwok, R.C.L.; Yip, P.S.F. Effect of Renal Disease on the Standardized Mortality Ratio and Life Expectancy of Patients With Systemic Lupus Erythematosus. *Arthritis Rheum.* **2013**, *65*, 2154–2160. [CrossRef] [PubMed]
12. Bajema, I.M.; Wilhelmus, S.; Alpers, C.E.; Bruijn, J.A.; Colvin, R.B.; Cook, H.T.; D'Agati, V.D.; Ferrario, F.; Haas, M.; Jennette, J.C.; et al. Revision of the International Society of Nephrology/Renal Pathology Society classification for lupus nephritis: Clarification of definitions, and modified National Institutes of Health activity and chronicity indices. *Kidney Int.* **2018**, *93*, 789–796. [CrossRef] [PubMed]
13. Arazi, A.; Rao, D.A.; Berthier, C.C.; Davidson, A.; Liu, Y.; Hoover, P.J.; Chicoine, A.; Eisenhaure, T.M.; Jonsson, A.H.; Li, S. The immune cell landscape in kidneys of patients with lupus nephritis. *Nat. Immunol.* **2019**, *20*, 902–914. [CrossRef] [PubMed]
14. Tsokos, G.C.; Boulougoura, A.; Kasinath, V.; Endo, U.; Abdi, R.; Li, H. The immunoregulatory roles of non-haematopoietic cells in the kidney. *Nat. Rev. Nephrol.* **2023**, 1–12. [CrossRef] [PubMed]
15. Anders, H.-J.; Saxena, R.; Zhao, M.-h.; Parodis, I.; Salmon, J.E.; Mohan, C. Lupus nephritis. *Nat. Rev. Dis. Primers* **2020**, *6*, 7. [CrossRef] [PubMed]
16. Lorenz, G.; Lech, M.; Anders, H.-J. Toll-like receptor activation in the pathogenesis of lupus nephritis. *Clin. Immunol.* **2017**, *185*, 86–94. [CrossRef] [PubMed]

17. Kaul, A.; Gordon, C.; Crow, M.K.; Touma, Z.; Urowitz, M.B.; van Vollenhoven, R.; Ruiz-Irastorza, G.; Hughes, G. Systemic lupus erythematosus. *Nat. Rev. Dis. Primers* **2016**, *2*, 16039. [CrossRef] [PubMed]
18. Migliorini, A.; Anders, H.-J. A novel pathogenetic concept—Antiviral immunity in lupus nephritis. *Nat. Rev. Nephrol.* **2012**, *8*, 183–189. [CrossRef]
19. Devarapu, S.; Lorenz, G.; Kulkarni, O.; Anders, H.-J.; Mulay, S. Cellular and molecular mechanisms of autoimmunity and lupus nephritis. *Int. Rev. Cell Mol. Biol.* **2017**, *332*, 43–154.
20. Hiepe, F.; Dörner, T.; Hauser, A.E.; Hoyer, B.F.; Mei, H.; Radbruch, A. Long-lived autoreactive plasma cells drive persistent autoimmune inflammation. *Nat. Rev. Rheumatol.* **2011**, *7*, 170–178. [CrossRef]
21. Hiepe, F.; Radbruch, A. Plasma cells as an innovative target in autoimmune disease with renal manifestations. *Nat. Rev. Nephrol.* **2016**, *12*, 232–240. [CrossRef]
22. Huang, X.; Chen, W.; Ren, G.; Zhao, L.; Guo, J.; Gong, D.; Zeng, C.; Hu, W.; Liu, Z. Autologous hematopoietic stem cell transplantation for refractory lupus nephritis. *Clin. J. Am. Soc. Nephrol. CJASN* **2019**, *14*, 719. [CrossRef]
23. Alexander, T.; Sarfert, R.; Klotsche, J.; Kühl, A.A.; Rubbert-Roth, A.; Lorenz, H.-M.; Rech, J.; Hoyer, B.F.; Cheng, Q.; Waka, A. The proteasome inhibitior bortezomib depletes plasma cells and ameliorates clinical manifestations of refractory systemic lupus erythematosus. *Ann. Rheum. Dis.* **2015**, *74*, 1474–1478. [CrossRef]
24. Der, E.; Suryawanshi, H.; Morozov, P.; Kustagi, M.; Goilav, B.; Ranabothu, S.; Izmirly, P.; Clancy, R.; Belmont, H.M.; Koenigsberg, M. Tubular cell and keratinocyte single-cell transcriptomics applied to lupus nephritis reveal type I IFN and fibrosis relevant pathways. *Nat. Immunol.* **2019**, *20*, 915–927. [CrossRef]
25. Bethunaickan, R.; Berthier, C.C.; Zhang, W.; Eksi, R.; Li, H.D.; Guan, Y.; Kretzler, M.; Davidson, A. Identification of stage-specific genes associated with lupus nephritis and response to remission induction in (NZB× NZW) F1 and NZM2410 mice. *Arthritis Rheumatol.* **2014**, *66*, 2246–2258. [CrossRef]
26. Anders, H.-J. Nephropathic autoantigens in the spectrum of lupus nephritis. *Nat. Rev. Nephrol.* **2019**, *15*, 595–596. [CrossRef]
27. Doria, A.; Gatto, M. Nephritogenic-antinephritogenic antibody network in lupus glomerulonephritis. *Lupus* **2012**, *21*, 1492–1496. [CrossRef]
28. Stojan, G.; Petri, M. Anti-C1q in systemic lupus erythematosus. *Lupus* **2016**, *25*, 873–877. [CrossRef]
29. Kotzen, E.S.; Roy, S.; Jain, K. Antiphospholipid syndrome nephropathy and other thrombotic microangiopathies among patients with systemic lupus erythematosus. *Adv. Chronic Kidney Dis.* **2019**, *26*, 376–386. [CrossRef]
30. Sciascia, S.; Cuadrado, M.J.; Khamashta, M.; Roccatello, D. Renal involvement in antiphospholipid syndrome. *Nat. Rev. Nephrol.* **2014**, *10*, 279–289. [CrossRef]
31. Ryu, M.; Migliorini, A.; Miosge, N.; Gross, O.; Shankland, S.; Brinkkoetter, P.T.; Hagmann, H.; Romagnani, P.; Liapis, H.; Anders, H.J. Plasma leakage through glomerular basement membrane ruptures triggers the proliferation of parietal epithelial cells and crescent formation in non-inflammatory glomerular injury. *J. Pathol.* **2012**, *228*, 482–494. [CrossRef] [PubMed]
32. Turner-Stokes, T.; Wilson, H.R.; Morreale, M.; Nunes, A.; Cairns, T.; Cook, H.T.; Pusey, C.D.; Tarzi, R.M.; Lightstone, L. Positive antineutrophil cytoplasmic antibody serology in patients with lupus nephritis is associated with distinct histopathologic features on renal biopsy. *Kidney Int.* **2017**, *92*, 1223–1231. [CrossRef]
33. Fanouriakis, A.; Kostopoulou, M.; Cheema, K.; Anders, H.-J.; Aringer, M.; Bajema, I.; Boletis, J.; Frangou, E.; Houssiau, F.A.; Hollis, J.; et al. 2019 Update of the Joint European League Against Rheumatism and European Renal Association–European Dialysis and Transplant Association (EULAR/ERA–EDTA) recommendations for the management of lupus nephritis. *Ann. Rheum. Dis.* **2020**, *79*, 713–723. [CrossRef] [PubMed]
34. Trendelenburg, M.; Lopez-Trascasa, M.; Potlukova, E.; Moll, S.; Regenass, S.; Fremeaux-Bacchi, V.; Martinez-Ara, J.; Jancova, E.; Picazo, M.L.; Honsova, E. High prevalence of anti-C1q antibodies in biopsy-proven active lupus nephritis. *Nephrol. Dial. Transplant.* **2006**, *21*, 3115–3121. [CrossRef] [PubMed]
35. Gargiulo, M.D.L.Á.; Khoury, M.; Gómez, G.; Grimaudo, S.; Suárez, L.; Collado, M.V.; Sarano, J. Cut-off values of immunological tests to identify patients at high risk of severe lupus nephritis. *Medicina* **2018**, *78*, 329–335.
36. Pesickova, S.S.; Rysava, R.; Lenicek, M.; Vitek, L.; Potlukova, E.; Hruskova, Z.; Jancova, E.; Honsova, E.; Zavada, J.; Trendelenburg, M.; et al. Prognostic value of anti-CRP antibodies in lupus nephritis in long-term follow-up. *Arthritis Res. Ther.* **2015**, *17*, 371. [CrossRef]
37. Bonanni, A.; Vaglio, A.; Bruschi, M.; Sinico, R.A.; Cavagna, L.; Moroni, G.; Franceschini, F.; Allegri, L.; Pratesi, F.; Migliorini, P.; et al. Multi-antibody composition in lupus nephritis: Isotype and antigen specificity make the difference. *Autoimmun. Rev.* **2015**, *14*, 692–702. [CrossRef]
38. Huang, Y.; Chen, L.; Chen, K.; Huang, F.; Feng, Y.; Xu, Z.; Wang, W. Anti-α-enolase antibody combined with β2 microglobulin evaluated the incidence of nephritis in systemic lupus erythematosus patients. *Lupus* **2019**, *28*, 365–370. [CrossRef]
39. Bruschi, M.; Sinico, R.A.; Moroni, G.; Pratesi, F.; Migliorini, P.; Galetti, M.; Murtas, C.; Tincani, A.; Madaio, M.; Radice, A.; et al. Glomerular Autoimmune Multicomponents of Human Lupus Nephritis In Vivo: α: -Enolase and Annexin AI. *J. Am. Soc. Nephrol.* **2014**, *25*, 2483. [CrossRef]
40. Bruschi, M.; Moroni, G.; Sinico, R.A.; Franceschini, F.; Fredi, M.; Vaglio, A.; Cavagna, L.; Petretto, A.; Pratesi, F.; Migliorini, P.; et al. Serum IgG2 antibody multicomposition in systemic lupus erythematosus and lupus nephritis (Part 1): Cross-sectional analysis. *Rheumatology* **2021**, *60*, 3176–3188. [CrossRef]

41. Babaei, M.; Rezaieyazdi, Z.; Saadati, N.; Saghafi, M.; Sahebari, M.; Naghibzadeh, B.; Esmaily, H. Serum alpha–actinin antibody status in systemic lupus erythematosus and its potential in the diagnosis of lupus nephritis. *Casp. J. Intern. Med.* **2016**, *7*, 272.
42. Cortés-Hernández, J.; Ordi-Ros, J.; Labrador, M.; Buján, S.; Balada, E.; Segarra, A.; Vilardell-Tarrés, M. Antihistone and anti–double-stranded deoxyribonucleic acid antibodies are associated with renal disease in systemic lupus erythematosus. *Am. J. Med.* **2004**, *116*, 165–173. [CrossRef]
43. Sun, X.Y.; Shi, J.; Han, L.; Su, Y.; Li, Z.G. Anti-histones antibodies in systemic lupus erythematosus: Prevalence and frequency in neuropsychiatric lupus. *J. Clin. Lab. Anal.* **2008**, *22*, 271–277. [CrossRef] [PubMed]
44. Ehrenstein, M.R.; Katz, D.R.; Griffiths, M.H.; Papadaki, L.; Winkler, T.H.; Kalden, J.R.; Isenberg, D.A. Human IgG anti-DNA antibodies deposit in kidneys and induce proteinuria in SCID mice. *Kidney Int.* **1995**, *48*, 705–711. [CrossRef] [PubMed]
45. Hakkim, A.; Fürnrohr, B.G.; Amann, K.; Laube, B.; Abed, U.A.; Brinkmann, V.; Herrmann, M.; Voll, R.E.; Zychlinsky, A. Impairment of neutrophil extracellular trap degradation is associated with lupus nephritis. *Proc. Natl. Acad. Sci. USA* **2010**, *107*, 9813–9818. [CrossRef]
46. Kalaaji, M.; Fenton, K.A.; Mortensen, E.S.; Olsen, R.; Sturfelt, G.; Alm, P.; Rekvig, O.P. Glomerular apoptotic nucleosomes are central target structures for nephritogenic antibodies in human SLE nephritis. *Kidney Int.* **2007**, *71*, 664–672. [CrossRef]
47. Hedberg, A.; Fismen, S.; Fenton, K.A.; Mortensen, E.S.; Rekvig, O.P. Deposition of chromatin-IgG complexes in skin of nephritic MRL-lpr/lpr mice is associated with increased local matrix metalloprotease activities. *Exp. Dermatol.* **2010**, *19*, e265–e274. [CrossRef]
48. Grootscholten, C.; Dieker, J.W.; McGrath, F.D.; Roos, A.; Derksen, R.H.; van der Vlag, J.; Daha, M.R.; Berden, J.H. A prospective study of anti-chromatin and anti-C1q autoantibodies in patients with proliferative lupus nephritis treated with cyclophosphamide pulses or azathioprine/methylprednisolone. *Ann. Rheum. Dis.* **2007**, *66*, 693–696. [CrossRef]
49. Wang, Y.; Huang, X.; Cai, J.; Xie, L.; Wang, W.; Tang, S.; Yin, S.; Gao, X.; Zhang, J.; Zhao, J.; et al. Clinicopathologic Characteristics and Outcomes of Lupus Nephritis With Antineutrophil Cytoplasmic Antibody: A Retrospective Study. *Medicine* **2016**, *95*, e2580. [CrossRef]
50. Wang, S.; Shang, J.; Xiao, J.; Zhao, Z. Clinicopathologic characteristics and outcomes of lupus nephritis with positive antineutrophil cytoplasmic antibody. *Ren. Fail.* **2020**, *42*, 244–254. [CrossRef]
51. Zhang, T.; Duran, V.; Vanarsa, K.; Mohan, C. Targeted urine proteomics in lupus nephritis–a meta-analysis. *Expert Rev. Proteom.* **2020**, *17*, 767–776. [CrossRef]
52. Rovin, B.H. The chemokine network in systemic lupus erythematous nephritis. *FBL* **2008**, *13*, 904–922. [CrossRef]
53. Phatak, S.; Chaurasia, S.; Mishra, P.; Gupta, R.; Agrawal, V.; Aggarwal, A.; Misra, R. Urinary B cell activating factor (BAFF) and a proliferation-inducing ligand (APRIL): Potential biomarkers of active lupus nephritis. *Clin. Exp. Immunol.* **2017**, *187*, 376–382. [CrossRef]
54. Guimarães, J.d.A.R.; Furtado, S.d.C.a.o.; Lucas, A.C.d.S.; Mori, B.; Barcellos, J.F.M. Diagnostic test accuracy of novel biomarkers for lupus nephritis—An overview of systematic reviews. *PLoS ONE* **2022**, *17*, e0275016. [CrossRef]
55. Rahmé, Z.; Franco, C.; Cruciani, C.; Pettorossi, F.; Zaramella, A.; Realdon, S.; Iaccarino, L.; Frontini, G.; Moroni, G.; Doria, A.; et al. Characterization of Serum Cytokine Profiles of Patients with Active Lupus Nephritis. *Int. J. Mol. Sci.* **2023**, *24*, 14883. [CrossRef]
56. Wu, H.; Zeng, J.; Yin, J.; Peng, Q.; Zhao, M.; Lu, Q. Organ-specific biomarkers in lupus. *Autoimmun. Rev.* **2017**, *16*, 391–397. [CrossRef]
57. Petri, M.; Stohl, W.; Chatham, W.; McCune, W.J.; Chevrier, M.; Ryel, J.; Recta, V.; Zhong, J.; Freimuth, W. Association of plasma B lymphocyte stimulator levels and disease activity in systemic lupus erythematosus. *Arthritis Rheum. Off. J. Am. Coll. Rheumatol.* **2008**, *58*, 2453–2459. [CrossRef]
58. Hegazy, M.; Darwish, H.; Darweesh, H.; El-Shehaby, A.; Emad, Y. Raised serum level of APRIL in patients with systemic lupus erythematosus: Correlations with disease activity indices. *Clin. Immunol.* **2010**, *135*, 118–124. [CrossRef]
59. Parodis, I.; Zickert, A.; Sundelin, B.; Axelsson, M.; Gerhardsson, J.; Svenungsson, E.; Malmström, V.; Gunnarsson, I. Evaluation of B lymphocyte stimulator and a proliferation inducing ligand as candidate biomarkers in lupus nephritis based on clinical and histopathological outcome following induction therapy. *Lupus Sci. Med.* **2015**, *2*, e000061. [CrossRef] [PubMed]
60. Levy, R.A.; Gonzalez-Rivera, T.; Khamashta, M.; Fox, N.L.; Jones-Leone, A.; Rubin, B.; Burriss, S.W.; Gairy, K.; Maurik, A.v.; Roth, D.A. 10 Years of belimumab experience: What have we learnt? *Lupus* **2021**, *30*, 1705–1721. [CrossRef] [PubMed]
61. Treamtrakanpon, W.; Tantivitayakul, P.; Benjachat, T.; Somparn, P.; Kittikowit, W.; Eiam-ong, S.; Leelahavanichkul, A.; Hirankarn, N.; Avihingsanon, Y. APRIL, a proliferation-inducing ligand, as a potential marker of lupus nephritis. *Arthritis Res. Ther.* **2012**, *14*, R252. [CrossRef]
62. Antonelli, A.; Ferrari, S.M.; Giuggioli, D.; Ferrannini, E.; Ferri, C.; Fallahi, P. Chemokine (C–X–C motif) ligand (CXCL)10 in autoimmune diseases. *Autoimmun. Rev.* **2014**, *13*, 272–280. [CrossRef] [PubMed]
63. Puapatanakul, P.; Chansritrakul, S.; Susantitaphong, P.; Ueaphongsukkit, T.; Eiam-Ong, S.; Praditpornsilpa, K.; Kittanamongkolchai, W.; Avihingsanon, Y. Interferon-inducible protein 10 and disease activity in systemic lupus erythematosus and lupus nephritis: A systematic review and meta-analysis. *Int. J. Mol. Sci.* **2019**, *20*, 4954. [CrossRef] [PubMed]
64. Biesen, R.; Demir, C.; Barkhudarova, F.; Grün, J.R.; Steinbrich-Zöllner, M.; Backhaus, M.; Häupl, T.; Rudwaleit, M.; Riemekasten, G.; Radbruch, A. Sialic acid–binding Ig-like lectin 1 expression in inflammatory and resident monocytes is a potential biomarker for monitoring disease activity and success of therapy in systemic lupus erythematosus. *Arthritis Rheum.* **2008**, *58*, 1136–1145. [CrossRef] [PubMed]

65. Chun, H.-Y.; Chung, J.-W.; Kim, H.-A.; Yun, J.-M.; Jeon, J.-Y.; Ye, Y.-M.; Kim, S.-H.; Park, H.-S.; Suh, C.-H. Cytokine IL-6 and IL-10 as biomarkers in systemic lupus erythematosus. *J. Clin. Immunol.* **2007**, *27*, 461–466. [CrossRef] [PubMed]
66. Choy, E.H.; De Benedetti, F.; Takeuchi, T.; Hashizume, M.; John, M.R.; Kishimoto, T. Translating IL-6 biology into effective treatments. *Nat. Rev. Rheumatol.* **2020**, *16*, 335–345. [CrossRef] [PubMed]
67. Jakiela, B.; Kosałka, J.; Plutecka, H.; Węgrzyn, A.S.; Bazan-Socha, S.; Sanak, M.; Musiał, J. Urinary cytokines and mRNA expression as biomarkers of disease activity in lupus nephritis. *Lupus* **2018**, *27*, 1259–1270. [CrossRef] [PubMed]
68. Glass, W.G.; Sarisky, R.T.; Vecchio, A.M.D. Not-so-sweet sixteen: The role of IL-16 in infectious and immune-mediated inflammatory diseases. *J. Interferon Cytokine Res.* **2006**, *26*, 511–520. [CrossRef]
69. Roth, S.; Agthe, M.; Eickhoff, S.; Möller, S.; Karsten, C.; Borregaard, N.; Solbach, W.; Laskay, T. Secondary necrotic neutrophils release interleukin-16C and macrophage migration inhibitory factor from stores in the cytosol. *Cell Death Discov.* **2015**, *1*, 15056. [CrossRef]
70. Fava, A.; Rao, D.A.; Mohan, C.; Zhang, T.; Rosenberg, A.; Fenaroli, P.; Belmont, H.M.; Izmirly, P.; Clancy, R.; Trujillo, J.M. Urine proteomics and renal single-cell transcriptomics implicate interleukin-16 in lupus nephritis. *Arthritis Rheumatol.* **2022**, *74*, 829–839. [CrossRef]
71. El-Banawy, H.S.; Gaber, E.W.; Maharem, D.A.; Matrawy, K.A. Angiopoietin-2, endothelial dysfunction and renal involvement in patients with systemic lupus erythematosus. *J. Nephrol.* **2012**, *25*, 541–550. [CrossRef] [PubMed]
72. Stanley, S.; Vanarsa, K.; Soliman, S.; Habazi, D.; Pedroza, C.; Gidley, G.; Zhang, T.; Mohan, S.; Der, E.; Suryawanshi, H. Comprehensive aptamer-based screening identifies a spectrum of urinary biomarkers of lupus nephritis across ethnicities. *Nat. Commun.* **2020**, *11*, 2197. [CrossRef] [PubMed]
73. Vanarsa, K.; Soomro, S.; Zhang, T.; Strachan, B.; Pedroza, C.; Nidhi, M.; Cicalese, P.; Gidley, C.; Dasari, S.; Mohan, S.; et al. Quantitative planar array screen of 1000 proteins uncovers novel urinary protein biomarkers of lupus nephritis. *Ann. Rheum. Dis.* **2020**, *79*, 1349–1361. [CrossRef] [PubMed]
74. Wu, T.; Du, Y.; Han, J.; Singh, S.; Xie, C.; Guo, Y.; Zhou, X.J.; Ahn, C.; Saxena, R.; Mohan, C. Urinary Angiostatin—A Novel Putative Marker of Renal Pathology Chronicity in Lupus Nephritis. *Mol. Cell. Proteom.* **2013**, *12*, 1170–1179. [CrossRef] [PubMed]
75. Soliman, S.; Mohamed, F.A.; Ismail, F.M.; Stanley, S.; Saxena, R.; Mohan, C. Urine angiostatin and VCAM-1 surpass conventional metrics in predicting elevated renal pathology activity indices in lupus nephritis. *Int. J. Rheum. Dis.* **2017**, *20*, 1714–1727. [CrossRef]
76. Raslan, H.Z.; Sibaii, H.; El-Zayat, S.R.; Hassan, H.; El-Kassaby, M. Increased level of B cell differentiation factor in systemic lupus erythematosus patients. *J. Genet. Eng. Biotechnol.* **2018**, *16*, 467–471. [CrossRef] [PubMed]
77. Zhu, Y.; Xue, Z.; Di, L. Regulation of MiR-146a and TRAF6 in the diagnosis of lupus nephritis. *Med. Sci. Monit. Int. Med. J. Exp. Clin. Res.* **2017**, *23*, 2550. [CrossRef] [PubMed]
78. Yang, Z.; Zhang, Z.; Qin, B.; Wu, P.; Zhong, R.; Zhou, L.; Liang, Y. Human epididymis protein 4: A novel biomarker for lupus nephritis and chronic kidney disease in systemic lupus erythematosus. *J. Clin. Lab. Anal.* **2016**, *30*, 897–904. [CrossRef]
79. Xia, Y.-R.; Li, Q.-R.; Wang, J.-P.; Guo, H.-S.; Bao, Y.-Q.; Mao, Y.-M.; Wu, J.; Pan, H.-F.; Ye, D.-Q. Diagnostic value of urinary monocyte chemoattractant protein-1 in evaluating the activity of lupus nephritis: A meta-analysis. *Lupus* **2020**, *29*, 599–606. [CrossRef]
80. Liu, L.; Wang, R.; Ding, H.; Tian, L.; Gao, T.; Bao, C. The utility of urinary biomarker panel in predicting renal pathology and treatment response in Chinese lupus nephritis patients. *PLoS ONE* **2020**, *15*, e0240942. [CrossRef]
81. Singh, R.; Usha; Rathore, S.S.; Behura, S.K.; Singh, N.K. Urinary MCP-1 as diagnostic and prognostic marker in patients with lupus nephritis flare. *Lupus* **2012**, *21*, 1214–1218. [CrossRef] [PubMed]
82. Rovin, B.H.; Song, H.; Birmingham, D.J.; Hebert, L.A.; Yu, C.Y.; Nagaraja, H.N. Urine chemokines as biomarkers of human systemic lupus erythematosus activity. *J. Am. Soc. Nephrol. JASN* **2004**, *16*, 467–473. [CrossRef] [PubMed]
83. Urrego-Callejas, T.; Álvarez, S.S.; Arias, L.F.; Reyes, B.O.; Vanegas-García, A.L.; González, L.A.; Muñoz-Vahos, C.H.; Vásquez, G.; Quintana, L.F.; Gómez-Puerta, J.A. Urinary levels of ceruloplasmin and monocyte chemoattractant protein-1 correlate with extra-capillary proliferation and chronic damage in patients with lupus nephritis. *Clin. Rheumatol.* **2021**, *40*, 1853–1859. [CrossRef] [PubMed]
84. Susianti, H.; Iriane, V.M.; Dharmanata, S.; Handono, K.; Widijanti, A.; Gunawan, A.; Kalim, H. Analysis of urinary TGF-β1, MCP-1, NGAL, and IL-17 as biomarkers for lupus nephritis. *Pathophysiology* **2015**, *22*, 65–71. [CrossRef] [PubMed]
85. Dedong, H.; Feiyan, Z.; Jie, S.; Xiaowei, L.; Shaoyang, W. Analysis of interleukin-17 and interleukin-23 for estimating disease activity and predicting the response to treatment in active lupus nephritis patients. *Immunol. Lett.* **2019**, *210*, 33–39. [CrossRef] [PubMed]
86. Mohan, C.; Zhang, T.; Putterman, C. Pathogenic cellular and molecular mediators in lupus nephritis. *Nat. Rev. Nephrol.* **2023**, *19*, 491–508. [CrossRef] [PubMed]
87. Salem, M.N.; Taha, H.A.; Abd El-Fattah El-Feqi, M.; Eesa, N.N.; Mohamed, R.A. Urinary TNF-like weak inducer of apoptosis (TWEAK) as a biomarker of lupus nephritis. *Z. Für Rheumatol.* **2018**, *77*, 71–77. [CrossRef]
88. Wang, Z.-H.; Dai, Z.-W.; Dong, Y.-Y.; Wang, H.; Yuan, F.-F.; Wang, B.; Ye, D.-Q. Urinary Tumor Necrosis Factor–Like Weak Inducer of Apoptosis as a Biomarker for Diagnosis and Evaluating Activity in Lupus Nephritis: A Meta-analysis. *JCR J. Clin. Rheumatol.* **2021**, *27*, 272–277. [CrossRef]

89. Stanley, S.; Mok, C.C.; Vanarsa, K.; Habazi, D.; Li, J.; Pedroza, C.; Saxena, R.; Mohan, C. Identification of Low-Abundance Urinary Biomarkers in Lupus Nephritis Using Electrochemiluminescence Immunoassays. *Arthritis Rheumatol.* **2019**, *71*, 744–755. [CrossRef]
90. Wu, C.-Y.; Yang, H.-Y.; Chien, H.-P.; Tseng, M.-H.; Huang, J.-L. Urinary clusterin—A novel urinary biomarker associated with pediatric lupus renal histopathologic features and renal survival. *Pediatr. Nephrol.* **2018**, *33*, 1189–1198. [CrossRef]
91. Gupta, R.; Aggarwal, A.; Sinha, S.; Rajasekhar, L.; Yadav, A.; Gaur, P.; Misra, R.; Negi, V. Urinary osteoprotegerin: A potential biomarker of lupus nephritis disease activity. *Lupus* **2016**, *25*, 1230–1236. [CrossRef] [PubMed]
92. Urrego, T.; Ortiz-Reyes, B.; Vanegas-García, A.L.; Muñoz, C.H.; González, L.A.; Vásquez, G.; Gómez-Puerta, J.A. Utility of urinary transferrin and ceruloplasmin in patients with systemic lupus erythematosus for differentiating patients with lupus nephritis. *Reumatol. Clínica (Engl. Ed.)* **2020**, *16*, 17–23. [CrossRef]
93. Springer, T.A. Adhesion receptors of the immune system. *Nature* **1990**, *346*, 425–434. [CrossRef] [PubMed]
94. Parodis, I.; Gokaraju, S.; Zickert, A.; Vanarsa, K.; Zhang, T.; Habazi, D.; Botto, J.; Serdoura Alves, C.; Giannopoulos, P.; Larsson, A.; et al. ALCAM and VCAM-1 as urine biomarkers of activity and long-term renal outcome in systemic lupus erythematosus. *Rheumatology* **2020**, *59*, 2237–2249. [CrossRef] [PubMed]
95. Ding, H.; Lin, C.; Cai, J.; Guo, Q.; Dai, M.; Mohan, C.; Shen, N. Urinary activated leukocyte cell adhesion molecule as a novel biomarker of lupus nephritis histology. *Arthritis Res. Ther.* **2020**, *22*, 1–9. [CrossRef]
96. Howe, H.S.; Kong, K.O.; Thong, B.Y.; Law, W.G.; Chia, F.L.; Lian, T.Y.; Lau, T.C.; Chng, H.H.; Leung, B.P. Urine s VCAM-1 and s ICAM-1 levels are elevated in lupus nephritis. *Int. J. Rheum. Dis.* **2012**, *15*, 13–16. [CrossRef]
97. Wang, Y.; Tao, Y.; Liu, Y.; Zhao, Y.; Song, C.; Zhou, B.; Wang, T.; Gao, L.; Zhang, L.; Hu, H. Rapid detection of urinary soluble intercellular adhesion molecule-1 for determination of lupus nephritis activity. *Medicine* **2018**, *97*, e11287. [CrossRef]
98. Mok, C.C.; Soliman, S.; Ho, L.Y.; Mohamed, F.A.; Mohamed, F.I.; Mohan, C. Urinary angiostatin, CXCL4 and VCAM-1 as biomarkers of lupus nephritis. *Arthritis Res. Ther.* **2018**, *20*, 1–10. [CrossRef]
99. Singh, S.; Wu, T.; Xie, C.; Vanarsa, K.; Han, J.; Mahajan, T.; Oei, H.B.; Ahn, C.; Zhou, X.J.; Putterman, C.; et al. Urine VCAM-1 as a marker of renal pathology activity index in lupus nephritis. *Arthritis Res. Ther.* **2012**, *14*, R164. [CrossRef]
100. Gupta, R.; Yadav, A.; Aggarwal, A. Urinary soluble CD163 is a good biomarker for renal disease activity in lupus nephritis. *Clin. Rheumatol.* **2021**, *40*, 941–948. [CrossRef]
101. Lei, R.; Vu, B.; Kourentzi, K.; Soomro, S.; Danthanarayana, A.N.; Brgoch, J.; Nadimpalli, S.; Petri, M.; Mohan, C.; Willson, R.C. A novel technology for home monitoring of lupus nephritis that tracks the pathogenic urine biomarker ALCAM. *Front. Immunol.* **2022**, *13*, 1044743. [CrossRef] [PubMed]
102. Gasparin, A.A.; de Andrade, N.P.B.; Hax, V.; Palominos, P.E.; Siebert, M.; Marx, R.; Schaefer, P.G.; Veronese, F.V.; Monticielo, O.A. Urinary soluble VCAM-1 is a useful biomarker of disease activity and treatment response in lupus nephritis. *BMC Rheumatol.* **2020**, *4*, 67. [CrossRef] [PubMed]
103. Yu, K.Y.C.; Yung, S.; Chau, M.K.M.; Tang, C.S.O.; Yap, D.Y.H.; Tang, A.H.N.; Ying, S.K.Y.; Lee, C.K.; Chan, T.M. Clinico-pathological associations of serum VCAM-1 and ICAM-1 levels in patients with lupus nephritis. *Lupus* **2021**, *30*, 1039–1050. [CrossRef] [PubMed]
104. Satirapoj, B.; Kitiyakara, C.; Leelahavanichkul, A.; Avihingsanon, Y.; Supasyndh, O. Urine neutrophil gelatinase-associated lipocalin to predict renal response after induction therapy in active lupus nephritis. *BMC Nephrol.* **2017**, *18*, 263. [CrossRef] [PubMed]
105. Mirioglu, S.; Cinar, S.; Yazici, H.; Ozluk, Y.; Kilicaslan, I.; Gul, A.; Ocal, L.; Inanc, M.; Artim-Esen, B. Serum and urine TNF-like weak inducer of apoptosis, monocyte chemoattractant protein-1 and neutrophil gelatinase-associated lipocalin as biomarkers of disease activity in patients with systemic lupus erythematosus. *Lupus* **2020**, *29*, 379–388. [CrossRef] [PubMed]
106. Mok, C.C.; Ding, H.H.; Kharboutli, M.; Mohan, C. Axl, Ferritin, Insulin-Like Growth Factor Binding Protein 2, and Tumor Necrosis Factor Receptor Type II as Biomarkers in Systemic Lupus Erythematosus. *Arthritis Care Res.* **2016**, *68*, 1303–1309. [CrossRef] [PubMed]
107. Parodis, I.; Ding, H.; Zickert, A.; Cosson, G.; Fathima, M.; Grönwall, C.; Mohan, C.; Gunnarsson, I. Serum Axl predicts histology-based response to induction therapy and long-term renal outcome in lupus nephritis. *PLoS ONE* **2019**, *14*, e0212068. [CrossRef]
108. Wu, T.; Ding, H.; Han, J.; Arriens, C.; Wei, C.; Han, W.; Pedroza, C.; Jiang, S.; Anolik, J.; Petri, M.; et al. Antibody-Array-Based Proteomic Screening of Serum Markers in Systemic Lupus Erythematosus: A Discovery Study. *J. Proteome Res.* **2016**, *15*, 2102–2114. [CrossRef]
109. Mejia-Vilet, J.M.; Zhang, X.L.; Cruz, C.; Cano-Verduzco, M.L.; Shapiro, J.P.; Nagaraja, H.N.; Morales-Buenrostro, L.E.; Rovin, B.H. Urinary Soluble CD163: A Novel Noninvasive Biomarker of Activity for Lupus Nephritis. *J. Am. Soc. Nephrol.* **2020**, *31*, 1335–1347. [CrossRef]
110. Zhang, T.; Li, H.; Vanarsa, K.; Gidley, G.; Mok, C.C.; Petri, M.; Saxena, R.; Mohan, C. Association of urine sCD163 with proliferative lupus nephritis, fibrinoid necrosis, cellular crescents and intrarenal M2 macrophages. *Front. Immunol.* **2020**, *11*, 671. [CrossRef]
111. Inthavong, H.; Vanarsa, K.; Castillo, J.; Hicks, M.J.; Mohan, C.; Wenderfer, S.E. Urinary CD163 is a marker of active kidney disease in childhood-onset lupus nephritis. *Rheumatology* **2023**, *62*, 1335–1342. [CrossRef] [PubMed]

112. Mejia-Vilet, J.M.; Shapiro, J.P.; Zhang, X.L.; Cruz, C.; Zimmerman, G.; Méndez-Pérez, R.A.; Cano-Verduzco, M.L.; Parikh, S.V.; Nagaraja, H.N.; Morales-Buenrostro, L.E.; et al. Association Between Urinary Epidermal Growth Factor and Renal Prognosis in Lupus Nephritis. *Arthritis Rheumatol.* **2021**, *73*, 244–254. [CrossRef] [PubMed]
113. Patyna, S.; Buettner, S.; Eckes, T.; Obermueller, N.; Bartel, C.; Braner, A.; Trautmann, S.; Thomas, D.; Geiger, H.; Pfeilschifter, J. Blood ceramides as novel markers for renal impairment in systemic lupus erythematosus. *Prostaglandins Other Lipid Mediat.* **2019**, *144*, 106348. [CrossRef] [PubMed]
114. Checa, A.; Idborg, H.; Zandian, A.; Sar, D.G.; Surowiec, I.; Trygg, J.; Svenungsson, E.; Jakobsson, P.; Nilsson, P.; Gunnarsson, I. Dysregulations in circulating sphingolipids associate with disease activity indices in female patients with systemic lupus erythematosus: A cross-sectional study. *Lupus* **2017**, *26*, 1023–1033. [CrossRef] [PubMed]
115. Leffler, J.; Bengtsson, A.A.; Blom, A.M. The complement system in systemic lupus erythematosus: An update. *Ann. Rheum. Dis.* **2014**, *73*, 1601–1606. [CrossRef] [PubMed]
116. Weinstein, A.; Alexander, R.V.; Zack, D.J. A review of complement activation in SLE. *Curr. Rheumatol. Rep.* **2021**, *23*, 1–8. [CrossRef] [PubMed]
117. Troldborg, A.; Jensen, L.; Deleuran, B.; Stengaard-Pedersen, K.; Thiel, S.; Jensenius, J.C. The C3dg fragment of complement is superior to conventional C3 as a diagnostic biomarker in systemic lupus erythematosus. *Front. Immunol.* **2018**, *9*, 581. [CrossRef]
118. Pillemer, S.; Austi, H., 3rd; Tsokos, G.; Balow, J. Lupus nephritis: Association between serology and renal biopsy measures. *J. Rheumatol.* **1988**, *15*, 284–288.
119. Martin, M.; Smolag, K.I.; Björk, A.; Gullstrand, B.; Okrój, M.; Leffler, J.; Jönsen, A.; Bengtsson, A.A.; Blom, A.M. Plasma C4d as marker for lupus nephritis in systemic lupus erythematosus. *Arthritis Res. Ther.* **2017**, *19*, 1–9. [CrossRef]
120. Martin, M.; Trattner, R.; Nilsson, S.C.; Björk, A.; Zickert, A.; Blom, A.M.; Gunnarsson, I. Plasma C4d correlates with C4d deposition in kidneys and with treatment response in lupus nephritis patients. *Front. Immunol.* **2020**, *11*, 582737. [CrossRef]
121. Hu, X.; Liu, H.; Du, J.; Chen, Y.; Yang, M.; Xie, Y.; Chen, J.; Yan, S.; Ouyang, S.; Gong, Z. The clinical significance of plasma CFHR 1–5 in lupus nephropathy. *Immunobiology* **2019**, *224*, 339–346. [CrossRef] [PubMed]
122. Te, J.L.; Dozmorov, I.M.; Guthridge, J.M.; Nguyen, K.L.; Cavett, J.W.; Kelly, J.A.; Bruner, G.R.; Harley, J.B.; Ojwang, J.O. Identification of unique microRNA signature associated with lupus nephritis. *PLoS ONE* **2010**, *5*, e10344. [CrossRef] [PubMed]
123. Dai, Y.; Sui, W.; Lan, H.; Yan, Q.; Huang, H.; Huang, Y. Comprehensive analysis of microRNA expression patterns in renal biopsies of lupus nephritis patients. *Rheumatol. Int.* **2009**, *29*, 749–754. [CrossRef] [PubMed]
124. Wei, Q.; Mi, Q.S.; Dong, Z. The regulation and function of microRNAs in kidney diseases. *IUBMB Life* **2013**, *65*, 602–614. [CrossRef] [PubMed]
125. Roointan, A.; Gholaminejad, A.; Shojaie, B.; Hudkins, K.L.; Gheisari, Y. Candidate MicroRNA Biomarkers in Lupus Nephritis: A Meta-analysis of Profiling Studies in Kidney, Blood and Urine Samples. *Mol. Diagn. Ther.* **2023**, *27*, 141–158. [CrossRef] [PubMed]
126. Perez-Hernandez, J.; Martinez-Arroyo, O.; Ortega, A.; Galera, M.; Solis-Salguero, M.A.; Chaves, F.J.; Redon, J.; Forner, M.J.; Cortes, R. Urinary exosomal miR-146a as a marker of albuminuria, activity changes and disease flares in lupus nephritis. *J. Nephrol.* **2021**, *34*, 1157–1167. [CrossRef]
127. Garcia-Vives, E.; Solé, C.; Moliné, T.; Vidal, M.; Agraz, I.; Ordi-Ros, J.; Cortés-Hernández, J. The urinary exosomal miRNA expression profile is predictive of clinical response in lupus nephritis. *Int. J. Mol. Sci.* **2020**, *21*, 1372. [CrossRef]
128. Nakhjavani, M.; Etemadi, J.; Pourlak, T.; Mirhosaini, Z.; Vahed, S.Z.; Abediazar, S. Plasma levels of miR-21, miR-150, miR-423 in patients with lupus nephritis. *Iran. J. Kidney Dis.* **2019**, *13*, 198.
129. Vahed, S.Z.; Nakhjavani, M.; Etemadi, J.; Jamshidi, H.; Jadidian, N.; Pourlak, T.; Abediazar, S. Altered levels of immune-regulatory microRNAs in plasma samples of patients with lupus nephritis. *BioImpacts BI* **2018**, *8*, 177.
130. Solé, C.; Cortés-Hernández, J.; Felip, M.L.; Vidal, M.; Ordi-Ros, J. miR-29c in urinary exosomes as predictor of early renal fibrosis in lupus nephritis. *Nephrol. Dial. Transplant.* **2015**, *30*, 1488–1496. [CrossRef]
131. Wu, G.-C.; Li, J.; Leng, R.-X.; Li, X.-P.; Li, X.-M.; Wang, D.-G.; Pan, H.-F.; Ye, D.-Q. Identification of long non-coding RNAs GAS5, linc0597 and lnc-DC in plasma as novel biomarkers for systemic lupus erythematosus. *Oncotarget* **2017**, *8*, 23650. [CrossRef] [PubMed]
132. Charras, A.; Haldenby, S.; Smith, E.M.D.; Egbivwie, N.; Olohan, L.; Kenny, J.G.; Schwarz, K.; Roberts, C.; Al-Abadi, E.; Armon, K.; et al. Panel sequencing links rare, likely damaging gene variants with distinct clinical phenotypes and outcomes in juvenile-onset SLE. *Rheumatology* **2022**, *62*, SI210–SI225. [CrossRef] [PubMed]
133. Brown, G.J.; Cañete, P.F.; Wang, H.; Medhavy, A.; Bones, J.; Roco, J.A.; He, Y.; Qin, Y.; Cappello, J.; Ellyard, J.I.; et al. TLR7 gain-of-function genetic variation causes human lupus. *Nature* **2022**, *605*, 349–356. [CrossRef] [PubMed]
134. Vinuesa, C.G.; Shen, N.; Ware, T. Genetics of SLE: Mechanistic insights from monogenic disease and disease-associated variants. *Nat. Rev. Nephrol.* **2023**, *19*, 558–572. [CrossRef]
135. Barturen, G.; Babaei, S.; Català-Moll, F.; Martínez-Bueno, M.; Makowska, Z.; Martorell-Marugán, J.; Carmona-Sáez, P.; Toro-Domínguez, D.; Carnero-Montoro, E.; Teruel, M.; et al. Integrative Analysis Reveals a Molecular Stratification of Systemic Autoimmune Diseases. *Arthritis Rheumatol.* **2021**, *73*, 1073–1085. [CrossRef]
136. Zhang, C.; Han, X.; Sun, L.; Yang, S.; Peng, J.; Chen, Y.; Jin, Y.; Xu, F.; Liu, Z.; Zhou, Q. Novel loss-of-function mutations in TNFAIP3 gene in patients with lupus nephritis. *Clin. Kidney J.* **2022**, *15*, 2027–2038. [CrossRef]

137. Aeschlimann, F.A.; Batu, E.D.; Canna, S.W.; Go, E.; Gül, A.; Hoffmann, P.; Leavis, H.L.; Ozen, S.; Schwartz, D.M.; Stone, D.L.; et al. A20 haploinsufficiency (HA20): Clinical phenotypes and disease course of patients with a newly recognised NF-kB-mediated autoinflammatory disease. *Ann. Rheum. Dis.* **2018**, *77*, 728–735. [CrossRef]
138. Li, G.M.; Liu, H.M.; Guan, W.Z.; Xu, H.; Wu, B.B.; Sun, L. Expanding the spectrum of A20 haploinsufficiency in two Chinese families: Cases report. *BMC Med. Genet.* **2019**, *20*, 124. [CrossRef]
139. Mohan, C.; Putterman, C. Genetics and pathogenesis of systemic lupus erythematosus and lupus nephritis. *Nat. Rev. Nephrol.* **2015**, *11*, 329–341. [CrossRef]
140. Lanata, C.M.; Nititham, J.; Taylor, K.E.; Chung, S.A.; Torgerson, D.G.; Seldin, M.F.; Pons-Estel, B.A.; Tusié-Luna, T.; Tsao, B.P.; Morand, E.F.; et al. Genetic contributions to lupus nephritis in a multi-ethnic cohort of systemic lupus erythematous patients. *PLoS ONE* **2018**, *13*, e0199003. [CrossRef]
141. Bolin, K.; Sandling, J.K.; Zickert, A.; Jönsen, A.; Sjöwall, C.; Svenungsson, E.; Bengtsson, A.A.; Eloranta, M.L.; Rönnblom, L.; Syvänen, A.C.; et al. Association of STAT4 polymorphism with severe renal insufficiency in lupus nephritis. *PLoS ONE* **2013**, *8*, e84450. [CrossRef] [PubMed]
142. Bolin, K.; Imgenberg-Kreuz, J.; Leonard, D.; Sandling, J.K.; Alexsson, A.; Pucholt, P.; Haarhaus, M.L.; Almlöf, J.C.; Nititham, J.; Jönsen, A.; et al. Variants in BANK1 are associated with lupus nephritis of European ancestry. *Genes Immun.* **2021**, *22*, 194–202. [CrossRef] [PubMed]
143. Chung, S.A.; Brown, E.E.; Williams, A.H.; Ramos, P.S.; Berthier, C.C.; Bhangale, T.; Alarcon-Riquelme, M.E.; Behrens, T.W.; Criswell, L.A.; Graham, D.C.; et al. Lupus nephritis susceptibility loci in women with systemic lupus erythematosus. *J. Am. Soc. Nephrol.* **2014**, *25*, 2859–2870. [CrossRef] [PubMed]
144. Wang, Z.; Hu, D.; Pei, G.; Zeng, R.; Yao, Y. Identification of driver genes in lupus nephritis based on comprehensive bioinformatics and machine learning. *Front. Immunol.* **2023**, *14*, 1288699. [CrossRef]
145. Yavuz, S.; Pucholt, P.; Sandling, J.K.; Bianchi, M.; Leonard, D.; Bolin, K.; Imgenberg-Kreuz, J.; Eloranta, M.L.; Kozyrev, S.V.; Lanata, C.M.; et al. Mer-tyrosine kinase: A novel susceptibility gene for SLE related end-stage renal disease. *Lupus Sci. Med.* **2022**, *9*, e000752. [CrossRef] [PubMed]
146. Seitz, H.M.; Camenisch, T.D.; Lemke, G.; Earp, H.S.; Matsushima, G.K. Macrophages and dendritic cells use different Axl/Mertk/Tyro3 receptors in clearance of apoptotic cells. *J. Immunol.* **2007**, *178*, 5635–5642. [CrossRef] [PubMed]
147. Sather, S.; Kenyon, K.D.; Lefkowitz, J.B.; Liang, X.; Varnum, B.C.; Henson, P.M.; Graham, D.K. A soluble form of the Mer receptor tyrosine kinase inhibits macrophage clearance of apoptotic cells and platelet aggregation. *Blood* **2007**, *109*, 1026–1033. [CrossRef] [PubMed]
148. Rothlin, C.V.; Ghosh, S.; Zuniga, E.I.; Oldstone, M.B.; Lemke, G. TAM receptors are pleiotropic inhibitors of the innate immune response. *Cell* **2007**, *131*, 1124–1136. [CrossRef]
149. Lee, Y.-J.; Han, J.-Y.; Byun, J.; Park, H.-J.; Park, E.-M.; Chong, Y.H.; Cho, M.-S.; Kang, J.L. Inhibiting Mer receptor tyrosine kinase suppresses STAT1, SOCS1/3, and NF-κB activation and enhances inflammatory responses in lipopolysaccharide-induced acute lung injury. *J. Leukoc. Biol.* **2012**, *91*, 921–932. [CrossRef]
150. Adomati, T.; Cham, L.B.; Hamdan, T.A.; Bhat, H.; Duhan, V.; Li, F.; Ali, M.; Lang, E.; Huang, A.; Naser, E. Dead cells induce innate anergy via mertk after acute viral infection. *Cell Rep.* **2020**, *30*, 3671–3681.e5. [CrossRef]
151. Keller, A.D.; Maniatis, T. Identification and characterization of a novel repressor of beta-interferon gene expression. *Genes Dev.* **1991**, *5*, 868–879. [CrossRef]
152. Freedman, B.I.; Langefeld, C.D.; Andringa, K.K.; Croker, J.A.; Williams, A.H.; Garner, N.E.; Birmingham, D.J.; Hebert, L.A.; Hicks, P.J.; Segal, M.S. End-stage renal disease in African Americans with lupus nephritis is associated with APOL1. *Arthritis Rheumatol.* **2014**, *66*, 390–396. [CrossRef] [PubMed]
153. Freedman, B.I.; Kopp, J.B.; Langefeld, C.D.; Genovese, G.; Friedman, D.J.; Nelson, G.W.; Winkler, C.A.; Bowden, D.W.; Pollak, M.R. The apolipoprotein L1 (APOL1) gene and nondiabetic nephropathy in African Americans. *J. Am. Soc. Nephrol. JASN* **2010**, *21*, 1422. [CrossRef] [PubMed]
154. Lin, C.P.; Adrianto, I.; Lessard, C.J.; Kelly, J.A.; Kaufman, K.M.; Guthridge, J.M.; Freedman, B.I.; Anaya, J.-M.; Alarcón-Riquelme, M.E.; Pons-Estel, B.A. Role of MYH9 and APOL1 in African and non-African populations with lupus nephritis. *Genes Immun.* **2012**, *13*, 232–238. [CrossRef] [PubMed]
155. Niu, Z.; Zhang, P.; Tong, Y. Value of HLA-DR genotype in systemic lupus erythematosus and lupus nephritis: A meta-analysis. *Int. J. Rheum. Dis.* **2015**, *18*, 17–28. [CrossRef]
156. Chen, L.; Wang, Y.F.; Liu, L.; Bielowka, A.; Ahmed, R.; Zhang, H.; Tombleson, P.; Roberts, A.L.; Odhams, C.A.; Cunninghame Graham, D.S.; et al. Genome-wide assessment of genetic risk for systemic lupus erythematosus and disease severity. *Hum. Mol. Genet.* **2020**, *29*, 1745–1756. [CrossRef] [PubMed]
157. Kwon, Y.C.; Ha, E.; Kwon, H.H.; Park, D.J.; Shin, J.M.; Joo, Y.B.; Chung, W.T.; Yoo, D.H.; Lee, H.S.; Kim, K.; et al. Higher Genetic Risk Loads Confer More Diverse Manifestations and Higher Risk of Lupus Nephritis in Systemic Lupus Erythematosus. *Arthritis Rheumatol.* **2023**, *75*, 1566–1572. [CrossRef]
158. Webber, D.; Cao, J.; Dominguez, D.; Gladman, D.D.; Levy, D.M.; Ng, L.; Paterson, A.D.; Touma, Z.; Urowitz, M.B.; Wither, J.E.; et al. Association of systemic lupus erythematosus (SLE) genetic susceptibility loci with lupus nephritis in childhood-onset and adult-onset SLE. *Rheumatology* **2020**, *59*, 90–98. [CrossRef]

159. Hedrich, C.M.; Tsokos, G.C. Epigenetic mechanisms in systemic lupus erythematosus and other autoimmune diseases. *Trends Mol. Med.* **2011**, *17*, 714–724. [CrossRef]
160. Crispín, J.C.; Hedrich, C.M.; Tsokos, G.C. Gene-function studies in systemic lupus erythematosus. *Nat. Rev. Rheumatol.* **2013**, *9*, 476–484. [CrossRef]
161. Ding, H.; Shen, Y.; Hong, S.M.; Xiang, C.; Shen, N. Biomarkers for systemic lupus erythematosus—A focus on organ Damage. *Expert Rev. Clin. Immunol.* **2023**, *20*, 39–58. [CrossRef] [PubMed]
162. Gómez-Puerta, J.A.; Ortiz-Reyes, B.; Urrego, T.; Vanegas-García, A.L.; Muñoz, C.H.; González, L.A.; Cervera, R.; Vásquez, G. Urinary neutrophil gelatinase-associated lipocalin and monocyte chemoattractant protein 1 as biomarkers for lupus nephritis in Colombian SLE patients. *Lupus* **2017**, *27*, 637–646. [CrossRef] [PubMed]
163. Birmingham, D.J.; Bitter, J.E.; Ndukwe, E.G.; Dials, S.; Gullo, T.R.; Conroy, S.; Nagaraja, H.N.; Rovin, B.H.; Hebert, L.A. Relationship of Circulating Anti-C3b and Anti-C1q IgG to Lupus Nephritis and Its Flare. *Clin. J. Am. Soc. Nephrol.* **2016**, *11*, 47–53. [CrossRef] [PubMed]
164. Fatemi, A.; Samadi, G.; Sayedbonakdar, Z.; Smiley, A. Anti-C1q antibody in patients with lupus nephritic flare: 18-month follow-up and a nested case-control study. *Mod. Rheumatol.* **2016**, *26*, 233–239. [CrossRef] [PubMed]
165. Tan, Y.; Song, D.; Wu, L.-h.; Yu, F.; Zhao, M.-h. Serum levels and renal deposition of C1q complement component and its antibodies reflect disease activity of lupus nephritis. *BMC Nephrol.* **2013**, *14*, 63. [CrossRef] [PubMed]
166. Pang, Y.; Tan, Y.; Li, Y.; Zhang, J.; Guo, Y.; Guo, Z.; Zhang, C.; Yu, F.; Zhao, M.-h. Serum A08 C1q antibodies are associated with disease activity and prognosis in Chinese patients with lupus nephritis. *Kidney Int.* **2016**, *90*, 1357–1367. [CrossRef]
167. Yap, D.Y.H.; Yung, S.; Zhang, Q.; Tang, C.; Chan, T.M. Serum level of proximal renal tubular epithelial cell-binding immunoglobulin G in patients with lupus nephritis. *Lupus* **2015**, *25*, 46–53. [CrossRef]
168. Tang, C.; Fang, M.; Tan, G.; Zhang, S.; Yang, B.; Li, Y.; Zhang, T.; Saxena, R.; Mohan, C.; Wu, T. Discovery of novel circulating immune complexes in lupus nephritis using immunoproteomics. *Front. Immunol.* **2022**, *13*, 850015. [CrossRef]
169. Ichinose, K.; Kitamura, M.; Sato, S.; Fujikawa, K.; Horai, Y.; Matsuoka, N.; Tsuboi, M.; Nonaka, F.; Shimizu, T.; Fukui, S.; et al. Podocyte foot process width is a prediction marker for complete renal response at 6 and 12 months after induction therapy in lupus nephritis. *Clin. Immunol.* **2018**, *197*, 161–168. [CrossRef]
170. Calich, A.L.; Borba, E.F.; Ugolini-Lopes, M.R.; da Rocha, L.F.; Bonfá, E.; Fuller, R. Serum uric acid levels are associated with lupus nephritis in patients with normal renal function. *Clin. Rheumatol.* **2018**, *37*, 1223–1228. [CrossRef]
171. Hafez, E.A.; Hassan, S.A.E.-m.; Teama, M.A.M.; Badr, F.M. Serum uric acid as a predictor for nephritis in Egyptian patients with systemic lupus erythematosus. *Lupus* **2020**, *30*, 378–384. [CrossRef] [PubMed]
172. Chen, Y.M.; Hung, W.T.; Liao, Y.W.; Hsu, C.Y.; Hsieh, T.Y.; Chen, H.H.; Hsieh, C.W.; Lin, C.T.; Lai, K.L.; Tang, K.T.; et al. Combination immunosuppressant therapy and lupus nephritis outcome: A hospital-based study. *Lupus* **2019**, *28*, 658–666. [CrossRef] [PubMed]
173. Liu, X.-R.; Qi, Y.-Y.; Zhao, Y.-F.; Cui, Y.; Wang, X.-Y.; Zhao, Z.-Z. Albumin-to-globulin ratio (AGR) as a potential marker of predicting lupus nephritis in Chinese patients with systemic lupus erythematosus. *Lupus* **2021**, *30*, 412–420. [CrossRef] [PubMed]
174. Petri, M.; Barr, E.; Magder, L.S. Risk of renal failure within 10 or 20 years of systemic lupus erythematosus diagnosis. *J. Rheumatol.* **2021**, *48*, 222–227. [CrossRef] [PubMed]
175. Selvaraja, M.; Abdullah, M.; Arip, M.; Chin, V.K.; Shah, A.; Amin Nordin, S. Elevated interleukin-25 and its association to Th2 cytokines in systemic lupus erythematosus with lupus nephritis. *PLoS ONE* **2019**, *14*, e0224707. [CrossRef] [PubMed]
176. Reyes-Martínez, F.; Pérez-Navarro, M.; Rodríguez-Matías, A.; Soto-Abraham, V.; Gutierrez-Reyes, G.; Medina-Avila, Z.; Valdez-Ortiz, R. Assessment of urinary TWEAK levels in Mexican patients with untreated lupus nephritis: An exploratory study. *Nefrología* **2018**, *38*, 152–160. [CrossRef] [PubMed]
177. Elsaid, D.S.; Abdel Noor, R.A.; Shalaby, K.A.; Haroun, R.A.-H. Urinary Tumor Necrosis Factor-Like Weak Inducer of Apoptosis (uTWEAK) and Urinary Monocyte Chemo-attractant Protein-1 (uMCP-1): Promising Biomarkers of Lupus Nephritis Activity? *Saudi J. Kidney Dis. Transplant.* **2021**, *32*, 19–29. [CrossRef]
178. Choe, J.-Y.; Kim, S.-K. Serum TWEAK as a biomarker for disease activity of systemic lupus erythematosus. *Inflamm. Res.* **2016**, *65*, 479–488. [CrossRef]
179. Wolf, B.J.; Spainhour, J.C.; Arthur, J.M.; Janech, M.G.; Petri, M.; Oates, J.C. Development of biomarker models to predict outcomes in lupus nephritis. *Arthritis Rheumatol.* **2016**, *68*, 1955–1963. [CrossRef]
180. Nordin, F.; Shaharir, S.S.; Abdul Wahab, A.; Mustafar, R.; Abdul Gafor, A.H.; Mohamed Said, M.S.; Rajalingham, S.; Shah, S.A. Serum and urine interleukin-17A levels as biomarkers of disease activity in systemic lupus erythematosus. *Int. J. Rheum. Dis.* **2019**, *22*, 1419–1426. [CrossRef]
181. Vincent, F.B.; Kandane-Rathnayake, R.; Hoi, A.Y.; Slavin, L.; Godsell, J.D.; Kitching, A.R.; Harris, J.; Nelson, C.L.; Jenkins, A.J.; Chrysostomou, A.; et al. Urinary B-cell-activating factor of the tumour necrosis factor family (BAFF) in systemic lupus erythematosus. *Lupus* **2018**, *27*, 2029–2040. [CrossRef] [PubMed]
182. Endo, N.; Tsuboi, N.; Furuhashi, K.; Shi, Y.; Du, Q.; Abe, T.; Hori, M.; Imaizumi, T.; Kim, H.; Katsuno, T.; et al. Urinary soluble CD163 level reflects glomerular inflammation in human lupus nephritis. *Nephrol. Dial. Transplant.* **2016**, *31*, 2023–2033. [CrossRef] [PubMed]

183. Davies, J.C.; Carlsson, E.; Midgley, A.; Smith, E.M.D.; Bruce, I.N.; Beresford, M.W.; Hedrich, C.M.; BILAG-BR and MRC MASTERPLANS Consortia. A panel of urinary proteins predicts active lupus nephritis and response to rituximab treatment. *Rheumatology* **2021**, *60*, 3747–3759. [CrossRef] [PubMed]
184. Chalmers, S.A.; Ayilam Ramachandran, R.; Garcia, S.J.; Der, E.; Herlitz, L.; Ampudia, J.; Chu, D.; Jordan, N.; Zhang, T.; Parodis, I.; et al. The CD6/ALCAM pathway promotes lupus nephritis via T cell–mediated responses. *J. Clin. Investig.* **2022**, *132*. [CrossRef] [PubMed]
185. Ren, Y.; Xie, J.; Lin, F.; Luo, W.; Zhang, Z.; Mao, P.; Zhong, R.; Liang, Y.; Yang, Z. Serum human epididymis protein 4 is a predictor for developing nephritis in patients with systemic lupus erythematosus: A prospective cohort study. *Int. Immunopharmacol.* **2018**, *60*, 189–193. [CrossRef]
186. Ding, H.; Kharboutli, M.; Saxena, R.; Wu, T. Insulin-like growth factor binding protein-2 as a novel biomarker for disease activity and renal pathology changes in lupus nephritis. *Clin. Exp. Immunol.* **2016**, *184*, 11–18. [CrossRef]
187. Wu, T.; Xie, C.; Han, J.; Ye, Y.; Singh, S.; Zhou, J.; Li, Y.; Ding, H.; Li, Q.-z.; Zhou, X. Insulin-like growth factor binding protein-4 as a marker of chronic lupus nephritis. *PLoS ONE* **2016**, *11*, e0151491. [CrossRef]
188. Smith, M.A.; Henault, J.; Karnell, J.L.; Parker, M.L.; Riggs, J.M.; Sinibaldi, D.; Taylor, D.K.; Ettinger, R.; Grant, E.P.; Sanjuan, M.A.; et al. SLE Plasma Profiling Identifies Unique Signatures of Lupus Nephritis and Discoid Lupus. *Sci. Rep.* **2019**, *9*, 14433. [CrossRef]
189. Parodis, I.; Ding, H.; Zickert, A.; Arnaud, L.; Larsson, A.; Svenungsson, E.; Mohan, C.; Gunnarsson, I. Serum soluble tumour necrosis factor receptor-2 (sTNFR2) as a biomarker of kidney tissue damage and long-term renal outcome in lupus nephritis. *Scand. J. Rheumatol.* **2017**, *46*, 263–272. [CrossRef]
190. Hutcheson, J.; Ye, Y.; Han, J.; Arriens, C.; Saxena, R.; Li, Q.-Z.; Mohan, C.; Wu, T. Resistin as a potential marker of renal disease in lupus nephritis. *Clin. Exp. Immunol.* **2015**, *179*, 435–443. [CrossRef]
191. Menke, J.; Amann, K.; Cavagna, L.; Blettner, M.; Weinmann, A.; Schwarting, A.; Kelley, V.R. Colony-Stimulating Factor-1: A Potential Biomarker for Lupus Nephritis. *J. Am. Soc. Nephrol.* **2015**, *26*, 379–389. [CrossRef] [PubMed]
192. Cheng, F.J.; Zhou, X.J.; Zhao, Y.F.; Zhao, M.H.; Zhang, H. Human neutrophil peptide 1–3, a component of the neutrophil extracellular trap, as a potential biomarker of lupus nephritis. *Int. J. Rheum. Dis.* **2015**, *18*, 533–540. [CrossRef] [PubMed]
193. Davies, J.C.; Midgley, A.; Carlsson, E.; Donohue, S.; Bruce, I.N.; Beresford, M.W.; Hedrich, C.M. Urine and serum S100A8/A9 and S100A12 associate with active lupus nephritis and may predict response to rituximab treatment. *RMD Open* **2020**, *6*, e001257. [CrossRef] [PubMed]
194. Fang, Y.G.; Chen, N.N.; Cheng, Y.B.; Sun, S.J.; Li, H.X.; Sun, F.; Xiang, Y. Urinary neutrophil gelatinase-associated lipocalin for diagnosis and estimating activity in lupus nephritis: A meta-analysis. *Lupus* **2015**, *24*, 1529–1539. [CrossRef] [PubMed]
195. Brunner, H.I.; Bennett, M.R.; Mina, R.; Suzuki, M.; Petri, M.; Kiani, A.N.; Pendl, J.; Witte, D.; Ying, J.; Rovin, B.H.; et al. Association of noninvasively measured renal protein biomarkers with histologic features of lupus nephritis. *Arthritis Rheum.* **2012**, *64*, 2687–2697. [CrossRef] [PubMed]
196. Torres-Salido, M.T.; Cortés-Hernández, J.; Vidal, X.; Pedrosa, A.; Vilardell-Tarrés, M.; Ordi-Ros, J. Neutrophil gelatinase-associated lipocalin as a biomarker for lupus nephritis. *Nephrol. Dial. Transplant.* **2014**, *29*, 1740–1749. [CrossRef] [PubMed]
197. El Shahawy, M.S.; Hemida, M.H.; Abdel-Hafez, H.A.; El-Baz, T.Z.; Lotfy, A.-W.M.; Emran, T.M. Urinary neutrophil gelatinase-associated lipocalin as a marker for disease activity in lupus nephritis. *Scand. J. Clin. Lab. Investig.* **2018**, *78*, 264–268. [CrossRef]
198. Gao, Y.; Wang, B.; Cao, J.; Feng, S.; Liu, B. Elevated Urinary Neutrophil Gelatinase-Associated Lipocalin Is a Biomarker for Lupus Nephritis: A Systematic Review and Meta-Analysis. *BioMed Res. Int.* **2020**, *2020*, 2768326. [CrossRef]
199. Li, Y.-J.; Wu, H.-H.; Liu, S.-H.; Tu, K.-H.; Lee, C.-C.; Hsu, H.-H.; Chang, M.-Y.; Yu, K.-H.; Chen, W.; Tian, Y.-C. Polyomavirus BK, BKV microRNA, and urinary neutrophil gelatinase-associated lipocalin can be used as potential biomarkers of lupus nephritis. *PLoS ONE* **2019**, *14*, e0210633. [CrossRef]
200. Qin, L.; Stanley, S.; Ding, H.; Zhang, T.; Truong, V.T.T.; Celhar, T.; Fairhurst, A.-M.; Pedroza, C.; Petri, M.; Saxena, R.; et al. Urinary pro-thrombotic, anti-thrombotic, and fibrinolytic molecules as biomarkers of lupus nephritis. *Arthritis Res. Ther.* **2019**, *21*, 176. [CrossRef]
201. Choe, J.Y.; Park, S.H.; Kim, S.K. Urine β2-microglobulin is associated with clinical disease activity and renal involvement in female patients with systemic lupus erythematosus. *Lupus* **2014**, *23*, 1486–1493. [CrossRef] [PubMed]
202. Go, D.J.; Lee, J.Y.; Kang, M.J.; Lee, E.Y.; Lee, E.B.; Yi, E.C.; Song, Y.W. Urinary vitamin D-binding protein, a novel biomarker for lupus nephritis, predicts the development of proteinuric flare. *Lupus* **2018**, *27*, 1600–1615. [CrossRef] [PubMed]
203. Torres-Salido, M.T.; Sanchis, M.; Solé, C.; Moliné, T.; Vidal, M.; Vidal, X.; Solà, A.; Hotter, G.; Ordi-Ros, J.; Cortés-Hernández, J. Urinary neuropilin-1: A predictive biomarker for renal outcome in lupus nephritis. *Int. J. Mol. Sci.* **2019**, *20*, 4601. [CrossRef] [PubMed]
204. Khoshmirsafa, M.; Kianmehr, N.; Falak, R.; Mowla, S.J.; Seif, F.; Mirzaei, B.; Valizadeh, M.; Shekarabi, M. Elevated expression of miR-21 and miR-155 in peripheral blood mononuclear cells as potential biomarkers for lupus nephritis. *Int. J. Rheum. Dis.* **2019**, *22*, 458–467. [CrossRef] [PubMed]
205. Alves, I.; Santos-Pereira, B.; Dalebout, H.; Santos, S.; Vicente, M.M.; Campar, A.; Thepaut, M.; Fieschi, F.; Strahl, S.; Boyaval, F.; et al. Protein Mannosylation as a Diagnostic and Prognostic Biomarker of Lupus Nephritis: An Unusual Glycan Neoepitope in Systemic Lupus Erythematosus. *Arthritis Rheumatol.* **2021**, *73*, 2069–2077. [CrossRef] [PubMed]

206. Wantanasiri, P.; Satirapoj, B.; Charoenpitakchai, M.; Aramwit, P. Periostin: A novel tissue biomarker correlates with chronicity index and renal function in lupus nephritis patients. *Lupus* **2015**, *24*, 835–845. [CrossRef]
207. Wang, S.; Wu, M.; Chiriboga, L.; Zeck, B.; Belmont, H.M. Membrane attack complex (mac) deposition in lupus nephritis is associated with hypertension and poor clinical response to treatment. *Semin. Arthritis Rheum.* **2018**, *48*, 256–262. [CrossRef]
208. Ding, Y.; Yu, X.; Wu, L.; Tan, Y.; Qu, Z.; Yu, F. The spectrum of C4d deposition in renal biopsies of lupus nephritis patients. *Front. Immunol.* **2021**, *12*, 654652. [CrossRef]
209. Arbuckle, M.R.; McClain, M.T.; Rubertone, M.V.; Scofield, R.H.; Dennis, G.J.; James, J.A.; Harley, J.B. Development of autoantibodies before the clinical onset of systemic lupus erythematosus. *N. Engl. J. Med.* **2003**, *349*, 1526–1533. [CrossRef]
210. Munroe, M.E.; Lu, R.; Zhao, Y.D.; Fife, D.A.; Robertson, J.M.; Guthridge, J.M.; Niewold, T.B.; Tsokos, G.C.; Keith, M.P.; Harley, J.B.; et al. Altered type II interferon precedes autoantibody accrual and elevated type I interferon activity prior to systemic lupus erythematosus classification. *Ann. Rheum. Dis.* **2016**, *75*, 2014–2021. [CrossRef]
211. Bhargava, R.; Lehoux, S.; Maeda, K.; Tsokos, M.G.; Krishfield, S.; Ellezian, L.; Pollak, M.; Stillman, I.E.; Cummings, R.D.; Tsokos, G.C. Aberrantly glycosylated IgG elicits pathogenic signaling in podocytes and signifies lupus nephritis. *JCI Insight* **2021**, *6*, e147789. [CrossRef] [PubMed]
212. Kim, H.; Kim, T.; Kim, M.; Lee, H.Y.; Kim, Y.; Kang, M.S.; Kim, J. Activation of the alternative complement pathway predicts renal outcome in patients with lupus nephritis. *Lupus* **2020**, *29*, 862–871. [CrossRef] [PubMed]
213. Leatherwood, C.; Speyer, C.B.; Feldman, C.H.; D'Silva, K.; Gómez-Puerta, J.A.; Hoover, P.J.; Waikar, S.S.; McMahon, G.M.; Rennke, H.G.; Costenbader, K.H. Clinical characteristics and renal prognosis associated with interstitial fibrosis and tubular atrophy (IFTA) and vascular injury in lupus nephritis biopsies. *Semin. Arthritis Rheum.* **2019**, *49*, 396–404. [CrossRef] [PubMed]

Disclaimer/Publisher's Note: The statements, opinions and data contained in all publications are solely those of the individual author(s) and contributor(s) and not of MDPI and/or the editor(s). MDPI and/or the editor(s) disclaim responsibility for any injury to people or property resulting from any ideas, methods, instructions or products referred to in the content.

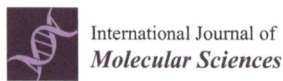

Review

Mitochondrial Dysfunction in Systemic Lupus Erythematosus with a Focus on Lupus Nephritis

Matthieu Halfon [1,*], Aurel T. Tankeu [1] and Camillo Ribi [2]

1. Transplantation Center, Lausanne University Hospital, Rue du Bugnon 44, CH-1010 Lausanne, Switzerland; aurel.tankeu-tiakouang@chuv.ch
2. Division of Immunology and Allergy, Lausanne University Hospital, CH-1010 Lausanne, Switzerland; camillo.ribi@chuv.ch
* Correspondence: matthieu.halfon@chuv.ch

Abstract: Systemic lupus erythematosus (SLE) is an autoimmune disease affecting mostly women of child-bearing age. Immune dysfunction in SLE results from disrupted apoptosis which lead to an unregulated interferon (IFN) stimulation and the production of autoantibodies, leading to immune complex formation, complement activation, and organ damage. Lupus nephritis (LN) is a common and severe complication of SLE, impacting approximately 30% to 40% of SLE patients. Recent studies have demonstrated an alteration in mitochondrial homeostasis in SLE patients. Mitochondrial dysfunction contributes significantly to SLE pathogenesis by enhancing type 1 IFN production through various pathways involving neutrophils, platelets, and T cells. Defective mitophagy, the process of clearing damaged mitochondria, exacerbates this cycle, leading to increased immune dysregulation. In this review, we aim to detail the physiopathological link between mitochondrial dysfunction and disease activity in SLE. Additionally, we will explore the potential role of mitochondria as biomarkers and therapeutic targets in SLE, with a specific focus on LN. In LN, mitochondrial abnormalities are observed in renal cells, correlating with disease progression and renal fibrosis. Studies exploring cell-free mitochondrial DNA as a biomarker in SLE and LN have shown promising but preliminary results, necessitating further validation and standardization. Therapeutically targeting mitochondrial dysfunction in SLE, using drugs like metformin or mTOR inhibitors, shows potential in modulating immune responses and improving clinical outcomes. The interplay between mitochondria, immune dysregulation, and renal involvement in SLE and LN underscores the need for comprehensive research and innovative therapeutic strategies. Understanding mitochondrial dynamics and their impact on immune responses offers promising avenues for developing personalized treatments and non-invasive biomarkers, ultimately improving outcomes for LN patients.

Keywords: lupus; kidney; mitochondria; mitochondrial DNA; mitophagy; interferon; lupus nephritis

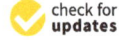

Citation: Halfon, M.; Tankeu, A.T.; Ribi, C. Mitochondrial Dysfunction in Systemic Lupus Erythematosus with a Focus on Lupus Nephritis. *Int. J. Mol. Sci.* **2024**, *25*, 6162. https://doi.org/ 10.3390/ijms25116162

Academic Editor: Ioannis Parodis

Received: 1 May 2024
Revised: 30 May 2024
Accepted: 31 May 2024
Published: 3 June 2024

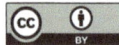

Copyright: © 2024 by the authors. Licensee MDPI, Basel, Switzerland. This article is an open access article distributed under the terms and conditions of the Creative Commons Attribution (CC BY) license (https:// creativecommons.org/licenses/by/ 4.0/).

1. Introduction

Systemic lupus erythematosus (SLE) stands out as an archetypal autoimmune disease, affecting predominantly women of child-bearing age, with an incidence ranging from 1.4 to 10 cases per 100,000 people annually. Its prevalence varies significantly among different ethnic groups, with the lowest rates observed in Asian descents and the highest among Afro-Caribbean populations [1]. In Europe, the estimated prevalence ranges from 40 to 80 people per 100,000 individuals [2]. The underlying autoimmune dysregulation is due to a combination of genetic and environmental factors [3]. Key genes primarily involved in SLE pathogenesis include elements within the toll-like receptor (TLR), type-I interferon (IFN-I), consisting of IFN-alpha and IFN-Beta, and complement pathways [3]. It is noteworthy that elements from both the innate and adaptive immune systems contribute to the immune dysfunction in SLE. A defining characteristic of this condition is the disruption of normal apoptosis mechanisms, leading to inappropriate cellular death and the impaired clearance of cellular debris. This leads to the accumulation of cellular remnants, fostering a loss of immune tolerance and the subsequent generation of autoantibodies. These autoantibodies form immune complexes that initiate complement activation, culminating in organ damage [4].

Given their susceptibility to immune complexes, the kidneys are frequently affected in SLE. Lupus nephritis (LN) serves as the initial presentation of SLE in approximately 16% of patients and appears in SLE with an overall prevalence ranging from 30% to 40% [5]. Furthermore, a significant proportion of SLE patients (20% to 50%) are at risk of developing LN within the first year following their initial diagnosis of SLE [5]. Despite recent breakthroughs in the development of new therapeutics, it is crucial to acknowledge that the remission rate for LN remains low, from 30% to 70% [6–11]. This fact holds significant importance because achieving remission in LN is intricately linked to the risk of progressing to end-stage kidney disease (ESKD). Even with optimal treatment, a notable subset of patients (5% to 20%) will ultimately develop ESKD which is associated with a substantial burden [12].

Recent experimental studies, conducted on animal models and human subjects, have provided compelling evidence of altered immune cell metabolism contributing to SLE pathogenesis. Indeed, immune cells in SLE exhibit heightened metabolic demands [13–15]. Given that mitochondria are the central hub for cellular metabolism, it is postulated that these organelles play a pivotal role in the development and amplification of the immune dysfunction in SLE. Defects in mitochondrial pathways, such as compromised mitophagy mechanisms and impaired mitochondrial DNA (mtDNA), have been recently considered key players in the pathogenesis of lupus. Mitochondrial dysfunctions were linked to the heightened production of IFN-I, a critical cytokine in SLE. In lupus-prone mice, the inhibition of glycolysis has been shown to result in a significant reduction in the production of autoantibodies and a decrease in T cell activation [16,17]. On the other side, mitochondrial dysfunction is seen in various kidney diseases, in the setting of acute kidney injury but also in chronic kidney disease [18–20].

In this review, our primary emphasis is on elucidating the interplay between mitochondria and the activation/amplification of SLE, with focus on LN. Additionally, we explore the usefulness of mitochondrial products as biomarkers and as targets for therapeutic interventions in SLE.

2. Mitochondria Anatomy, Role, and Functions

Mitochondria are small intracellular compartments with unique anatomical and physiological characteristics, ranging in size from 0.5 to 3 μm. Their main role is energy production in the cell through an electron transport chain (ETC) and oxidative phosphorylation (OXPHOS) [21]. Mitochondria exist in almost all eukaryotic cells and are thought to have bacterial origin [22]. Indeed, similarly to bacteria, mitochondria are surrounded by a double-stranded membrane, possess their own genome known as mtDNA, and rely on specific ribosomes that are vulnerable to antibiotics [23]. The double membrane consists of an outer layer (OMM) and an inner layer separated by the intermembrane space. The inner mitochondrial membrane (IMM) forms numerous folds called cristae, which extend into the free space demarcated by the double membrane, called the mitochondrial matrix. The location of the mtDNA close to the IMM and the cristae, together with the lack of introns and histones, makes it highly susceptible to intrinsic aggression, mostly due to reactive oxygen species (ROS) generated by mitochondria complexes during OXPHOS. Given all the above and due to a less effective DNA repair system, mtDNA has a higher mutation rate (10–20 times higher) than for nuclear DNA, and alterations in its sequence (mutations, insertion, and deletions) and structure (rearrangements and breaks) are frequent. In humans, the number of copies of mtDNA per mitochondria varies from 5 to 10 [24]. The multiple copies of mtDNA within a cell and its high susceptibility to alterations favors the coexistence of several mtDNA populations (wild type and mutated mtDNA) in the same cell. This phenomenon is called heteroplasmy, as opposed to homoplasmy which is the existence of unique types of mtDNA within the cell (less frequent). The proportion of mutated mtDNA in relation to total mtDNA determines the heteroplasmy rate [25].

Similarly, to mtDNA, mitochondrial macromolecules (lipids and proteins) can be damaged by ROS, leading to mitochondrial dysfunction. Healthy mitochondria are critical for cell survival, while dysfunctional mitochondria promote apoptosis through Ca2+ and cytochrome *c* release to the cytosol [26]. The cellular population of mitochondria (mitochondria mass and quality) is regulated through fine-tuned processes, including the generation of new mitochondria through biogenesis (new mitochondria formation), the fusion or fission of existing mitochondria, and the degradation of damaged mitochondria by mitophagy [27] (Figure 1).

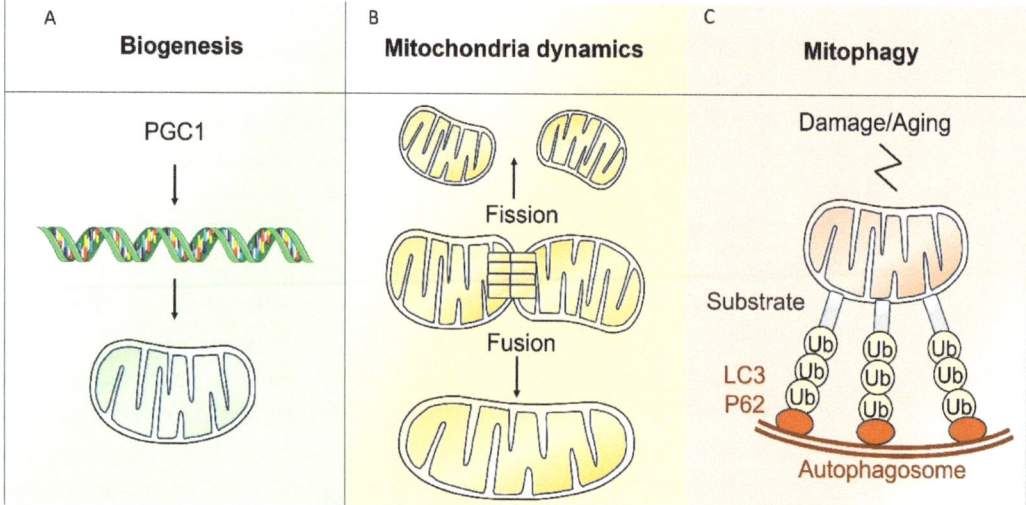

Figure 1. Quality control mechanism in mitochondria. Figure legend: (**A**) Biogenesis: activation of peroxisome proliferator-activated receptor-γ coactivator-1α (PGC1) due to stress factors, then activation of mt DNA transcription leading to formation of new mitochondria. (**B**) Mitochondria dynamic: fission of a mitochondrion resulting in two separate mitochondria. Fusion: Two mitochondria fusion at the outer and inner membrane interfaces. This process allows for exchange of mtDNA, proteins, or metabolites and improves overall mitochondria respiratory function and efficiency. (**C**) Mitophagy: degradation of the mitochondria with the ubiquitin pathway into the phagosome.

In response to specific needs or stresses such as exercise, cold, or fasting, mitochondria biogenesis is activated through its master regulator: the peroxisome proliferator-activated receptor-γ coactivator-1α (PGC-1α), which activates mtDNA transcription and increases in the expression of mitochondrial transcription factor A (TFAM), the final effector of mtDNA transcription and replication [27,28]. Mitochondrial fission is the division of a mitochondrion into two distinct mitochondria. This process plays a role in inheritance and mitochondrial partitioning during cell division, apoptosis, and mitophagy [29]. Mitochondrial fission in mammals is coordinated by a GTPase dynamin-related protein 1 (DRP1), which act in conjunction with mitochondrial fission 1 (FIS1), and mitochondrial fission factor (MFF). DRP1, a cytosolic protein composed of four domains, is recruited by its adaptors present on the OMM, (MFF and FIS1), where it undergoes the formation of an oligomeric ring structure around the mitochondrion, further constricting it. Then, the GTP hydrolysis of DRP1 completes the mitochondrion cleavage process.

Defective or damaged mitochondria that lost their membrane potential are inclined to release high amounts of Ca^{2+} and cytochrome c to the cytosol, which promotes cell apoptosis [26]. To prevent this, dysfunctional mitochondria are degraded through a specific autophagy-dependent process known as mitophagy.

Mitophagy can be classified into receptor-dependent (also called Parkin-independent) mitophagy and ubiquitin-dependent (or Parkin-dependent) mitophagy [26,30]. In mammals, receptor-dependent mitophagy is a three-step process starting with the activation of receptors located on the OMM (FUNDC1, NIX/BNIP3L, BNIP3, or Bcl2L13), followed by the binding of the autophagosome marker LC3, which initiates the development of the phagophore membrane and forms the autophagosome, and finally, the fusion of the autophagosome with the lysosome for cargo degradation [26].

Ubiquitin is a protein involved in protein and organelle degradation through ubiquitination, which is the conjugation of ubiquitin to proteins mediated by three enzymes: ubiquitin-activating enzymes (E1), ubiquitin-conjugating enzymes (E2), and ubiquitin-protein ligases (E3) [31]. The ubiquitin proteasome system (UPS) is a proteasome-mediated degradation machinery that removes proteins from various cellular compartments. Autophagy and UPS represent the main intracellular proteolysis machineries that enforce protein and organelle quality control in the cell [30].

Both systems utilize ubiquitin signaling to tag their targets, thus cooperating in the elimination of damaged and dysfunctional mitochondria. By tagging substrates to be degraded by autophagy or by UPS, ubiquitin is therefore a common signal for protein or organelle degradation [26]. One of the most well-characterized ubiquitin-dependent autophagy is the mitophagy pathway; it involves the PTEN-induced putative kinase 1 (PINK1) and the E3 ubiquitin-protein ligase Parkin [32]. Here, the initial step is the accumulation of PINK1 at the OMM following the loss of mitochondria membrane potential. PINK1 accumulation phosphorylates and activates Parkin that is recruited to the OMM where it ubiquitinates OMM proteins using its E3 ligase activity. Ubiquitinylated OMM proteins are recognized by specific adaptors, allowing the engulfment of mitochondria and formation of autophagosomes with the recruitment of LC3 via an LC3-interacting region (LIR) motif [32]. The fusion and degradation of autophagosomes with lysosomes are then consistent with receptor-mediated mitophagy [26]. Mitophagy is highly responsive to the dynamics of endogenous metabolites, including iron-, calcium-, glycolysis-TCA-, NAD+ -, amino acids-, fatty acids-, and cAMP-associated metabolites [33]. For instance, the disruption of mitochondrial membrane potential is a potent mitophagy activator, but SIRT3, a mitochondrial sirtuin and NAD + metabolic sensor, has been shown to restore the proton gradient, playing a role in maintaining mitochondrial membrane potential in response to mitochondrial stress, therefore reducing mitophagy [34,35]. Mitophagy can start with fission, which help in the fragmentation of mitochondria before their degradation. It has been shown that the mitochondrial recruitment of Drp1 is a crucial step to initiate mitophagy [36]. HRES-1/Rab4 promotes the lysosomal degradation of Drp1; therefore, HRES-1/Rab4 induces the accumulation of mitochondria by inhibiting mitophagy [37].

3. Mitochondrial Dysfunction: A Trigger and Amplifier of Type I Interferon

Type I IFNs represent a group of inflammatory cytokines that play a pivotal role in the body's defense against viral infections, primarily by the activation of TLRs in response to viral particles. Through pleiotropic mechanisms, IFN-I activates both T and B-cells [38]. For decades, SLE has been recognized as a quintessential interferonopathy. This designation stems from the robust expression of IFN-I seen in most SLE patients. The high IFN-I signature in SLE has long been attributed to activated plasmacytoid dendritic cells (pDCs). These pDCs are implicated in the proliferation and survival of autoreactive lymphocytes, which significantly contribute to the production of autoantibodies and the formation of immune complexes. However, recent findings in SLE challenge the notion that pDCs are the primary source of IFN [39]. Neutrophils undergoing NETosis have emerged as significant IFN producers via the stimulator of interferon gene (STING) pathway, notably contributing to the IFN gene signature observed in the kidneys of patients suffering from LN [40]. Also, a novel concept involves "local" IFN release by non-hematopoietic cells such as epithelial or proximal tubular cells in the kidney, releasing IFN [41,42]. This local, non-circulating IFN production may contribute to the diverse phenotypes observed in SLE. Of note, GDF-15, a cytokine released locally by various organs in cases of mitochondrial stress, is known to regulate IFN production [43].

A substantial proportion of individuals with SLE exhibit an upregulation of type I IFN-regulated genes, collectively referred to as the "IFN-I signature," both in their blood and affected tissues. IFN-I signatures correlate with SLE activity. They have been used in clinical trials to stratify patient groups for treatments targeting the IFN-I pathway, such as anifrolumab, an IgG1κ monoclonal antibody (mAb) blocking the IFN-I receptor subunit 1. Anifrolumab was recently approved for the treatment of SLE, which underscores the value of targeting IFN-I pathways in SLE. Other approaches, such as targeting pDCs as potential source of INF-I in SLE, are currently under investigation, such as the mAB litifilimab, which targets the blood dendritic cell antigen 2 (BDCA2) [44,45]. A summary of the current drugs used to treat LN is provided in Table 1.

IFN-I production is amplified by dysregulated mitochondrial homeostasis through various mechanisms. First and foremost, mtDNA itself acts as a danger-associated molecular pattern (DAMP) due to its unmethylated CpG sequence's structural resemblance to bacterial DNA. This structural similarity to bacterial DNA enables TLR9 activation, ultimately leading to the release of IFN-I [46]. In SLE, high levels of circulating oxidized mtDNA (oxmtDNA) have been identified within circulating neutrophils. What is particularly intriguing is that oxmtDNA has been found to possess a heightened propensity for internalization by pDCs, thus potentially contributing to the IFN-I signature seen in SLE [47,48]. Under normal physiological conditions, oxmtDNA undergoes a process of degradation within the lysosome. The endocytosis of oxmtDNA into the lysosome is facilitated by its dissociation from TFAM. Caielli and colleagues have demonstrated that autoantibodies targeting ribonucleotide proteins (anti-RNP) may obstruct TFAM phosphorylation, which in turn prevents oxmtDNA dissociation, rendering it resistant to degradation. This disruption in the natural degradation of oxmtDNA degradation may contribute to the vicious circle characterizing immune dysregulation in SLE [47] (Figure 2).

Another contributor to the immune dysfunction in SLE is the formation of extracellular traps, first described in neutrophils and termed "NETosis" [49]. Extracellular trap formation (ETF) is primarily used as a defense mechanism against pathogens. Cells capable of ETF extrude proteins and DNA to form a biological "web", intended to trap microorganisms. In neutrophils, NETosis was thought to be ineluctably associated with cell death (suicidal or lytic NETosis). Recently, another type of NETosis was reported, where cell functions are preserved (vital NETosis) [50]. It has been observed that IFN-I can trigger NETosis in SLE. On the other hand, oxmtDNA is a major component of extruded cell material during NETosis [48]. ETF thus may constitute another amplifying loop, where oxmtDNA enhances IFN-I production, while IFN-I-regulated genes promote ETF with the release of additional oxmtDNA. Finally, mitochondrial reactive oxygen (mtROS) species also act as DAMPs and may enhance IFN-I production by provoking the oligomerization of mitochondrial antiviral stimulator (MAVS) and ETF [51].

Table 1. Summary of the principal drugs used to treat lupus nephritis.

Standard Therapy for Lupus Nephritis			
Drugs	Mechanism of action	Indication	Comments
Cyclophosphamide with corticosteroid *	Alkylating agent: reduces number of lymphocytes (both B and T cells)	Induction phase	Two regimens: Eurolupus protocol: IV cyclophosphamide 500 mg every 2 weeks for a total of six doses (3 months). NIH protocol: IV cyclophosphamide 500–1000 mg/m² once a month for 6 months.
Mycophenolate mofetil with corticosteroid *	Inhibits the synthesis of guanine nucleotides	Both induction and maintenance phase	MMF 2–3 g per day, divided into two doses (1–1.5 g twice daily) for induction phase. MMF 1–2 g per day, divided into two doses (0.5–1 g twice daily) for maintenance phase.
Belimumab with SOC	Monoclonal antibody that inhibits the BAFF pathway	Both induction and maintenance phase	Use as a corticoid-sparing agent for articular SLE. Duration of treatment: two years (*BLISS-LN study*).

Non-Standard Therapy for Lupus Nephritis			
Drugs	Mechanism of action	Indication	Comments
Rituximab	Monoclonal antibody that targets CD20 protein, which is expressed on the surface of pre-B and mature B lymphocytes	Induction phase or as rescue therapy	Could be used as monotherapy for inducing remission in pure Lupus nephritis Class V. Could be used in conjunction with low dose of MMF for induction remission in active LN (Rituxilup protocol).
Voclosporin with MMF and low dose of corticoid	Calcineurin inhibitor: inhibition of T cell activation	Both induction and maintenance phase	Duration of treatment up to three years (Aurora 2 study).
Obinutuzumab with MMF and low dose of corticoid	Monoclonal antibody that targets CD20 protein. More potent than rituximab and notably enhances antibody-dependent cellular cytotoxicity and cellular apoptosis	Induction phase	Obinutuzumab 1000 mg at day 1, then weeks 2, 24, and 26.
Tacrolimus with low dose of MMF and lose dose of corticoid	Calcineurin inhibitor: inhibition of T cell activation	Induction and maintenance phase	Part of the multitarget therapy. MMF 1–1.5 g twice daily. Tacrolimus: 2–4 mg daily, adjusted based on blood levels and clinical response.

* Considered standard of care (SOC), BAFF: B-cell activating factor, MMF: Mycophenolate mofetil, NIH: National Institutes of Health.

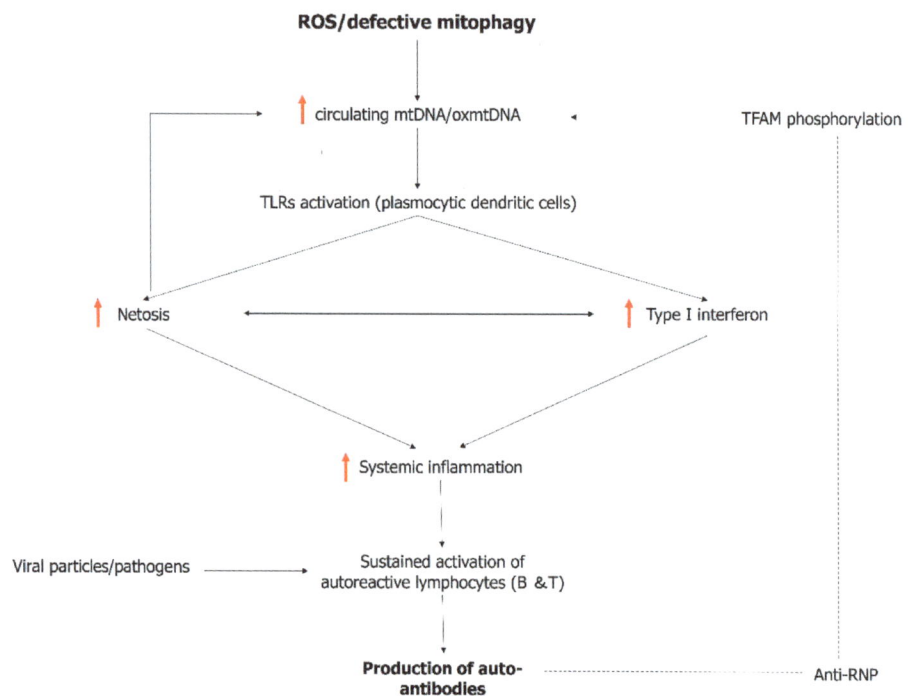

Figure 2. Interplay between mitochondrial dysregulation and inflammation in systemic lupus erythematosus. Red arrow = increase.

Neutrophils are not the only cells capable of ETF and sources of extracellular mitochondrial material. It was recently shown that platelets activated by immune complexes also release mitochondrial material [52]. Furthermore, recent findings have revealed that mtDNA that has leaked into the cytosole may also serve as a proinflammatory stimulus, boosting the cell's IFN-I expression [53]. The leakage of mtDNA to the cytosol occurs through pores in the OMM and activates the BAX/BAK pathways and subsequently caspase-9, thereby initiating the apoptosis cascade [54]. An alternative mechanism for the cytosolic release of mtDNA has also been described by Kim and colleagues [55]. They describe that the oligomerization of the voltage-dependent anion-selective channel 1 (VDAC1) is responsible for allowing mtDNA to leak into the cytosol, particularly under conditions of oxidative stress observed in lupus-prone mouse models.

Mitophagy prevents the release of mitochondrial materials into the extracellular environment, which is pivotal in maintaining cellular homeostasis. In SLE, various findings hint at defective mitophagy. Impaired mitophagy likely contributes to the release of mitochondrial components to the cytosol and the extracellular compartment, thus amplifying SLE immune dysregulation and, in particular, heightened IFN-I response.

CD4+ T cells in individuals with SLE exhibit an elevated mitochondrial mass, primarily attributed to a dysfunction in mitophagy [56]. Among the mechanisms contributing to this impaired mitophagy in CD4+ T cells is the overexpression of HRES-1/Rab4, a GTPase enzyme that promotes the degradation of Drp1 [14]. CD8+ T cells also have mitochondrial impairment. Elevated CD38 expression in CD8 + l T cells leads to decreased mitochondrial endocytosis by inhibiting sirtuin protein activity. Furthermore, it reduces V-ATPase activity, hindering lysosomal acidification due to diminished NAD+ levels. Consequently, the inability to internalize or degrade mitochondria within lysosomes contributes to the accumulation of dysfunctional mitochondria, increased mitochondrial mass, and the disruption of cellular function [57]. This accumulation further triggers the release of DAMPs like mtDNA and mitochondrial ROS, subsequently activating the STING pathway and inducing IFN production. Importantly, it is worth noting that IFN itself can enhance the expression of CD38 [56]. Mitophagy dysfunction is not confined to immune cells in SLE. Caielli and colleagues have recently revealed that a unique population of red blood cells, distinct to SLE patients, retains their mitochondria. This unusual phenomenon results from a disruption in the metabolic pathway responsible for transitioning between glycolysis and oxidative phosphorylation in mitochondria. Indeed, this transition is essential for activating the ubiquitin–proteasome system, which plays a pivotal role in mitophagy regulation [58]. Furthermore, in some SLE patients, there are antibodies that can bind to and opsonize red blood cells. When these opsonized red blood cells are encountered by myeloid cells, the mitochondria within them serve as DAMPs and are a potential source of IFN release [58].

4. Mitochondrial Dysfunction in Lupus Nephritis

Mitochondrial damage is associated with the progressive decline of renal function in chronic kidney diseases (CKDs) related to various conditions and LN in particular. Recent research by Luan and colleagues, employing electron microscopy in kidney biopsies, has unveiled several mitochondrial abnormalities in LN patients, including fission occurring within podocytes [59]. Furthermore, a connection between mtDNA and ETF in the kidney was established by Wang et al., who demonstrated the deposition of mtDNA within NETs found in the kidney biopsies of patients experiencing active LN [60].

Specific expression patterns in mitochondrial genes are seen in LN, progressing to renal fibrosis. Particularly, circular RNA originating from the mitochondrial gene MTND5 exhibits downregulation in LN-afflicted renal cells. Circular RNAs, a recently identified class of non-coding RNA fragments, are recognized for their role in regulating protein expression by modulating microRNAs, thereby influencing either the inhibition or activation of their function. In the case of circular MTND5, it normally downregulates microRNA6812, which is known to facilitate the activation of genes associated with fibrosis [59]. Moreover, a recent study by Tian et al. closely linked defective mitophagy to podocyte injuries, suggesting it could play a role in proteinuria in LN. First, they demonstrated that the podocyte expression of nestin was inversely correlated with proteinuria in LN. Furthermore, the expression of nestin was also linked to the expression of nephrin, a key protein of the glomerular basal membrane. Finally, they showed that nestin could regulate nephrin by inducing mitophagy through the PINK1 pathway [61].

Expanding on these observations, numerous authors have delved into the exploration of mitochondrial DNA as a surrogate marker for mitochondrial dysfunction in the context of LN. Notably, there has been a surge of enthusiasm surrounding the assessment of cell-free mitochondrial DNA as a potential biomarker.

In a cohort study comparing 80 SLE patients to 43 healthy controls, Hui-tin Lee and colleagues discovered that compared to the healthy controls, SLE patients exhibited higher levels of relative cell-free nuclear DNA (CFnDNA) and lower levels of relative cell-free mitochondrial DNA (CFmtDNA). Within SLE, individuals with active disease, indicated by an SLEDAI > 8, demonstrated even lower levels of CFmtDNA. Patients with LN showed a trend toward lower CFmtDNA compared to non-renal SLE. To explain this difference between mtDNA and nuclear DNA, the authors suggest that SLE patients were undergoing more vital NETosis than lytic NETosis, the former releasing a higher amount of nuclear DNA than mtDNA into the circulation. Furthermore, it is important to note that during NETosis, mitochondrial DNA becomes entrapped in the NET and is not freely found in the plasma [62]. The observation of lower CFmtDNA in LN is interesting, considering the pivotal role NETosis plays in this pathology [63–65]. Others have found a positive association between the total-mtDNA-to-CFmtDNA ratio and renal damage in SLE (eGFR < 60 mL/min). In this study, a lower CFmtDNA copy number was associated with proteinuria. The cell-free DNA profile failed, however, to discriminate patients with proliferative LN (Class III A and Class IV A) [66]. Another study conducted by Hui-Tin and colleagues delves into the "qualitative" dimension of mtDNA in SLE [67]. Their focus centers on the heteroplasmy of the D310 region, specifically examining variations in the number of cysteine and thymidine (D310 polymorphism) in the mtDNA of leukocytes. This particular mutation is the most prevalent, and its presence in this region raises suspicions of potential interference with the replication of mitochondrial DNA [68,69]. Their findings revealed that SLE patients exhibited a higher degree of D310 heteroplasmy compared to a control group. Moreover, there was a noticeable trend towards increased heteroplasmy with the progression of disease activity in the SLE group, as measured by the SLEDAI, and this corresponded to lower mtDNA copy numbers and a reduced expression of mitochondrial RNA genes. Moreover, patients with renal involvement demonstrated an even greater degree of D310 heteroplasmy [67].

In another study, Wang et al. demonstrated the presence of antibodies against mtDNA in 41% of patients within their cohort. Furthermore, these antibodies exhibited higher positivity in patients classified under Class III or IV A compared to Class III or IV C, although it is crucial to note the limited number of patients within Class III or IV C (N = 3) [60].

Collectively, these studies underscore the potential of mtDNA as a marker in SLE, particularly in the context of LN, offering promise for diagnostic applications. However, a cautious approach is warranted in interpreting these findings due to the existing heterogeneity in mtDNA quantification methods. Presently, these results lack validation in large cohorts and lack a robust direct comparison with the histology of renal biopsies from SLE patients, underscoring the necessity for circumspection when drawing definitive conclusions and assessing clinical utility. Furthermore, considering the intricate interplay between mitochondrial damage and interferon production, a comparison with classic interferon markers, such as the "interferon gene signature", could provide valuable insights for a comprehensive assessment.

5. Mitochondria as Therapeutic Targets in SLE

Given the close relationship between mitochondria and interferon production in SLE, mitochondria stand out as a potential new target for therapy. Remarkably, there are currently affordable and readily available drugs that specifically target mitochondrial dysfunction, such as metformin or mTOR inhibitors. These drugs hold promise in modulating mitochondrial function and could potentially offer therapeutic benefits in managing SLE by targeting this critical cellular pathway.

Indeed, Lai et al. conducted a study on patients experiencing persistent lupus activity, examining the effects of sirolimus. The rationale behind this investigation was the known impact of mTOR inhibitors, such as sirolimus, on mitophagy. This effect is believed to occur due to their interaction with HRES-1/Rab4 expression [14]. In Lai's study, it was found that 55% of patients treated with sirolimus experienced a reduction in SLEDAI and BILAG scores during the study period. However, it is crucial to note that over 25% of patients were excluded from the final analysis due to intolerance and non-compliance, potentially introducing bias into the results. Furthermore, the exclusion of patients with proteinuria raises questions about the potential role of sirolimus in LN since mTOR inhibitors have been associated with inducing proteinuria and focal segmental glomerulosclerosis. This limitation suggests a restricted scope regarding its application in LN management [70]. However, Wang et al. recently studied the efficacy of UMI-77, a molecule that restores mitophagy, in LN [71]. UMI-77 potentiates mitophagy by blocking the interaction between MCL-1 and Bax/Bak pathways, allowing MCL-1 to interact with LC3 and induce mitophagy. In their study on lupus-prone mice, the authors demonstrated that the kidneys of lupus mice treated with UMI-77 exhibited less glomerular inflammation, a reduced infiltration of inflammatory cells, fewer crescent formations, less fibrosis, and fewer immune complex deposits compared to the control. Interestingly, the effect of UMI-77 was not directly on the mitochondria of podocytes or tubular cells but rather on plasmacytoid dendritic cells, restoring their mitochondrial homeostasis and thereby contributing to reducing T cell infiltration in the kidney. Their study not only provides proof of concept for the role of mitophagy in LN but also serves as a salient milestone that will pave the way for further research on mitophagy as a therapeutic target of SLE [71]. In animal model studies, drugs known to enhance mitochondrial metabolism, such as idebenone (an analogue of coenzyme Q10) or mitoQ, have demonstrated improvements in renal histology [51,72]. These improvements were evident in reduced fibrosis, diminishing immune deposits on glomeruli. In vivo, those molecules also diminish NET formation and markers of IFN. However, most studies focusing on targeting mitochondria in LN remain in the preliminary stages, suggesting a long and extensive journey before their translation into clinical utility. A summary of the mitochondrial-targeting drugs in development for SLE is provided in Table 2.

Table 2. Current mitochondrial-targeting drugs assessed in systematic lupus erythematosus.

Drug	Mechanism of Action on Mitochondria	Efficacy in SLE
Metformin	Inhibits the mitochondrial enzyme complex: mitochondrial glycerophosphate dehydrogenase	Increased renal function and reduced glomerular inflammation in a murine lupus model. No effect on lupus flare in a small, randomized control study.
Sirolimus	Restoration of mitophagy by interaction with HRES-1/Rab4 expression	Decrease in BILAG and in total dose of corticoid in patients with persistent SLE activity in a single-arm trial.
MitoQ	Mitochondrial antioxidant	Reduced NET formation, serum IFN-I, reduced immune complex deposit in kidneys in a murine model.
Idebenone	Analogue of coenzyme Q10	Decreased glomerular inflammation and fibrosis and decreased NET formation in murine model.
UMI-77	Inducer of mitophagy by interacting with the BAK/BAX pathway	Reduced glomerular inflammation, notably by decreasing T cell infiltration in the kidney in a murine model of LN.

BILAG: British Isles Lupus Assessment Group. IFN: interferon. LN: lupus nephritis.

6. Conclusions

LN stands as a complex disease, currently hindered by a limited array of new treatments. Its characterization is marked by the absence of non-invasive biomarkers, which are crucial for diagnosing active disease or assessing treatment response. The emerging role of mitochondria as a pivotal nexus for various essential mechanisms in the pathophysiology of LN represents an area yet to be fully explored and understood. Research in this domain holds the promise of eventually paving the way for more personalized and precisely tailored therapies in LN.

Author Contributions: M.H. and A.T.T. wrote the manuscript; C.R. critically review the manuscript. All authors have read and agreed to the published version of the manuscript.

Funding: The study was funded by a grant of from the Department of Medicine and Laboratory of Lausanne university hospital.

Conflicts of Interest: The authors declare no conflict of interest.

References

1. D'Cruz, D.P.; Khamashta, M.A.; Hughes, G.R. Systemic lupus erythematosus. *Lancet* **2007**, *369*, 587–596. [CrossRef] [PubMed]
2. Barber, M.R.W.; Drenkard, C.; Falasinnu, T.; Hoi, A.; Mak, A.; Kow, N.Y.; Svenungsson, E.; Peterson, J.; Clarke, A.E.; Ramsey-Goldman, R. Global epidemiology of systemic lupus erythematosus. *Nat. Rev. Rheumatol.* **2021**, *17*, 515–532. [CrossRef] [PubMed]
3. Wong, M.; Tsao, B.P. Current topics in human SLE genetics. *Springer Semin. Immunopathol.* **2006**, *28*, 97–107. [CrossRef] [PubMed]
4. Foster, M.H. T cells and B cells in lupus nephritis. *Semin. Nephrol.* **2007**, *27*, 47–58. [CrossRef] [PubMed]
5. Cameron, J.S. Lupus nephritis. *J. Am. Soc. Nephrol.* **1999**, *10*, 413–424. [CrossRef]
6. Bono, L.; Cameron, J.S.; Hicks, J.A. The very long-term prognosis and complications of lupus nephritis and its treatment. *QJM* **1999**, *92*, 211–218. [CrossRef]

7. Rovin, B.H.; Furie, R.; Latinis, K.; Looney, R.J.; Fervenza, F.C.; Sanchez-Guerrero, J.; Maciuca, R.; Zhang, D.; Garg, J.P.; Brunetta, P.; et al. Efficacy and safety of rituximab in patients with active proliferative lupus nephritis: The Lupus Nephritis Assessment with Rituximab study. *Arthritis Rheum.* **2012**, *64*, 1215–1226. [CrossRef]
8. Furie, R.; Rovin, B.H.; Houssiau, F.; Malvar, A.; Teng, Y.K.O.; Contreras, G.; Amoura, Z.; Yu, X.; Mok, C.-C.; Santiago, M.B.; et al. Two-Year, Randomized, Controlled Trial of Belimumab in Lupus Nephritis. *N. Engl. J. Med.* **2020**, *383*, 1117–1128. [CrossRef] [PubMed]
9. Rovin, B.H.; Teng, Y.K.O.; Ginzler, E.M.; Arriens, C.; Caster, D.J.; Romero-Diaz, J.; Gibson, K.; Kaplan, J.; Lisk, L.; Navarra, S.; et al. Efficacy and safety of voclosporin versus placebo for lupus nephritis (AURORA 1): A double-blind, randomised, multicentre, placebo-controlled, phase 3 trial. *Lancet* **2021**, *397*, 2070–2080. [CrossRef]
10. Rovin, B.; Furie, R. B-cell depletion and response in a randomized, controlled trial of obinutuzumab for proliferative lupus nephritis. *Ann Rheum Dis.* **2022**, *81*, 100–107. [CrossRef]
11. Halfon, M.; Bachelet, D.; Hanouna, G.; Dema, B.; Pellefigues, C.; Manchon, P.; Laouenan, C.; Charles, N.; Daugas, E. CD62L on blood basophils: A first pre-treatment predictor of remission in severe lupus nephritis. *Nephrol. Dial. Transplant.* **2021**, *36*, 2256–2262. [CrossRef] [PubMed]
12. Ioannidis, J.P.; Boki, K.A.; Katsorida, M.E.; Drosos, A.A.; Skopouli, F.N.; Boletis, J.N.; Moutsopoulos, H.M. Remission, relapse, and re-remission of proliferative lupus nephritis treated with cyclophosphamide. *Kidney Int.* **2000**, *57*, 258–264. [CrossRef] [PubMed]
13. Li, W.; Gong, M.; Park, Y.P.; Elshikha, A.S.; Choi, S.C.; Brown, J.; Kanda, N.; Yeh, W.-I.; Peters, L.; Titov, A.A.; et al. Lupus susceptibility gene Esrrg modulates regulatory T cells through mitochondrial metabolism. *JCI Insight* **2021**, *6*, e143540. [CrossRef] [PubMed]
14. Caza, T.N.; Fernandez, D.R.; Talaber, G.; Oaks, Z.; Haas, M.; Madaio, M.P.; Lai, Z.W.; Miklossy, G.; Singh, R.R.; Chudakov, D.M.; et al. HRES-1/Rab4-mediated depletion of Drp1 impairs mitochondrial homeostasis represents a target for treatment in, S.L.E. *Ann. Rheum. Dis.* **2014**, *73*, 1888–1897. [CrossRef]
15. Ma, L.; Roach, T.; Morel, L. Immunometabolic alterations in lupus: Where do they come from and where do we go from there? *Curr. Opin. Immunol.* **2022**, *78*, 102245. [CrossRef] [PubMed]
16. Zou, X.; Choi, S.C.; Zeumer-Spataro, L.; Scindia, Y.; Moser, E.K.; Morel, L. Metabolic regulation of follicular helper T cell differentiation in a mouse model of lupus. *Immunol. Lett.* **2022**, *247*, 13–21. [CrossRef] [PubMed]
17. Choi, S.C.; Titov, A.A.; Abboud, G.; Seay, H.R.; Brusko, T.M.; Roopenian, D.C.; Salek-Ardakani, S.; Morel, L. Inhibition of glucose metabolism selectively targets autoreactive follicular helper T cells. *Nat. Commun.* **2018**, *9*, 4369. [CrossRef] [PubMed]
18. Doke, T.; Susztak, K. The multifaceted role of kidney tubule mitochondrial dysfunction in kidney disease development. *Trends Cell Biol.* **2022**, *32*, 841–853. [CrossRef] [PubMed]
19. Emma, F.; Montini, G.; Parikh, S.M.; Salviati, L. Mitochondrial dysfunction in inherited renal disease and acute kidney injury. *Nat. Rev. Nephrol.* **2016**, *12*, 267–280. [CrossRef]
20. Galvan, D.L.; Green, N.H.; Danesh, F.R. The hallmarks of mitochondrial dysfunction in chronic kidney disease. *Kidney Int.* **2017**, *92*, 1051–1057. [CrossRef]
21. Miyazono, Y.; Hirashima, S.; Ishihara, N.; Kusukawa, J.; Nakamura, K.I.; Ohta, K. Uncoupled mitochondria quickly shorten along their long axis to form indented spheroids, instead of rings, in a fission-independent manner. *Sci. Rep.* **2018**, *8*, 350. [CrossRef] [PubMed]
22. Vafai, S.B.; Mootha, V.K. Mitochondrial disorders as windows into an ancient organelle. *Nature* **2012**, *491*, 374–383. [CrossRef]
23. Habbane, M.; Montoya, J.; Rhouda, T.; Sbaoui, Y.; Radallah, D.; Emperador, S. Human Mitochondrial DNA: Particularities and Diseases. *Biomedicines* **2021**, *9*, 1364. [CrossRef]
24. Spelbrink, J.N. Functional organization of mammalian mitochondrial DNA in nucleoids: History, recent developments, and future challenges. *IUBMB Life* **2010**, *62*, 19–32. [CrossRef]
25. Rensch, T.; Villar, D.; Horvath, J.; Odom, D.T.; Flicek, P. Mitochondrial heteroplasmy in vertebrates using ChIP-sequencing data. *Genome Biol.* **2016**, *17*, 139. [CrossRef]
26. Tan, T.; Zimmermann, M.; Reichert, A.S. Controlling quality and amount of mitochondria by mitophagy: Insights into the role of ubiquitination and deubiquitination. *Biol. Chem.* **2016**, *397*, 637–647. [CrossRef] [PubMed]
27. Popov, L.D. Mitochondrial biogenesis: An update. *J. Cell. Mol. Med.* **2020**, *24*, 4892–4899. [CrossRef] [PubMed]
28. Atici, A.E.; Crother, T.R.; Noval Rivas, M. Mitochondrial quality control in health and cardiovascular diseases. *Front. Cell Dev. Biol.* **2023**, *11*, 1290046. [CrossRef]
29. Adebayo, M.; Singh, S.; Singh, A.P.; Dasgupta, S. Mitochondrial fusion and fission: The fine-tune balance for cellular homeostasis. *FASEB J.* **2021**, *35*, e21620. [CrossRef]
30. Sulkshane, P.; Ram, J.; Thakur, A.; Reis, N.; Kleifeld, O.; Glickman, M.H. Ubiquitination and receptor-mediated mitophagy converge to eliminate oxidation-damaged mitochondria during hypoxia. *Redox Biol.* **2021**, *45*, 102047. [CrossRef]
31. Guo, H.J.; Rahimi, N.; Tadi, P. *Biochemistry, Ubiquitination*; StatPearls: Treasure Island, FL, USA, 2023.
32. Pattingre, S.; Turtoi, A. BAG Family Members as Mitophagy Regulators in Mammals. *Cells* **2022**, *11*, 681. [CrossRef] [PubMed]
33. Zhang, T.; Liu, Q.; Gao, W.; Sehgal, S.A.; Wu, H. The multifaceted regulation of mitophagy by endogenous metabolites. *Autophagy* **2022**, *18*, 1216–1239. [CrossRef] [PubMed]
34. Wan, W.; Hua, F.; Fang, P.; Li, C.; Deng, F.; Chen, S.; Ying, J.; Wang, X. Regulation of Mitophagy by Sirtuin Family Proteins: A Vital Role in Aging and Age-Related Diseases. *Front. Aging Neurosci.* **2022**, *14*, 845330. [CrossRef] [PubMed]

35. Li, Y.; Ma, Y.; Song, L.; Yu, L.; Zhang, L.; Zhang, Y.; Xing, Y.; Yin, Y.; Ma, H. SIRT3 deficiency exacerbates p53/Parkin-mediated mitophagy inhibition and promotes mitochondrial dysfunction: Implication for aged hearts. *Int. J. Mol. Med.* **2018**, *41*, 3517–3526. [CrossRef] [PubMed]
36. Li, W.; Feng, J.; Gao, C.; Wu, M.; Du, Q.; Tsoi, B.; Wang, Q.; Yang, D.; Shen, J. Nitration of Drp1 provokes mitophagy activation mediating neuronal injury in experimental autoimmune encephalomyelitis. *Free Radic. Biol. Med.* **2019**, *143*, 70–83. [CrossRef] [PubMed]
37. Talaber, G.; Miklossy, G.; Oaks, Z.; Liu, Y.; Tooze, S.A.; Chudakov, D.M.; Banki, K.; Perl, A. HRES-1/Rab4 promotes the formation of LC3(+) autophagosomes and the accumulation of mitochondria during autophagy. *PLoS ONE* **2014**, *9*, e84392. [CrossRef] [PubMed]
38. Ramaswamy, M.; Tummala, R.; Streicher, K.; Nogueira da Costa, A.; Brohawn, P.Z. The Pathogenesis, Molecular Mechanisms, and Therapeutic Potential of the Interferon Pathway in Systemic Lupus Erythematosus and Other Autoimmune Diseases. *Int. J. Mol. Sci.* **2021**, *22*, 11286. [CrossRef] [PubMed]
39. Psarras, A.; Wittmann, M.; Vital, E.M. Emerging concepts of type I interferons in SLE pathogenesis and therapy. *Nat. Rev. Rheumatol.* **2022**, *18*, 575–590. [CrossRef]
40. Denny, M.F.; Yalavarthi, S.; Zhao, W.; Thacker, S.G.; Anderson, M.; Sandy, A.R.; McCune, W.J.; Kaplan, M.J. A distinct subset of proinflammatory neutrophils isolated from patients with systemic lupus erythematosus induces vascular damage and synthesizes type I IFNs. *J. Immunol.* **2010**, *184*, 3284–3297. [CrossRef]
41. Skopelja-Gardner, S.; Tai, J.; Sun, X.; Tanaka, L.; Kuchenbecker, J.A.; Snyder, J.M.; Kubes, P.; Mustelin, T.; Elkon, K.B. Acute skin exposure to ultraviolet light triggers neutrophil-mediated kidney inflammation. *Proc. Natl. Acad. Sci. USA* **2021**, *118*, e2019097118. [CrossRef]
42. Castellano, G.; Cafiero, C.; Divella, C.; Sallustio, F.; Gigante, M.; Pontrelli, P.; De Palma, G.; Rossini, M.; Grandaliano, G.; Gesualdo, L. Local synthesis of interferon-alpha in lupus nephritis is associated with type I interferons signature and LMP7 induction in renal tubular epithelial cells. *Arthritis Res Ther.* **2015**, *17*, 72. [CrossRef] [PubMed]
43. Reyes, J.; Zhao, Y.; Pandya, K.; Yap, G.S. Growth differentiation factor-15 is an IFN-gamma regulated mediator of infection-induced weight loss and the hepatic FGF21 response. *Brain Behav. Immun.* **2024**, *116*, 24–33. [CrossRef]
44. Morand, E.F.; Furie, R.; Tanaka, Y.; Bruce, I.N.; Askanase, A.D.; Richez, C.; Bae, S.C.; Brohawn, P.Z.; Pineda, L.; Berglind, A.; et al. Trial of Anifrolumab in Active Systemic Lupus Erythematosus. *N. Engl. J. Med.* **2020**, *382*, 211–221. [CrossRef] [PubMed]
45. Furie, R.A.; van Vollenhoven, R.F.; Kalunian, K.; Navarra, S.; Romero-Diaz, J.; Werth, V.P.; Huang, X.; Clark, G.; Carroll, H.; Meyers, A.; et al. Trial of Anti-BDCA2 Antibody Litifilimab for Systemic Lupus Erythematosus. *N. Engl. J. Med.* **2022**, *387*, 894–904. [CrossRef] [PubMed]
46. Zhang, Q.; Raoof, M.; Chen, Y.; Sumi, Y.; Sursal, T.; Junger, W.; Brohi, K.; Itagaki, K.; Hauser, C.J. Circulating mitochondrial DAMPs cause inflammatory responses to injury. *Nature* **2010**, *464*, 104–107. [CrossRef] [PubMed]
47. Caielli, S.; Athale, S.; Domic, B.; Murat, E.; Chandra, M.; Banchereau, R.; Baisch, J.; Phelps, K.; Clayton, S.; Gong, M.; et al. Oxidized mitochondrial nucleoids released by neutrophils drive type I interferon production in human lupus. *J. Exp. Med.* **2016**, *213*, 697–713. [CrossRef] [PubMed]
48. Lood, C.; Blanco, L.P.; Purmalek, M.M.; Carmona-Rivera, C.; De Ravin, S.S.; Smith, C.K.; Malech, H.L.; Ledbetter, J.A.; Elkon, K.B.; Kaplan, M.J. Neutrophil extracellular traps enriched in oxidized mitochondrial DNA are interferogenic and contribute to lupus-like disease. *Nat. Med.* **2016**, *22*, 146–153. [CrossRef] [PubMed]
49. Frangou, E.; Vassilopoulos, D.; Boletis, J.; Boumpas, D.T. An emerging role of neutrophils and NETosis in chronic inflammation and fibrosis in systemic lupus erythematosus (SLE) and ANCA-associated vasculitides (AAV): Implications for the pathogenesis and treatment. *Autoimmun. Rev.* **2019**, *18*, 751–760. [CrossRef] [PubMed]
50. Pieterse, E.; Rother, N.; Yanginlar, C.; Hilbrands, L.B.; van der Vlag, J. Neutrophils Discriminate between Lipopolysaccharides of Different Bacterial Sources and Selectively Release Neutrophil Extracellular Traps. *Front. Immunol.* **2016**, *7*, 484. [CrossRef]
51. Fortner, K.A.; Blanco, L.P.; Buskiewicz, I.; Huang, N.; Gibson, P.C.; Cook, D.L.; Pedersen, H.L.; Yuen, P.S.; Murphy, M.; Perl, A.; et al. Targeting mitochondrial oxidative stress with MitoQ reduces NET formation and kidney disease in lupus-prone MRL-lpr mice. *Lupus Sci. Med.* **2020**, *7*, e000387. [CrossRef]
52. Melki, I.; Allaeys, I.; Tessandier, N.; Levesque, T.; Cloutier, N.; Laroche, A.; Vernoux, N.; Becker, Y.; Benk-Fortin, H.; Zufferey, A.; et al. Platelets release mitochondrial antigens in systemic lupus erythematosus. *Sci. Transl. Med.* **2021**, *13*, eaav5928. [CrossRef] [PubMed]
53. West, A.P.; Shadel, G.S. Mitochondrial DNA in innate immune responses and inflammatory pathology. *Nat. Rev. Immunol.* **2017**, *17*, 363–375. [CrossRef] [PubMed]
54. Wolf, P.; Schoeniger, A.; Edlich, F. Pro-apoptotic complexes of BAX and BAK on the outer mitochondrial membrane. *Biochim. Biophys. Acta Mol. Cell Res.* **2022**, *1869*, 119317. [CrossRef] [PubMed]
55. Kim, J.; Gupta, R.; Blanco, L.P.; Yang, S.; Shteinfer-Kuzmine, A.; Wang, K.; Zhu, J.; Yoon, H.E.; Wang, X.; Kerkhofs, M.; et al. VDAC oligomers form mitochondrial pores to release mtDNA fragments and promote lupus-like disease. *Science* **2019**, *366*, 1531–1536. [CrossRef] [PubMed]
56. Caza, T.N.; Talaber, G.; Perl, A. Metabolic regulation of organelle homeostasis in lupus T cells. *Clin. Immunol.* **2012**, *144*, 200–213. [CrossRef] [PubMed]

57. Chen, P.M.; Katsuyama, E.; Satyam, A.; Li, H.; Rubio, J.; Jung, S.; Andrzejewski, S.; Becherer, J.D.; Tsokos, M.G.; Abdi, R.; et al. CD38 reduces mitochondrial fitness and cytotoxic T cell response against viral infection in lupus patients by suppressing mitophagy. *Sci. Adv.* **2022**, *8*, eabo4271. [CrossRef] [PubMed]
58. Caielli, S.; Cardenas, J.; de Jesus, A.A.; Baisch, J.; Walters, L.; Blanck, J.P.; Balasubramanian, P.; Stagnar, C.; Ohouo, M.; Hong, S.; et al. Erythroid mitochondrial retention triggers myeloid-dependent type I interferon in human, S.L.E. *Cell* **2021**, *184*, 4464–4479. [CrossRef] [PubMed]
59. Luan, J.; Jiao, C.; Ma, C.; Zhang, Y.; Hao, X.; Zhou, G.; Fu, J.; Qiu, X.; Li, H.; Yang, W.; et al. circMTND5 Participates in Renal Mitochondrial Injury and Fibrosis by Sponging MIR6812 in Lupus Nephritis. *Oxid. Med. Cell. Longev.* **2022**, *2022*, 2769487. [CrossRef] [PubMed]
60. Wang, H.; Li, T.; Chen, S.; Gu, Y.; Ye, S. Neutrophil Extracellular Trap Mitochondrial DNA and Its Autoantibody in Systemic Lupus Erythematosus and a Proof-of-Concept Trial of Metformin. *Arthritis Rheumatol.* **2015**, *67*, 3190–3200. [CrossRef]
61. Tian, Y.; Guo, H.; Miao, X.; Xu, J.; Yang, R.; Zhao, L.; Liu, J.; Yang, L.; Gao, F.; Zhang, W.; et al. Nestin protects podocyte from injury in lupus nephritis by mitophagy and oxidative stress. *Cell Death Dis.* **2020**, *11*, 319. [CrossRef]
62. Lee, H.T.; Lin, C.S.; Pan, S.C.; Chen, W.S.; Tsai, C.Y.; Wei, Y.H. The Role of Plasma Cell-Free Mitochondrial DNA and Nuclear DNA in Systemic Lupus Erythematosus. *Front. Biosci.* **2022**, *27*, 333. [CrossRef] [PubMed]
63. Hakkim, A.; Furnrohr, B.G.; Amann, K.; Laube, B.; Abed, U.A.; Brinkmann, V.; Herrmann, M.; Voll, R.E.; Zychlinsky, A. Impairment of neutrophil extracellular trap degradation is associated with lupus nephritis. *Proc. Natl. Acad. Sci. USA* **2010**, *107*, 9813–9818. [CrossRef] [PubMed]
64. Fenton, K. The effect of cell death in the initiation of lupus nephritis. *Clin. Exp. Immunol.* **2015**, *179*, 11–16. [CrossRef] [PubMed]
65. Knight, J.S.; Kaplan, M.J. Lupus neutrophils: 'NET' gain in understanding lupus pathogenesis. *Curr. Opin. Rheumatol.* **2012**, *24*, 441–450. [CrossRef] [PubMed]
66. Truszewska, A.; Wirkowska, A.; Gala, K.; Truszewski, P.; Krzemien-Ojak, L.; Perkowska-Ptasinska, A.; Mucha, K.; Pączek, L.; Foroncewicz, B. Cell-free DNA profiling in patients with lupus nephritis. *Lupus* **2020**, *29*, 1759–1772. [CrossRef] [PubMed]
67. Lee, H.T.; Lin, C.S.; Chen, W.S.; Liao, H.T.; Tsai, C.Y.; Wei, Y.H. Leukocyte mitochondrial DNA alteration in systemic lupus erythematosus and its relevance to the susceptibility to lupus nephritis. *Int. J. Mol. Sci.* **2012**, *13*, 8853–8868. [CrossRef] [PubMed]
68. Mambo, E.; Gao, X.; Cohen, Y.; Guo, Z.; Talalay, P.; Sidransky, D. Electrophile and oxidant damage of mitochondrial DNA leading to rapid evolution of homoplasmic mutations. *Proc. Natl. Acad. Sci. USA* **2003**, *100*, 1838–1843. [CrossRef] [PubMed]
69. Lee, H.C.; Wei, Y.H. Mitochondrial biogenesis and mitochondrial DNA maintenance of mammalian cells under oxidative stress. *Int. J. Biochem. Cell Biol.* **2005**, *37*, 822–834. [CrossRef] [PubMed]
70. Lai, Z.W.; Kelly, R.; Winans, T.; Marchena, I.; Shadakshari, A.; Yu, J.; Dawood, M.; Garcia, R.; Tily, H.; Francis, L.; et al. Sirolimus in patients with clinically active systemic lupus erythematosus resistant to, or intolerant of, conventional medications: A single-arm, open-label, phase 1/2 trial. *Lancet* **2018**, *391*, 1186–1196. [CrossRef]
71. Wang, H.; Shen, M.; Ma, Y.; Lan, L.; Jiang, X.; Cen, X.; Guo, G.; Zhou, Q.; Yuan, M.; Chen, J.; et al. Novel mitophagy inducer alleviates lupus nephritis by reducing myeloid cell activation and autoantigen presentation. *Kidney Int.* **2024**, *105*, 759–774. [CrossRef]
72. Blanco, L.P.; Pedersen, H.L.; Wang, X.; Lightfoot, Y.L.; Seto, N.; Carmona-Rivera, C.; Yu, Z.; Hoffmann, V.; Yuen, P.S.T.; Kaplan, M.J. Improved Mitochondrial Metabolism and Reduced Inflammation Following Attenuation of Murine Lupus With Coenzyme Q10 Analog Idebenone. *Arthritis Rheumatol.* **2020**, *72*, 454–464. [CrossRef] [PubMed]

Disclaimer/Publisher's Note: The statements, opinions and data contained in all publications are solely those of the individual author(s) and contributor(s) and not of MDPI and/or the editor(s). MDPI and/or the editor(s) disclaim responsibility for any injury to people or property resulting from any ideas, methods, instructions or products referred to in the content.

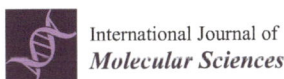

Review

Human and Murine Toll-like Receptor-Driven Disease in Systemic Lupus Erythematosus

Susannah von Hofsten [1], Kristin Andreassen Fenton [2] and Hege Lynum Pedersen [2,*]

1. Department of Medical Biology, Faculty of Health Sciences, UiT The Arctic University of Norway, 9019 Tromsø, Norway; susannah.hofsten@uit.no
2. Centre of Clinical Research and Education, University Hospital of North Norway, Department of Medical Biology, Faculty of Health Sciences, UiT The Arctic University of Norway, 9019 Tromsø, Norway; kristin.fenton@uit.no
* Correspondence: hege.lynum.pedersen@uit.no

Abstract: The pathogenesis of systemic lupus erythematosus (SLE) is linked to the differential roles of toll-like receptors (TLRs), particularly TLR7, TLR8, and TLR9. TLR7 overexpression or gene duplication, as seen with the Y-linked autoimmune accelerator (*Yaa*) locus or TLR7 agonist imiquimod, correlates with increased SLE severity, and specific TLR7 polymorphisms and gain-of-function variants are associated with enhanced SLE susceptibility and severity. In addition, the X-chromosome location of *TLR7* and its escape from X-chromosome inactivation provide a genetic basis for female predominance in SLE. The absence of TLR8 and TLR9 have been shown to exacerbate the detrimental effects of TLR7, leading to upregulated TLR7 activity and increased disease severity in mouse models of SLE. The regulatory functions of TLR8 and TLR9 have been proposed to involve competition for the endosomal trafficking chaperone UNC93B1. However, recent evidence implies more direct, regulatory functions of TLR9 on TLR7 activity. The association between age-associated B cells (ABCs) and autoantibody production positions these cells as potential targets for treatment in SLE, but the lack of specific markers necessitates further research for precise therapeutic intervention. Therapeutically, targeting TLRs is a promising strategy for SLE treatment, with drugs like hydroxychloroquine already in clinical use.

Keywords: systemic lupus erythematosus; toll-like receptor; mouse models

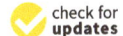

Citation: von Hofsten, S.; Fenton, K.A.; Pedersen, H.L. Human and Murine Toll-like Receptor-Driven Disease in Systemic Lupus Erythematosus. *Int. J. Mol. Sci.* **2024**, *25*, 5351. https://doi.org/10.3390/ijms25105351

Academic Editors: Christopher Sjöwall and Ioannis Parodis

Received: 26 April 2024
Revised: 10 May 2024
Accepted: 12 May 2024
Published: 14 May 2024

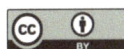

Copyright: © 2024 by the authors. Licensee MDPI, Basel, Switzerland. This article is an open access article distributed under the terms and conditions of the Creative Commons Attribution (CC BY) license (https://creativecommons.org/licenses/by/4.0/).

1. Introduction

Systemic lupus erythematosus (SLE) is an autoimmune systemic disease that affects various organs in the body. The disease is complex with heterogenous manifestations, and both genetic and environmental factors such as ultraviolet radiation, viral infections, and exposure to certain chemicals have been implicated in disease etiology. Characteristic of this disease are autoantibodies against DNA and an increased production of type I interferons (IFNs). The innate immune system is the first responder to infections and damage and is responsible for the interferon response. Most cells can produce type I IFNs. However, plasmacytoid dendritic cells (pDCs) are the most potent producers of these cytokines. In contrast, antibody production involves the adaptive immune response. Cells such as dendritic cells (DCs), T cells, and B cells are the main players in this response.

Several anti-nuclear autoantibodies (ANAs), such as anti-double-stranded DNA (dsDNA), anti-nucleosome (nuc), anti-Sm, anti-small nuclear riboprotein (snRNP), anti-Sjogrens syndrome antigen A (SSA/Ro), anti-Sjogrens syndrome antigen B (SSB/La), anti-phospholipid (PL), and anti-C1q antibodies have been implicated in SLE, but anti-dsDNA and anti-Sm are the only antibodies that are considered specific for SLE [1]. Immunoglobulin isotypes such as IgA, IgM, IgG, IgG1, igG2, IgG3, and IgG4 have all been observed in SLE, but only the IgG isotype is used in the classification criteria for diagnosis (reviewed in [1,2]).

Autoantibodies cause inflammation and may form immune complexes that can be deposited in organs and cause local inflammation and organ damage. In SLE, the kidneys are often affected, and patients may develop lupus nephritis (LN), which is a serious complication that can lead to kidney failure [3]. The predominance of nucleic acid-associated autoantigens in SLE is noteworthy and is probably due to the ability of these antigens to also bind to members of the toll-like receptor (TLR) family of pattern recognition receptors. Other nucleic acid sensors such as cytosolic dsRNA sensors, including melanoma differentiation-associated protein 5 (MDA5) and retinoic acid-inducible gene I (RIG-1), and DNA sensors such as cyclic GMP-AMP synthase (cGAS), interferon-gamma inducible 16 (IFI16), absent in melanoma 2 (AIM2), and DNA-dependent activator of IRFs (DAI) may also be involved in SLE.

TLRs are involved in shaping the immune response by recognizing pathogen-associated molecular patterns (PAMPs) and damage-associated molecular patterns (DAMPs). Several TLRs have been identified, including TLR1-TLR10 in humans, and TLR1-TLR13 in mice. However, the *Tlr10* gene is not functional in mice [4]. TLR1–TLR2, TLR2–TLR6, and possibly TLR2–TLR10 form heterodimers [5]. The TLRs can be divided by their localization in the cell, either on the cell surface or in endosomes, and by which ligand they bind (Figure 1).

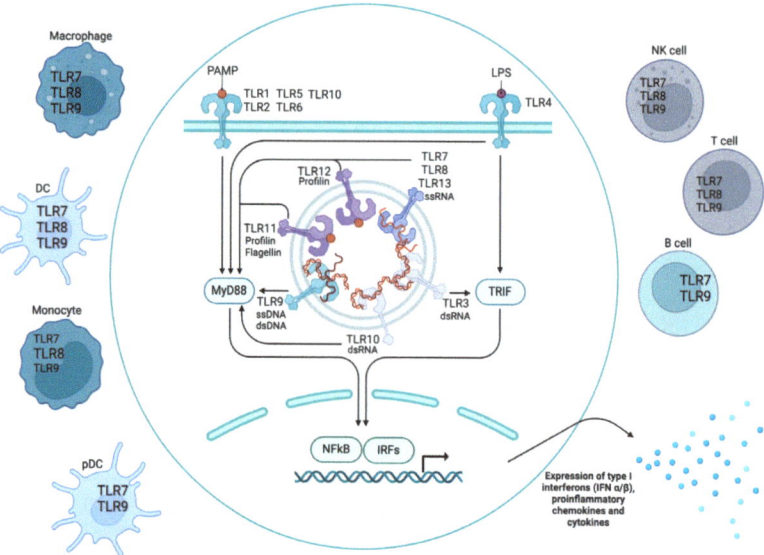

Figure 1. TLR signaling and expression in immune cells. TLRs are a class of proteins that are involved in immune responses upon recognizing molecules such as pathogen-associated molecular patterns (PAMPs), lipopolysaccharide (LPS), profilin, flagellin, ssDNA, dsDNA, ssRNA, and dsRNA. TLR1-TLR13 is found in mice, and TLR1-TLR10 is found in humans. The signaling pathways downstream of TLR activation are complex but can be roughly divided into MyD88-dependent and TIR domain-containing adapter-inducing IFN-β (TRIF)-dependent pathways. The myeloid differentiation factor 88 (MyD88)-dependent pathway is utilized by all TLRs except TLR3, while TLR4 can activate both pathways. Nuclear factor-kB (NFkB) comprises a family of transcription factors regulating genes involved in immune and inflammatory responses. Interferon regulatory factors (IRFs) regulate the transcription of interferons (IFNs), primarily type I IFNs. In the figure, the size of the TLR7-TLR9 letters in the different immune cells indicate their expression levels in these cells. Created with BioRender.com. DC, dendritic cell; pDC, plasmacytoid dendritic cell; NK, natural killer cell; ss, single-stranded; ds, double-stranded; IFN, interferon.

Due to their diversity, TLRs can bind to diverse ligands, making them important sensors of environmental stimuli such as bacterial and viral infections. In addition, other cellular pathways may interact with the TLR pathways in an autoimmune setting. For example, both MDA5 and cGAS were upregulated in in vitro matured splenic B cells from a TLR7 agonist-induced lupus model, while the MDA5 pathway was also activated without additional stimulation with CD40L [6].

Upon ligand binding, TLRs undergo conformational changes leading to the recruitment of adaptor proteins such as myeloid differentiation factor 88 (MyD88) and TIR domain-containing adapter-inducing IFN-β (TRIF). This recruitment initiates downstream signaling cascades, ultimately resulting in the activation of transcription factors like nuclear factor-kB (NFkB) and interferon regulatory factors (IRFs). These transcription factors induce the expression of inflammatory chemokines, cytokines, type I interferons (IFNs), and antimicrobial peptides [5]. Due to their role in sensing and regulating immune reactions, TLRs can have various implications in autoimmunity and SLE.

In this review, we focus on TLRs' role in human SLE and SLE mouse models, and their possible involvement in tolerance breakage. TLRs are expressed by different immune cells involved both in the innate and adaptive immune system, as well as platelets and epithelial cells. TLRs are well-known for their central role in autoimmunity and SLE.

2. Animal Mouse Models of SLE and LN and the Involvement of TLRs

Existing spontaneous mouse models of SLE and LN have been extensively reviewed during the past 10 years [7–12]. In addition, several genetically modified mice or other models with a lupus-like disease have been studied to determine the mechanism of SLE and LN in mice [7]. The genetically modified mouse models include knockout (KO), knock-in (KI), knock-down (KD), and transgenic (tg) mouse models.

2.1. Spontaneous Mouse Models of SLE and LN

The most common spontaneous mouse models used in research on the development of SLE and LN include the strains (NZBxNZW)F1 (NZBW), MRL/MpJ-Fas^{lpr} (MRL/lpr), BXSB/Yaa, and several congenic strains [13,14]. The MRL/lpr model contains a spontaneous lymphoproliferation (lpr) mutation caused by an alteration in the Fas gene causing a defect in FAS signaling and reduced cell death leading to lymphadenopathy. Several genetic modifications of this lupus model have been used to study the impact of TLRs on the development of autoimmune disease and are discussed later. The NZBW model, a hybrid of a New Zealand black (NZB) and a New Zealand white (NZW) mouse, developed a kidney disease resembling human LN with the development of glomerulonephritis [13,14]. Both NZB and NZW mice carry genes and develop an immunological phenotype with increased autoantibody production. However, it is only the hybrid that developed proteinuria. Several other recombinant inbred strains with an NZB or NZW background, called New Zealand mixed (NZM), have been developed to study the genetic background of murine lupus [15]. In addition, the crossing of NZB mice with several clinically normal mouse strains like SWR (SNF1 model) or SJL (NSF1 model), and the crossing of NZW with BXSB (WBF1 model), led to development of a clinical disease similar or milder to the NZBW model (reviewed in [11]). Common for most of the models is the production of autoantibodies to dsDNA and active proliferative nephritis, with a few exemptions like mild proliferative nephritis in SNF1 and WBF1 mice.

Other spontaneous mouse models include BXSB, BXD2, and (SWRxSJL)F1 mice that develop anti-dsDNA antibodies and Sm/U1snRNP antibodies. The (SWRxSJL)F1 mice may develop proteinuria at 20 weeks old with increased levels of IgG and IgA [16]. The BXSB and BXD2 models are recombinant inbreds derived from a mix of SB/Le and DBA/2J males with C57BL/6 (B6) females, respectively [17]. However, the BXSB model is unique as it mainly affects the males because of the presence of the Y-chromosome-linked autoimmune accelerator (*Yaa*). Mice with the *Yaa* locus have a duplication of the *Tlr7* gene. The *Yaa* is also important for the autoimmune phenotype in the Fc gamma receptor 2B (*FcgrIIB*)$^{-/-Yaa}$

mice [18]. The mice develop a more severe disease than $Fcgr IIB^{-/-}$ without the Yaa, but with less ANA production [18]. In addition, $Fcgr IIb^{-/-}$ mice on a B6 background develop spontaneous and fatal glomerulonephritis [19]. The 564Igi strain (B6.129S4(Cg)-Igktm1(Igk564)Tik Ightm1(Igh564)Tik/J)) mice have heavy and light chain genes encoding the 564 immunoglobulin (derived from an autoimmune SWRxNZB hybridoma) targeted to the heavy and light chain loci of C57BL/6 mice [20]. These mice produce anti-RNA antibodies.

2.2. Other Genetic Mice Models Mimicking the Pathogenesis of SLE and LN

The development of *Tlr7* tg mice confirmed that the *Yaa* gene is essential for developing an autoimmune phenotype in some spontaneous models of lupus [21]. The protein tyrosine phosphatase nonreceptor 22 (PTPN22) gene encodes the lymphoid tyrosine phosphatase (LYP) in humans, and the PEST domain-enriched tyrosine phosphatase (PEP) is the homologue in mice. The LYP protein is important in regulating the function of adaptive immunity cells, and polymorphism in this gene is associated with several autoimmune diseases including SLE [22]. PTPN22 expression in myeloid cells is important for regulation of multiple pattern recognition receptors [23]. Mouse models of *Pep* KO, *Pep* KI, *Pep* KD, or *Pep* tg mice show varying degrees of autoimmunity, and this is based on the selected strain used (reviewed in [24]).

DNase1l3 deficiency has been shown in both MRL/lpr and NZBW mice, as both strains are homozygous for a missense of this enzyme in the macrophages [25]. In a recent study of conditional knockout of *Dnase1l3* in macrophages, autoantibody production and mild kidney affection were observed [26]. Systemic KO models of *Dnase1l3* on either B6 or 129SvEv backgrounds induce ANAs, specifically anti-dsDNA antibodies in addition to anti-chromatin antibodies [27,28]. A double KO of *Dnase1l3*- and *FcgrIIb*-deficient mice showed early production of anti-dsDNA antibodies [28], while $Siglecg^{-/-}$ x $Dnase1l3^{-/-}$ double KO mice, but not $Siglecg^{-/-}$ x $Dnase1^{-/-}$ KO mice, produced autoantibodies only later in life [29]. However, $Dnase1^{-/-}$ mice produced ANAs, had glomerular immune complex deposits, and developed glomerulonephritis, demonstrating the importance of chromatin degradation to maintain tolerance against nuclear antigens [30,31].

LYN is an Src kinase associated with SLE. $Lyn^{-/-}$ mice showed increased levels of IgG and immune complex deposition and developed glomerulonephritis [32]. Other SLE symptoms included anemia, leukopenia, and thrombocytopenia. LYN is an inhibitor of IRF5 and thereby regulates signaling through TLRs [33]. Mice with a B-cell-specific deletion of CR6-interacting factor 1 (CRIF1), a nuclear transcriptional regulator and a mitochondrial inner membrane protein, had a lupus-like phenotype with anti-dsDNA antibody production and development of LN [34]. Depletion of CRIF1 has been shown to enhance activation trough TLR7 and TLR9 [35]. Deficiency in B-lymphocyte-induced maturation protein (BLIMP)-1 in dendritic cells (DCs) (*Prdm1*) led to a lupus-like phenotype with increased subsets of T follicular helper (Tfh) cells and plasma cells [36–38]. Another study showed that Blimp-1 directly suppressed interleukin-1 receptor-associated kinase 3 (*Irak3*) [39]. In a recent KI tg model, the gene *ERN1* encoding inositol-requiring enzyme 1α (IRE1α) carrying a heterozygous mutation led to a defect in IRE1α ribonuclease activity on X-box binding protein 1 (XBP1) splicing; the mice developed a broad panel of autoantibodies including antibodies against chromatin, Scl-100, or Sm/RNP [40].

Transcription factor E2F2-deficient mice with a mixed 129/sv x B6 background showed diffuse late onset SLE with systemic inflammatory infiltrates in the lung and liver, splenomegaly, immune complex deposition, and varying anti-dsDNA antibody titers [41]. However, backcrossing the original $E2f2^{-/-}$ mice into a pure B6 background eliminated the autoimmunity. Introducing an overexpression of the anti-apoptotic Bcl-2 protein in the B cells of these mice induced increased anti-DNA antibodies and development of mild glomerulonephritis [42]. Another study showed that E2F2 directly regulated the expression of MyD88, the adaptor of most of the TLRs, by binding to its promoter [43]. Phospholipase D family member 4 (PLD4) mutant mice (BALB/c *Pld4* thss/thss) developed anti-dsDNA and ANAs [44,45]. PLD4 is a 5′ exonuclease important for the degradation of single-stranded (ss) DNA in the endolysosomes, regulating ssDNA signaling through TLRs [46]. A gain-of-function mutation of another phospholipase Cγ2 (PLCγ2) in mice leads to an autoimmune phenotype [47].

Wiskott–Aldrich Syndrome (WAS) is a rare disease that is caused by WAS protein (WASP) deficiency and is characterized by diverse immune aberrations, including the production of autoantibodies. A mouse model has been developed where B cells, but not any other hematopoietic lineages, fail to express WASP [48]. This model has been termed $B^{WAS-/-}$, and the mice develop high titers of anti-DNA and anti-RNA antibodies [49]. The mechanism behind development of autoimmunity in this model has been related to the hyperresponsiveness of $WAS^{-/-}$ B cells to both BCR and TLR signals.

Taken together, there are several different genes that are either directly or indirectly linked to TLR signaling and are thus important for immune homeostasis. Figure 2 summarizes some of the most central genes and gene products linked to TLR signaling that may cause a lupus-like phenotype if mutated or knocked out.

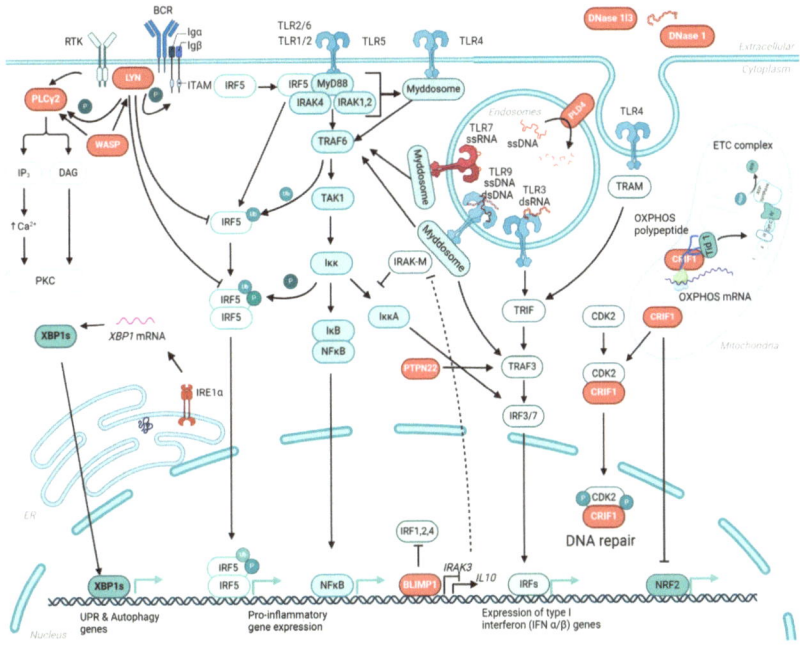

Figure 2. Overview of single-gene knockout (KO), knock-in (KI), or mutations in mice causing a lupus-like phenotype by influencing toll-like receptor (TLR) signaling and gene expression. Normal signaling pathways are shown with single-gene KO or mutations marked in red. *Tlr7* duplications in both spontaneous lupus models carrying the *Yaa* gene and in *TLR7* transgenic mice induce spontaneous autoimmunity. *Dnase1l3* and *Dnase1* KO mice have reduced clearance of circulating chromatin, thus increasing the antigens for TLRs. PLD4 mutant mice have increased signaling through TLRs due to reduced degradation of ssDNA in endosomes. CRIF1 deficiency influences CDK2-induced DNA repair, NRF2 binding, and formation of the ETC complex [50]. BLIMP1 normally controls the binding of IRF1, 2, and 4 and increases IL-10 expression. It also suppresses the expression of IRAK3 an inhibitor of IRF7 signaling [51]. PTPN22 inhibits various signaling pathways but acts as a selective promoter of type I interferon by promoting autoubiquitination of TRAF3 and phosphorylation of IRF3 and IRF7 [23]. LYN phosphorylates ITAM and PLCγ2 and inhibits IRF5 activation [52]. PLCγ2 activation via tyrosine kinases like LYN leads to increased Ca^{2+} signaling and a gain-of-function mutation, which was shown to cause hyperreactive external calcium entry [53]. WASP affects many parts of the BCR signaling pathways [54] and B-cell-specific WAS deficient mice

develop autoantibodies against both DNA and RNA [48]. IRE1α is an ER membrane protein important for transducing signals of misfolded protein accumulation in ER to the nucleus by splicing X-box binding 1 (*XBP1*) mRNA and leading to the production of stable transcription factor XBP1 (XBP1s) [55]. XBP1s targets various genes involved in multiple cellular functions [56]. Created with BioRender.com. KI, knock-in; KO, knockout; PLD4, phospholipase D family member 4; UPR, unfolded protein response; ssDNA, single-stranded DNA; ETC, electron transport chain; BCR, B-cell receptor; WAS, Wiskott–Aldrich syndrome; ER, endoplasmatic reticulum; IRF, interferon regulatory factors; CRIF, CR6-interacting factor 1; IRAK, interleukin-1 receptor-associated kinase; PTPN, protein tyrosine phosphatase nonreceptor 22; XBP1, X-box binding 1; PLCγ2, phospholipase Cγ2; BLIMP, B-lymphocyte-induced maturation protein.

2.3. Inducible SLE Mouse Models

Pristane (2,6,10,14 tetramethylpentadecane) has been used since the 1980s as an inducible model of LN in various healthy mice strains like BALB/c, SJL/J, and C57BL/6, as it results in immune complex-mediated glomerulonephritis (reviewed in [57]). It is also a good model for SLE in general since the mice may develop erosive arthritis, skin rash and, in more severe cases, pulmonary vasculitis and haemorrhage [58]. However, the choice of strain used is important as they show huge differences in their autoantibody profiles [59]. In addition, pristane may induce ANAs, anti-dsDNA, and anti-SnRNP antibodies and show an overproduction of type I IFN, which makes it very suitable as a model for SLE since high amounts of type I IFN are observed in 50% of SLE patients [60]. The model relies on the expression of TLR7 [61] and has been used to determine the role of other TLRs like TLR2 [62], TLR4 [63], and TLR9 [63,64], in addition to induction factors like BAFF [65] and tonicity-responsive enhancer-binding protein (TonEBP) [66] and signaling molecules and sensors like IRF7 [67], cGAS-STING pathway [68], and IRAK4 [69] in murine lupus. Pristane has also been used to accelerate the disease in NZBW and the SNF1 model [70,71]. Using pristane treatment in normal B6 and B6/lpr and B6/gld mice demonstrated the contribution of defects in the Fas or Fas ligand [72].

A newer inducible lupus model involved topical treatment with resiquimod or imiquimod creams containing TLR-7/8 or TLR7 ligand/agonist in wild-type (WT) mice. When applied three times a week for 4-8 weeks, it induced anti-dsDNA antibodies, glomerulonephritis, hepatitis, carditis, and photosensitivity in these mice [73]. The application of imiquimod to the skin is a prerequisite for inducing the disease, as oral administration and injection of imiquimod do not lead to the same immune cell activation. In graft-versus-host disease (GVHD) and chronic GVHD (cGVHD), donor lymphocytes are injected into a semi-allogenic recipient to induce a lupus-like syndrome [74]. Autoantibody-mediated (lupus-like) cGVHD in mice is caused by alloantibody secretion and deposition, in addition to B- and T-cell infiltrations in the affected tissues [75]. A recent study showed increased expression of TLR7 in mice with cGVHD [76]. Garimella et al. (2021) used syngeneic apoptotic cells to break B cell tolerance in C57Bl and UNC93B1 mutant mice that lacked signaling through TLR3, TLR7, and TLR9 [77]. They found reduced responses against known autoantigens in the mutant mice, showing the importance of endosomal TLR in tolerance breakage against lupus autoantigens.

2.4. Acceleration of Spontaneous Lupus Models and Humanized Mouse

Some of the spontaneous models develop SLE and LN over a long time (5–12 months) and the disease manifestations are very heterogenic with some mice never developing proteinuria, making the models difficult to use in treatment strategies to prevent LN. To solve this, several different compounds have been used to study the mechanism of SLE by accelerating different processes in spontaneous mouse models. This has also included the use of pristane and imiquimod, accelerating the development of proteinuria in NZBW and MRL/lpr mice [78]. Recently, resiquimod treatment of B6.Sle1.Sle2.Sle3 triple congenic mice induced an increased leaky gut, and this was shown to be due to TLR7/8 activation [79]. Other compounds normally not inducing SLE in healthy mice include poly IC [80], IFNα [81,82], mercury [81,82], respirable crystalline silica dust particles [83], LPS [83], and CpG [84] and these have also been used for this purpose.

Humanized mouse models of SLE involve transferring PBMC from SLE patients to immunodeficient mice or transferring human hematopoietic stems cells to immunodeficient mice with subsequent induction of lupus via intraperitoneal injection of pristane (reviewed in [85]). Other studies have introduced human genes into mice strains, like human *TLR8* in an SLE1.Yaa strain that induced fatal anemia [86]. In a recent study by Cakan et al. (2023) to study the role of TLR7 and TLR9 in induction of B-cell tolerance, they used NOD-scid-common gamma chain (γc) knockout (NSG) immunodeficient mice with CD34+ human fetal hematopoietic stem cells (HSCs) transduced with GFP-tagged lentivirus expressing shRNA to inhibit the expression of MYD88, TLR7, and TLR9 [87]. It was shown that TLR9 is important for maintaining central B-cell tolerance, as both TLR9 and MYD88 silencing resulted in increased polyreactive or ANA-producing B cells. In addition, the study demonstrated that CXCL4 production sequestered TLR9 ligands away from the late endosomes and thus inhibited TLR9 function in B cells.

3. TLR Signaling in SLE—An Update on Recent Findings

TLRs may contribute to the chronic activation of the immune system in patients with SLE or in lupus-prone or -induced mice. High mobility group box 1 (HMGB1) is a typical DAMP and can be released by apoptotic and necrotic cells. Higher levels of serum HMGB1 and anti-HMGB1 antibodies correlating with disease activity have been found in SLE patients [88–91]. HMGB1 can be recognized by TLR2, TLR4, and TLR5 [92,93]. Ma et al. (2018) identified TLR4+CXCR4+ plasma cells in peripheral blood and kidney tissue, correlating with anti-dsDNA levels in SLE patients and lupus-prone mice, and showed that TLR4 blockade in vitro reduced anti-dsDNA IgG secretion from these cells [94]. Also, in MRL/lpr mice, the expression of TLR4+CXCR4+ plasma cells was significantly increased. Interestingly, this cell population decreased upon Nrf2 overexpression [95], indicating a potential role in LN disease progression and revealing this pathway as a possible target for treatment. An investigation into the expression and interplay of HMGB1 and *TLR4* in patients with neuropsychiatric SLE (NPSLE), found either protein or mRNA expression to be increased in serum and PBMCs, respectively, but did not observe significant correlation between HMGB1 and *TLR4* expression and NPSLE-related seizures [96]. Several studies have also investigated the genetic association between *TLR2* and *TLR4* polymorphisms and SLE susceptibility [97–99]. However, the results from those studies have not provided evidence for *TLR2* and *TLR4* gene polymorphisms and SLE.

TLR5 recognizes bacterial flagellin. A recent study by Alajoleen et al. (2024) using TLR5-deficient MRL/lpr mice demonstrated a worsening of the disease, possibly due to an increased germinal center reaction and suppression of regulatory lymphocytes [100]. There have been very few studies on the role of TLR5 in SLE and LN. Both increased and decreased levels of TLR5 expression have been shown in different organs during murine lupus disease progression [101]. In addition, several studies on polymorphisms in SLE have indicated no association with *TLR5* polymorphisms even though an increase in *TLR5* gene expression was observed in LN biopsies [98,102,103]. However, Hou et al. (2023) recently identified a mutation in TLR5 in early-onset pediatric SLE with renal, hematological, and central nervous system involvement [104]. The new findings indicate that TLR5 influences important regulatory functions of the immune system, and more studies on its role in autoimmune diseases are required.

Among the TLRs, TLR3, TLR7, TLR8, TLR9, TLR10, and TLR13 (Figure 1) are specific for nucleic acids and perhaps most relevant to SLE. TLR3 recognizes dsRNA, while TLR7 and TLR8 recognize ssRNA. TLR9 identifies unmethylated CpG DNA. TLR13 is specific for rRNA regions, particularly certain 23S rRNA motifs found in bacteria [105,106]. Human TLR10 has been shown to bind to dsRNA in vitro at acidic pH, suggesting it has an endosomal location [107] in addition to having a plasma membrane localization [108]. The exact mechanisms of TLR10 are somewhat unclear and it is suspected to have both pro-

and anti-inflammatory properties (reviewed in [108]). Interestingly, in relation to SLE, Lee et al. (2018) showed that the binding of TLR10 to dsRNA activated the MyD88 signaling pathway and suppression of IRF7-dependent type I IFN expression as well as inhibition of TLR3 signaling through sequestering dsRNA from this receptor [107]. Engagement of TLRs is important in the pathogenesis of SLE, contributing to the production of type I IFNs and the activation of autoreactive B cells (reviewed in [109]).

Platelets also express TLRs. In SLE, platelets are activated, and their abnormal expression in blood can mirror disease activity. Platelets express FcγRs and TLRs TLR1-TLR4, TLR7, and TLR9 [110], indicating that different PAMPs, DAMPs, immune complexes, and nucleic acids can activate platelets (reviewed in [110–113]). When activated, platelets express CD40L and P-selectin on the cell surface, contributing to interaction with immune cells [113]. In addition, activated platelets release extracellular vesicles, leading to constituents such as HMGB1 and P-selectin being accessible to other cells not normally in contact with these components [110–113]. Activated platelets and extracellular vesicles can stimulate neutrophils to undergo neutrophil extracellular trap (NET)osis, pDCs to produce IFNα, B cells to produce autoantibodies, regulatory T cells to downregulate FOXP3, and maturation of monocytes to APCs [111], all factors that can contribute to disease progression in SLE. A recent study by Baroni Pietto et al. (2024) showed that platelets could contribute to inflammation in SLE patients [114], and similar findings are reviewed in [111]. Interestingly, Tay et al. (2024) found TLR7 expression in platelets to be important for platelet–low-density neutrophil (LDN) complexes. LDNs are a subset of neutrophils associated with SLE, while platelet-neutrophil complexes have been observed after platelet activation and are formed during inflammation.

The nucleic acid-sensing TLRs TLR7, TLR8, and TLR9 (Figure 1) have been well studied in relation to SLE. All three are located intracellularly in endosomes, but their expression varies between different subsets of immune cells, which in turn affects how they are implicated in SLE. T cells and natural killer cells express low amounts of all of them, while B cells and pDCs express both TLR7 and TLR9 [115]. Monocytes express low levels of TLR7 and TLR9, but instead express TLR8, which is absent in B cells and pDCs. DCs and macrophages express TLR7, TLR8, and TLR9 [116,117]. TLR7 and TLR9 have homologous ligands and functions in mice and humans, whereas TLR8 is not bound by ssRNA in mice and its murine ligand is yet to be identified [118]. For a while, it was thought that TLR8 may not be functional in mice. For this reason, many of the studies on TLR function in SLE have focused on TLR7 and TLR9. Still, it has been demonstrated that murine TLR8 could have regulatory functions that may be independent of ligand binding [116].

2.5. TLR Driven Autoantibody Production and Tolerance Breakage

In addition to stimulating a general inflammatory response by causing the production of inflammatory cytokines, TLRs can also be directly involved in the production of autoantibodies. An accepted description of how this may occur is through a specific form of T-independent B-cell activation where self-DNA or self-RNA binds to the BCR of a naïve B cell that expresses a BCR specific to DNA or RNA (Figure 3) [119,120]. This leads to internalization of the BCR-DNA/RNA complex in the endosome, which may fuse with another endosome containing TLRs. In this way, the internalized DNA or RNA may also bind to and activate TLR9 or TLR7, respectively. It has been demonstrated that this co-engagement of the BCR and a TLR is enough to activate B cells without help from T cells, in turn leading to the maturation of plasma cells producing antibodies that bind to DNA or RNA [121–125]. Likewise, proteins bound to DNA or RNA may also be internalized via binding to a BCR that is specific for that protein and bring with them DNA or RNA into an endosome, activating TLRs and causing the maturation of plasma cells producing autoantibodies like anti-Sm, anti-RNP, and anti-nucleosome. Normally, T-independent B-cell activation results only in the production of IgM antibodies. However, CpG binding to TLR9 on B cells can also activate antibody class switching to the Th1-like isotypes IgG2a, IgG2b, and IgG3, which are commonly seen in SLE [126,127]. One study even found that class switching of anti-DNA antibodies to IgG2a and IgG2b isotypes was impaired in TLR9-deficient mice [128]. Several studies have demonstrated the concept of TLR-BCR co-engagement, for instance by immunizing mice with protein antigens linked to CpG DNA, chromatin-containing immune complexes, or RNA-containing immune complexes, with subsequently enhanced production of antigen-specific antibodies [122,125,129]. They also confirmed the involvement of TLR9 or MyD88 in these results by knocking out or inhibiting them. This was recently confirmed by Cakan et al. (2023), as described above [87]. Furthermore, a recent study on the same concept investigating TLR4 and TLR5 also demonstrated that B-cell activation mediated by TLR-BCR co-engagement is T-cell independent, through performing similar studies using a mouse model which was devoid of T cells [130].

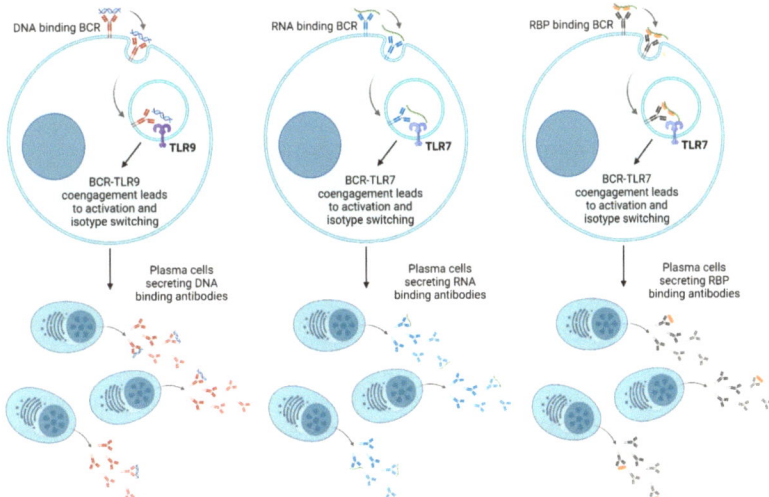

Figure 3. TLR-driven autoantibody production. Recognition of extracellular nucleic acids or proteins bound to nucleic acids by naïve B cells via the B-cell receptor (BCR) causes internalization of the BCR–antigen complex, which ends up in an endosome. Endosomal toll-like receptors (TLRs) like TLR7 and TLR9 may then also encounter the internalized nucleic acid-containing antigens. Co-engagement of BCR and TLR via antigens can lead to activation of the B cell and induce isotype switching to IgG. Consequently, a large number of autoantibody secreting plasma cells can be generated. Created with BioRender.com. RBP, RNA-binding protein.

Upon the initial discovery of TLR9, it was stated that TLR9 was able to discriminate between bacterial DNA and self-DNA because its ligand, unmethylated CpG DNA, is quite scarce in mammalians. However, unmethylated CpG DNA does exist in mammalian DNA as well, and several studies have demonstrated a dependence on TLR9 signaling to produce anti-DNA antibodies associated with SLE [49,124,131]. A more accepted notion today is that the intracellular location of the nucleic acid-sensing TLRs is the main mechanism of discriminating self from non-self. Indeed, since B cells generally do not endocytose extracellular material unless the BCR is bound, host-derived DNA or RNA, for instance originating from dead cells, would not normally come into contact with TLR9 or TLR7 in B cells and therefore would not activate them. In contrast, B cells carrying a nucleic acid-binding BCR naturally endocytose nucleic acids, possibly breaking self-tolerance in these cells [131]. Moreover, engagement of TLR9 can protect B cells from spontaneous or BCR-mediated apoptosis, contributing to tolerance breakage [132–134]. Further supporting the notion that TLR-BCR dual engagement is a key mechanism for the maturation of plasma cells producing nucleic acid-specific antibodies is the fact that global or B-cell-specific deletion of MyD88 in lupus-prone mice has been shown to suppress the production of all antinuclear antibodies [125,135–137]. More specifically, several studies have demonstrated that the specific deletion of TLR7 or TLR9, either globally or in B cells only, abrogated production of anti-RNA and anti-DNA antibodies, respectively [49,117,124,131,135,138].

2.6. Diverse Effects of Different TLRs on SLE Pathogenesis—TLR7 As the Main Driver of Disease

Despite the direct influence of both TLR7 and TLR9 on autoantibody production, as well as the fact that TLR7, TLR8, and TLR9 all activate the same signaling pathways, their roles in the pathogenesis of SLE are not equivalent. Numerous studies have implicated TLR7 as the main driver of SLE disease, while both TLR8 and TLR9 have been shown to have more regulatory roles where they contribute to dampening TLR7 signaling and thereby prevent autoimmunity [116,124,139]. This is demonstrated by the fact that knocking out either *Tlr8* or *Tlr9* in healthy C57BL/6 mice induced SLE-like autoimmune disease, while additional knockout of *Tlr7* eliminated disease symptoms, indicating that the disease development was dependent on TLR7 [116,140]. Single knockout of *Tlr7* in lupus-prone mice also ameliorated disease [124]. Moreover, gene duplication of *Tlr7*, as seen in mice bearing the Y-linked autoimmune accelerator (*Yaa*) locus, contributed to accelerating autoimmune disease. In addition, topical treatment of mice with the TLR7 agonist imiquimod also induced SLE-like disease [73].

Strong evidence supports the disease-promoting role of TLR7 in humans as well. The *Tlr7* gene is located on the X chromosome and the risk of developing SLE correlates with the number of X chromosomes an individual carries, demonstrated by the female predominance and increased incidence in men with Klinefelter syndrome (47, XXY) [141]. X-chromosome inactivation normally contributes to the silencing of one arbitrary X chromosome, but not all genes are affected, and it has been shown that *Tlr7* escapes X-chromosome inactivation in B cells, monocytes, and pDCs in both women and Klinefelter syndrome men [142]. Recently, it was demonstrated that the gene encoding TLR8, which is closely located to *Tlr7*, also escapes X-chromosome inactivation in immune cells in women and Klinefelter syndrome men [143]. Increased expression of TLR7, independent of gene copy number, has also been associated with more severe SLE disease in humans [144]. A specific *Tlr7* polymorphism (rs3853839-G) has been demonstrated to cause increased expression of TLR7 and is associated with SLE in humans [145–147]. Recently, a never-before-seen *Tlr7* gain-of-function gene variant ($Tlr7^{Y264H}$) was identified in a young girl suffering from SLE [148]. This variant of TLR7 was shown to have increased affinity to guanosine present in RNA and enhanced NF-κB activation. When introduced into C57BL/6 mice, the $Tlr7^{Y264H}$ gene induced an SLE-like disease.

2.7. Regulatory Functions of TLR8 and TLR9

As previously mentioned, global knockout of *Tlr9* induces or worsens lupus-like disease in several mouse models. This concept has been demonstrated in a number of different mouse models, including MRL/lpr, MRL/+, B6-lpr/lpr, B6.Nba2, FcγRIIB$^{-/-}$, Plcg2$^{Ali5/+}$, and pristane-treated BALB/c [64,124,149–153]. Similar to TLR9, TLR8 has also been implicated to have regulatory functions on TLR7 [116]. Thus, C57BL/6 mice who are deficient in both *Tlr8* and *Tlr9* suffered from more pronounced disease compared with mice lacking only one of these genes [140]. However, the same study demonstrated that TLR8 and TLR9 exerted their regulatory effects in different cell types. TLR8 seemed to mainly act in DCs, whereas TLR9 mainly exerted its regulatory functions in B cells [140].

An extensive amount of work has been conducted to study the relationship between TLR7 and TLR9 in B cells. It has been demonstrated that B-cell-specific knockout of *Tlr7* is enough to ameliorate disease in lupus-prone mice, while B-cell-specific knockout of *Tlr9* exacerbates disease [49,117]. One study showed that absence of TLR9 in B cells caused exacerbated nephritis, while overexpression of TLR9 in B cells caused reduction of both nephritis and proteinuria [117]. The latter was demonstrated in both MRL/lpr and FcγRIIB$^{-/-}$.Yaa mice [117]. In contrast, deletion of TLR9 in cDCs, pDCs, macrophages, or neutrophils had no effect on SLE disease parameters, further supporting the notion that it is the B-cell-intrinsic TLR9 which is protective in SLE. In line with this, deletion of TLR7 in

CD11c$^+$ cell populations mainly comprising DCs had no impact on SLE disease parameters in MRL/lpr mice [154]. However, B-cell-specific deletion of TLR7 did ameliorate disease, especially in TLR9-deficient mice.

Since exacerbation of SLE disease in $Tlr9^{-/-}$ mice depends on TLR7, it has been hypothesized that TLR9, either directly or indirectly, negatively regulates TLR7 activity. In that case, deletion of TLR9 would increase TLR7 activity and, in turn, cause worsened disease. In line with this, several studies have demonstrated higher expression of TLR7 and increased response to TLR7 ligands in $Tlr9$ knockout models [140,151,155]. For instance, B cells from $Tlr9^{-/-}$ and $Tlr8^{-/-}Tlr9^{-/-}$ C57BL/6 mice responded more strongly to the TLR7 ligand R848 than B cells from WT or $Tlr8^{-/-}$ mice [140]. B cells from $Tlr9^{-/-}$ B6.Nba2.Yaa mice also responded more strongly to imiquimod and expressed higher levels of TLR7 than B cells from $Tlr9^{+/+}$ mice [151].

One popular hypothesis explaining how TLR9 may indirectly regulate TLR7 activity suggests that deletion of TLR9 causes increased trafficking of TLR7 to late endosomes because TLR7 and TLR9 compete for the same shuttle mechanism [156]. UNC93B1 is an endoplasmatic reticulum (ER)-resident chaperone that controls trafficking of nucleic acid-sensing TLRs as well as TLR5, TLR11, and TLR12 from the ER to their respective locations in endosomes or on the cell surface [157,158]. Upon viral infection or TLR signaling, nucleic acid-sensing TLRs are transported to endosomes. TLR7 and TLR9 both bind to UNC93B1, which has the strongest affinity for TLR9 [159]. However, a mutation in UNC93B1 (D34A) causes enhanced affinity for TLR7 and, thus, enhanced trafficking of TLR7 to endolysosomes, which in turn induces TLR7-dependent systemic inflammation [156]. Based on these findings, it has been suggested that when TLR9 is absent, this causes less competition for binding to UNC93B1 and, thus, increased trafficking of TLR7 to endosomes, which could be the mechanism that drives the worsened disease seen in $Tlr9^{-/-}$ mice [156]. The same hypothesis has also been proposed for $Tlr8^{-/-}$ mice, as TLR8 is also shuttled to endosomes by UNC93B1 [140]. However, this theory has recently been challenged as it was demonstrated that the localization of TLR7 was the same in WT and $Tlr9^{-/-}$ mice, probably because the mere absence of TLR9 (or TLR8) does not increase the affinity of UNC93B1 for TLR7 [160]. TLR7 and TLR9 were also largely located in separate compartments, indicating that they should not compete with each other for binding to UNC93B1. Interestingly, unlike previously mentioned findings, the current study did not identify differences in expression and signaling of TLR7 between WT and $Tlr9^{-/-}$ mice. Instead, it was explored whether TLR9 could regulate TLR7 activity through other mechanisms. Point-mutated versions of TLR9 that lacked either ligand or MyD88 binding were expressed in MRL/lpr mice [160]. Both mutated versions of TLR9 increased survival compared with $Tlr9^{-/-}$ mice, suggesting that simply the presence of TLR9, despite being "dysfunctional", is protective. Furthermore, the TLR9 version that could bind ligand but did not signal through MyD88 was the most protective, suggesting that TLR9 has protective effects that are ligand-dependent but MyD88-independent. This also indicates that TLR9 signaling through MyD88 does promote disease, as would be expected [156].

Despite TLR8 not being so well studied as TLR9, several studies support the notion that TLR8 also has regulatory functions on TLR7. For instance, TLR8-deficient C57BL/6 mice showed increased expression of TLR7 in DCs, which was accompanied by increased responses to TLR7 agonists and increased NF-κB activation [116]. These mice also had elevated levels of both anti-RNA and anti-DNA antibodies. In contrast, $TLR7^{-/-}$ and $Tlr8^{-/-}Tlr7^{-/-}$ mice did not produce autoantibodies. The $Tlr8^{-/-}$ mice also had increased numbers of plasma cells, and $Tlr8^{-/-}$ DC had increased cytokine production compared with WT DCs. However, there was no difference in cytokine production by macrophages, supporting the fact that the effect of TLR8 on TLR7 is cell-type-specific. Another study, also based on C57BL/6, supported the finding that DCs express higher levels of TLR7 when TLR8 is knocked out [140]. These $Tlr8^{-/-}$ DCs also responded more strongly to the TLR7 ligand R848 compared with DCs from WT mice, and the same pattern was observed for pDCs. One study found that a high-fat diet exacerbated SLE in $Tlr8$ knockout mice, an effect which was dependent on TLR7 since it was abrogated in *Tlr7/8* KO mice [161]. Again, that study also found that *Tlr8* knockout mice expressed higher levels of TLR7 than WT mice in DCs as well as macrophages. Interestingly, in a human setting, a mutation in TLR8 was recently described and found to cause severe autoimmune disease in the monozygotic twins who carried it [162]. The mechanism behind the development of autoimmunity was found to be reduced ability of TLR8 to regulate TLR7 signaling, as well as increased binding of TLR8 to TLR7 ligands, which increased TLR7 signaling.

2.8. Regulation of TLR Signaling—Endosomal Trafficking and Glycosylation

In addition to TLR8 and TLR9 having regulatory functions affecting TLR7, several other proteins and signaling pathways can influence the levels of signaling by these TLRs in a cell (reviewed in [163]). One such protein is the previously mentioned UNC93B1, which has gained much attention during recent years and can influence TLR signaling in different ways. As mentioned, UNC93B1 is required for the trafficking of nucleic acid-sensing TLRs to endosomes. One study found that UNC93B1 must be glycosylated at a specific asparagine residue in order to recruit MyD88 and signal properly upon TLR9 activation. This glycosylation was not necessary for TLR7 signaling to function [164]. Another study identified a mutation in UNC93B1 (S282A) that abolished signaling in TLR9, but did not affect other TLRs [165]. The mutation did not alter TLR9 trafficking, but inhibited binding of TLR9 to its ligand. It was demonstrated that TLR9 needs to be released from UNC93B1 to be able to signal properly. Recently, Ni et al. (2024) showed that this release depended on the removal of a palmitoylation, initially added to TLR9 in the Golgi and necessary for its trafficking to endosomes [166]. Conversely, TLR7 does not need to be released in order to function. Indeed, another study discovered a different mutation in UNC93B1 (530-PKP/AAA-532) that caused enhanced signaling through TLR7 without affecting TLR7 trafficking [167]. Under normal conditions, the protein syntenin-1 binds to UNC93B1 after stimulation of TLR7 (but not other TLRs) and causes TLR7 to be taken up into intraluminal vesicles and exosomes, which is likely to dampen continued TLR7 signaling. K63-linked ubiquitinylation, which normally marks cargo for sorting into intraluminal vesicles, was markedly reduced in the mutated version of UNC93B1 and reduced ubiquitinylation correlated with enhanced TLR7 signaling. Phosphorylation of UNC93B1 at specific sites was required for recruitment of syntenin-1. Mice carrying the 530-PKP/AAA-532 mutation in UNC93B1 developed severe systemic inflammation and produced ANAs. However, upon knockout of *Tlr7*, the mice were rescued from disease, supporting the hypothesis that the mutation specifically affected TLR7 signaling [167]. In humans, a few different mutations in UNC93B1 that cause increased TLR7 signaling through various mechanisms have been identified in SLE patients and underscore the importance of a functional UNC93B1 [168,169].

Glycosylation of TLRs represents another way to regulate their signaling. One study using a CRISPR/Cas9 screening method identified the oligosaccharide transferase complex (OSTC) as indispensable for TLR5, TLR7, and TLR9 responses [170]. OSTC glycosylates proteins in the ER and its absence inhibits cell surface expression of TLR5. Although it has not been conclusively demonstrated, it was hypothesized that glycosylation by OSTC induces maturation and trafficking of TLR5, TLR7, and TLR9 from the ER. The activity of TLR3 has also been found to depend on glycosylation [171]. In addition, Neu1 sialidase, which cleaves sialic acid residues from glycosylated sites of TLRs, has been shown to be important for the activity of TLR2, TLR3, and TLR4 [172]. Overall, defects in glycosylation of a variety of immune cell-related proteins have been associated with SLE in both mice and humans [173].

2.9. Diverse Effects of TLR Signaling on Autoantibody Repertoire in Different Mouse Models of SLE

As previously mentioned, TLR7 and TLR9 have been specifically linked to the production of anti-RNA and anti-DNA antibodies, respectively. For instance, this has been shown in both the MRL/lpr mouse model and the $B^{WAS-/-}$ model. Interestingly, in both models, deletion of *Tlr9* not only suppressed the production of anti-DNA antibodies but also increased the production of anti-RNA antibodies [49,135]. One study using the MRL/lpr mouse model found that B-cell-specific deletion of TLR9 more or less completely inhibited the production of anti-DNA antibodies, while B-cell-specific overexpression of TLR9 increased the anti-DNA-to-anti-RNA antibody ratio [117]. However, the same study did not report this effect in the FcγRIIB$^{-/-}$·Yaa model. Indeed, results regarding the type and amount of antibodies produced in TLR knockout models vary considerably between different genetic backgrounds. For instance, $Plcg2^{Ali5/+}$-$Tlr9^{-/-}$ mice were shown to produce similar amounts of anti-DNA auto-antibodies as $Plcg2^{Ali5/+}$-$Tlr9^{+/+}$ mice, while anti-nucleosome antibodies were significantly decreased and anti-nucleolar antibodies were increased in $Tlr9^{-/-}$ mice [153]. Similarly, another study also found that development of anti-nucleosome antibodies was abrogated in B6-lpr/lpr mice when TLR9 was knocked out, whereas the anti-dsDNA antibody titer was significantly higher [150]. Increased levels of anti-dsDNA antibodies and decreased levels of anti-chromatin antibodies upon knockout of *Tlr9* have also been reported in B6.Nba2.Yaa mice [151]. One study that looked at the effect of diet on SLE pathogenesis in $Tlr8^{-/-}$ mice found that additional knockout of *Tlr7* significantly decreased the amount of anti-DNA antibodies, indicating that the production of anti-DNA antibodies depended on TLR7 [161]. Furthermore, treatment of mice with the TLR7 agonist imiquimod led to the production of both anti-DNA and anti-RNA antibodies, and production of anti-DNA antibodies was not abrogated by knocking out *Tlr9* in imiquimod-treated mice [73]. Taken together, these results suggest that TLR9 is not the only potential driver of anti-DNA antibody production in SLE.

2.10. Age-Associated B Cells as the Main Source of TLR Driven Autoantibody Production

A specific subset of B cells, referred to as age-associated B cells (ABCs), are highly dependent on TLR signaling and are also strongly associated with SLE (reviewed in [174,175]). Several studies have linked ABCs to SLE in both mice and humans, where they are thought to be the precursor cells to autoantibody-secreting cells [176]. In humans, ABCs are sometimes also referred to as atypical memory B cells or double-negative (DN) cells [174,177]. Large numbers of ABCs are found both in human SLE patients and several different murine SLE models. For instance, ABCs accumulate drastically in NZBW, MRL/lpr, $SLC^{-/-}$, and $Mer^{-/-}$ mice with disease onset [178,179]. Previously, it was shown that ABCs increased in individuals with enhanced TLR7 expression [148]. Differentiation of ABCs occurs upon engagement of TLR7 or TLR9, together with the BCR [175]. Dai et al. (2024), found the transcription factor ZEB2 to be essential for ABC differentiation in vitro and vital for ABC formation in TLR7-induced lupus disease, while mice deficient in *Zeb2* and *ZEB2* haploinsufficient persons had reduced numbers of ABCs [180]. In addition, cytokine signaling through IFNγ and IL-21, as well as stimulation of CD40, is necessary for differentiation of ABCs [175,177,181]. B cells that express a BCR specific for DNA, RNA, or nucleic acid-associated proteins are probably inclined to follow this differentiation program, as BCR-TLR co-engagement naturally occurs in these cells. Indeed, a recent study found that 3H9$^+$ mice, whose BCRs mainly bind to nucleosomes or dsDNA, had increased numbers of ABCs compared with control animals, suggesting the ABCs originated from the DNA-binding B cells [182]. Also, when *Tlr9* was knocked out in these mice, the ABC population decreased. The same study demonstrated that ABCs are a dynamic B-cell population that can develop into plasma cells or have a more memory-like phenotype and probably go through multiple rounds of reactivation. One of the hallmarks of ABCs is expression of the T-box transcription factor (T-bet). TLR9-BCR crosslinking has been found to stimulate activation of T-bet, which is involved in class switching to IgG2a and 2b isotypes [128,183]. Interestingly, a distinct feature of ABCs is their germinal center-independent extrafollicular response [148,180]. In a study by Caielli et al. (2018), it was found that the levels of IgG, IgA, and ABCs in the blood of SLE patients correlated with an increase in CD4 Th10 cells [109]. CD4 Th10 cells have been shown to be equally effective in inducing differentiation in B cells as Tfh cells [109] and have been identified in response to COVID-19 vaccines [184]. These cells induce differentiation of naïve and memory B cells into plasma cells with the help of IL-10 and succinate. Another study using human blood samples showed that a higher percentage of B cells from SLE patients expressed cell surface PLD4 compared with B cells from healthy donors [185]. Interestingly, these PLD4$^+$ B cells largely overlapped with the ABC population, and it was found that stimulation of TLR7 or TLR9 could upregulate cell surface PLD4, indicating that PLD4$^+$ B cells are probably TLR-stimulated autoreactive cells.

2.11. Targeting TLRs in the Treatment of SLE

Given the central role of TLR signaling in SLE disease, the past few decades have seen great interest in the development of drugs targeting the different TLRs [186,187]. Intriguingly, SLE drugs that are currently in clinical use in humans may also partly exert their effects by affecting TLR signaling. For instance, hydroxychloroquine, whose effect in cells is to increase the pH in acidic organelles, has been shown to prevent endosomal cleavage of TLR7, which in turn inhibits its function [188]. TLR9 is also cleaved in lysosomes and may likewise be inhibited by chloroquine [189]. Hydroxychloroquine has also been postulated to be able to inhibit presentation of autoantigens on MHC class II molecules through interfering with the formation of autoantigens in lysosomes [190]. In contrast, TLR signaling has been shown to dampen the effects of glucocorticoids, which are also commonly used to treat SLE patients [191]. Dual treatment with glucocorticoids and TLR antagonists may therefore be a promising strategy. Indeed, a recent preclinical study demonstrated that TLR7/8 inhibition increased the effect of glucocorticoids in lupus-prone mice and sensitized human PBMC against glucocorticoid treatment [192].

TLR antagonists also show potential as single agents. The targeting of TLR7/8 seems to be especially effective, and inhibitors of TLR7/8 are currently being tested in humans (NCT05638802, NCT05278663) [193]. Several other TLR-modulating drug candidates are also currently being developed and tested in murine models of SLE [194–196]. For instance, anti-TLR7 and anti-TLR9 antibodies have been tested in the NZBW model, where it was demonstrated that targeting TLR7 protected against LN while targeting of TLR9 had no effects [197]. In addition, a peptide derived from the core β sheet from TIRAP and conjugated to penetratin (a cell-penetrating peptide) was shown to block TLR4 signaling and subsequent cytokine response via inhibiting the MyD88 and TRIF-dependent pathways [198]. Clinical data from human trials with TLR antagonists are still relatively scarce, meaning that available reports on side effects are also limited. However, existing data imply that TLR antagonists are well tolerated and cause only mild side effects [193]. Inhibiting TLR activity has immunosuppressive effects. Thus, TLR antagonists may cause similar side effects to those of other immunosuppressive drugs, such as causing users to be more prone to infectious diseases and cancer [199]. Indeed, TLR agonists, including imiquimod, are used in cancer treatment [200], suggesting that TLR antagonism could instead have tumor-promoting effects. Hydroxychloroquine is considered safe and does not abrogate TLR signaling completely [190]. However, it can cause gastrointestinal problems like vomiting and diarrhea [201].

In addition, studies targeting pathways related to TLRs have been performed. For example, silencing HMGB1 expression in ovalbumin-induced asthmatic mice decreased expression of IgE and inflammatory factors [202]. In a review by Xue et al. (2021), different isoforms of HMGB1 are described with distinct physiological functions when released into the extracellular matrix, making it challenging to therapeutically target this protein [203]. The association between ABCs and autoantibody production in SLE has made these cells an interesting target for treatment of SLE. However, the markers currently used to identify this cell type are also shared by other immune cells and are therefore not specific enough to be used for targeting only ABCs [182]. Future work should therefore aim to identify ways of specifically targeting both ABCs and TLRs.

3. Conclusions and Future Directions

Due to its heterogenous nature, SLE is difficult to diagnose and treat efficiently, and animal models are invaluable for studying disease mechanisms and for testing novel therapeutics. Here, we have described various SLE mouse models, including spontaneous, genetically modified, inducible, and humanized models. Such models have contributed greatly to our knowledge about SLE and there are pronounced advantages to using mouse models when studying complex diseases.

The genetic and biological similarities between mice and humans are high as the genome of mice is 99% similar to the human genome, and the immune, endocrine, nervous, cardiovascular, and skeletal systems share similar complexity to the human systems. The reproducibility of mice and ease of breeding them, together with the use of modern sequencing and genomic engineering technologies to generate genetic alterations, allows us to utilize mouse models to research specific genetic targets of disease. However, mouse models do have limitations when compared with human SLE. Even though humans and mice are quite similar, we do not share the same immune system, and it is thus not possible to directly transfer results from mice to humans. The same goes for tolerance and response to treatment.

Current treatment of SLE often involves anti-inflammatory and immunosuppressive drugs, making the patients susceptible to infections. Environmental factors such as viruses and chemical elements resembling TLR ligands that can bind to and activate TLR and downstream signaling pathways may all contribute to SLE disease initiation and progression. As shown in an imiquimod-induced setting, both RNA and DNA sensing pathways may be activated in a TLR7-induced way without viral infection, indicating that other environmental stimuli such as chemicals can induce activation of cellular pathways involved in SLE. Evolutionarily developed bacterial and viral immune evasion strategies targeting TLR pathways may identify new compounds that can be used to stop or dampen any signaling aggravating the autoimmune disease.

The expression and interaction between the different TLRs, especially TLR7, TLR8, and TLR9, have a role in disease development in SLE. TLR7 acts as a disease-promoting factor, while TLR8 and TLR9 might have more regulating functions. Understanding these dynamics offers potential therapeutic targets for modulating immune responses in SLE and other autoimmune diseases. In addition, the dynamics between TLRs and other immune cells such as ABCs are important for disease etiology. Challenges remain in identifying the most appropriate targets for diagnosis, disease monitoring, and treatment. The fact that some of the TLRs have a tolerogenic function, such as TLR9, which may be responsible for the establishment of central B-cell tolerance, makes it an important target to restore B-cell tolerance in SLE and other autoimmune diseases. Thus, it is possible that dual inhibitors of TLR7 and TLR8 or TLR9 may be less effective than those that target only TLR7. It is therefore highly important to acquire more knowledge about the specific functions of individual TLRs.

In summary, understanding the interplay between environmental factors and pathway signaling and their involvement in SLE is necessary to provide insights into the mechanisms underlying disease flares and progression, potentially leading to the development of targeted therapies. Future studies using new technology and humanized mouse models have the potential to increase our knowledge of complex diseases such as SLE. However, while mouse models offer valuable insights and facilitate the exploration of specific genetic and molecular aspects of SLE, careful selection and interpretation of these models are crucial for advancing our understanding and treatment of SLE, exemplified by the different results regarding autoantibody repertoire in different SLE mouse models, both before and after knockout of TLRs.

Author Contributions: Conceptualization, S.v.H., K.A.F. and H.L.P.; methodology, S.v.H., K.A.F. and H.L.P.; writing—original draft preparation, S.v.H., K.A.F. and H.L.P.; writing—review and editing, S.v.H., K.A.F. and H.L.P.; visualization, S.v.H., K.A.F. and H.L.P.; supervision, K.A.F. and H.L.P.;

project administration, K.A.F. and H.L.P.; funding acquisition, K.A.F. and H.L.P. All authors have read and agreed to the published version of the manuscript.

Funding: This research was funded in whole or in part by Northern Norway Regional Health Authority (HNF1343-17 and HNF1427-18) and UiT The Arctic University of Norway.

Conflicts of Interest: The authors declare no conflicts of interest.

References

1. Aringer, M.; Costenbader, K.; Daikh, D.; Brinks, R.; Mosca, M.; Ramsey-Goldman, R.; Smolen, J.S.; Wofsy, D.; Boumpas, D.T.; Kamen, D.L.; et al. 2019 European League Against Rheumatism/American College of Rheumatology classification criteria for systemic lupus erythematosus. *Ann. Rheum. Dis.* **2019**, *78*, 1151–1159. [CrossRef] [PubMed]
2. Dema, B.; Charles, N. Autoantibodies in SLE: Specificities, Isotypes and Receptors. *Antibodies* **2016**, *5*, 2. [CrossRef] [PubMed]
3. Nowling, T.K.; Gilkeson, G.S. Mechanisms of tissue injury in lupus nephritis. *Arthritis Res. Ther.* **2011**, *13*, 250. [CrossRef] [PubMed]
4. Duan, T.; Du, Y.; Xing, C.; Wang, H.Y.; Wang, R.-F. Toll-Like Receptor Signaling and Its Role in Cell-Mediated Immunity. *Front. Immunol.* **2022**, *13*, 812774. [CrossRef] [PubMed]
5. Kawai, T.; Ikegawa, M.; Ori, D.; Akira, S. Decoding Toll-like receptors: Recent insights and perspectives in innate immunity. *Immunity* **2024**, *57*, 649–673. [CrossRef] [PubMed]
6. Su, Y.J.; Li, F.A.; Sheu, J.J.; Li, S.C.; Weng, S.W.; Shen, F.C.; Chang, Y.H.; Chen, H.Y.; Liou, C.W.; Lin, T.K.; et al. A Study on MDA5 Signaling in Splenic B Cells from an Imiquimod-Induced Lupus Mouse Model with Proteomics. *Cells* **2022**, *11*, 3350. [CrossRef] [PubMed]
7. Moore, E.; Putterman, C. Are lupus animal models useful for understanding and developing new therapies for human SLE? *J. Autoimmun.* **2020**, *112*, 102490. [CrossRef]
8. Du, Y.; Sanam, S.; Kate, K.; Mohan, C. Animal models of lupus and lupus nephritis. *Curr. Pharm. Des.* **2015**, *21*, 2320–2349. [CrossRef] [PubMed]
9. Li, W.; Titov, A.A.; Morel, L. An update on lupus animal models. *Curr. Opin. Rheumatol.* **2017**, *29*, 434–441. [CrossRef]
10. Richard, M.L.; Gilkeson, G. Mouse models of lupus: What they tell us and what they don't. *Lupus Sci. Med.* **2018**, *5*, e000199. [CrossRef]
11. Halkom, A.; Wu, H.; Lu, Q. Contribution of mouse models in our understanding of lupus. *Int. Rev. Immunol.* **2020**, *39*, 174–187. [CrossRef] [PubMed]
12. Katikaneni, D.; Morel, L.; Scindia, Y. Animal models of lupus nephritis: The past, present and a future outlook. *Autoimmunity* **2024**, *57*, 2319203. [CrossRef] [PubMed]
13. Helyer, B.J.; Howie, J.B. Renal disease associated with positive lupus erythematosus tests in a cross-bred strain of mice. *Nature* **1963**, *197*, 197. [CrossRef] [PubMed]
14. Dubois, E.L.; Horowitz, R.E.; Demopoulos, H.B.; Teplitz, R. NZB/NZW mice as a model of systemic lupus erythematosus. *JAMA* **1966**, *195*, 285–289. [CrossRef] [PubMed]
15. Morel, L. Mapping lupus susceptibility genes in the NZM2410 mouse model. *Adv. Immunol.* **2012**, *115*, 113–139. [CrossRef] [PubMed]
16. Vidal, S.; Gelpi, C.; Rodriguez-Sanchez, J.L. (SWR × SJL)F1 mice: A new model of lupus-like disease. *J. Exp. Med.* **1994**, *179*, 1429–1435. [CrossRef] [PubMed]
17. Andrews, B.S.; Eisenberg, R.A.; Theofilopoulos, A.N.; Izui, S.; Wilson, C.B.; McConahey, P.J.; Murphy, E.D.; Roths, J.B.; Dixon, F.J. Spontaneous murine lupus-like syndromes. Clinical and immunopathological manifestations in several strains. *J. Exp. Med.* **1978**, *148*, 1198–1215. [CrossRef]
18. Bolland, S.; Yim, Y.S.; Tus, K.; Wakeland, E.K.; Ravetch, J.V. Genetic modifiers of systemic lupus erythematosus in FcgammaRIIB(-/-) mice. *J. Exp. Med.* **2002**, *195*, 1167–1174. [CrossRef]
19. Ondee, T.; Surawut, S.; Taratummarat, S.; Hirankarn, N.; Palaga, T.; Pisitkun, P.; Pisitkun, T.; Leelahavanichkul, A. Fc Gamma Receptor IIB Deficient Mice: A Lupus Model with Increased Endotoxin Tolerance-Related Sepsis Susceptibility. *Shock* **2017**, *47*, 743–752. [CrossRef]
20. Han, J.H.; Umiker, B.R.; Kazimirova, A.A.; Fray, M.; Korgaonkar, P.; Selsing, E.; Imanishi-Kari, T. Expression of an anti-RNA autoantibody in a mouse model of SLE increases neutrophil and monocyte numbers as well as IFN-I expression. *Eur. J. Immunol.* **2014**, *44*, 215–226. [CrossRef]
21. Deane, J.A.; Pisitkun, P.; Barrett, R.S.; Feigenbaum, L.; Town, T.; Ward, J.M.; Flavell, R.A.; Bolland, S. Control of Toll-like Receptor 7 Expression Is Essential to Restrict Autoimmunity and Dendritic Cell Proliferation. *Immunity* **2007**, *27*, 801–810. [CrossRef] [PubMed]
22. Tizaoui, K.; Terrazzino, S.; Cargnin, S.; Lee, K.H.; Gauckler, P.; Li, H.; Shin, J.I.; Kronbichler, A. The role of PTPN22 in the pathogenesis of autoimmune diseases: A comprehensive review. *Semin. Arthritis Rheum.* **2021**, *51*, 513–522. [CrossRef]
23. Wang, Y.; Shaked, I.; Stanford, S.M.; Zhou, W.; Curtsinger, J.M.; Mikulski, Z.; Shaheen, Z.R.; Cheng, G.; Sawatzke, K.; Campbell, A.M.; et al. The autoimmunity-associated gene PTPN22 potentiates toll-like receptor-driven, type 1 interferon-dependent immunity. *Immunity* **2013**, *39*, 111–122. [CrossRef] [PubMed]

24. Zheng, J.; Petersen, F.; Yu, X. The role of PTPN22 in autoimmunity: Learning from mice. *Autoimmun. Rev.* **2014**, *13*, 266–271. [CrossRef] [PubMed]
25. Wilber, A.; O'Connor, T.P.; Lu, M.L.; Karimi, A.; Schneider, M.C. Dnase1l3 deficiency in lupus-prone MRL and NZB/W F1 mice. *Clin. Exp. Immunol.* **2003**, *134*, 46–52. [CrossRef] [PubMed]
26. Engavale, M.; Hernandez, C.J.; Infante, A.; LeRoith, T.; Radovan, E.; Evans, L.; Villarreal, J.; Reilly, C.M.; Sutton, R.B.; Keyel, P.A. Deficiency of macrophage-derived Dnase1L3 causes lupus-like phenotypes in mice. *J. Leukoc. Biol.* **2023**, *114*, 547–556. [CrossRef] [PubMed]
27. Sisirak, V.; Sally, B.; D'Agati, V.; Martinez-Ortiz, W.; Ozcakar, Z.B.; David, J.; Rashidfarrokhi, A.; Yeste, A.; Panea, C.; Chida, A.S.; et al. Digestion of Chromatin in Apoptotic Cell Microparticles Prevents Autoimmunity. *Cell* **2016**, *166*, 88–101. [CrossRef]
28. Weisenburger, T.; von Neubeck, B.; Schneider, A.; Ebert, N.; Schreyer, D.; Acs, A.; Winkler, T.H. Epistatic Interactions Between Mutations of Deoxyribonuclease 1-Like 3 and the Inhibitory Fc Gamma Receptor IIB Result in Very Early and Massive Autoantibodies Against Double-Stranded DNA. *Front. Immunol.* **2018**, *9*, 1551. [CrossRef] [PubMed]
29. Korn, M.A.; Steffensen, M.; Brandl, C.; Royzman, D.; Daniel, C.; Winkler, T.H.; Nitschke, L. Epistatic effects of Siglec-G and DNase1 or DNase1l3 deficiencies in the development of systemic lupus erythematosus. *Front. Immunol.* **2023**, *14*, 1095830. [CrossRef] [PubMed]
30. Napirei, M.; Karsunky, H.; Zevnik, B.; Stephan, H.; Mannherz, H.G.; Moroy, T. Features of systemic lupus erythematosus in Dnase1-deficient mice. *Nat. Genet.* **2000**, *25*, 177–181. [CrossRef]
31. Kenny, E.F.; Raupach, B.; Abu Abed, U.; Brinkmann, V.; Zychlinsky, A. Dnase1-deficient mice spontaneously develop a systemic lupus erythematosus-like disease. *Eur. J. Immunol.* **2019**, *49*, 590–599. [CrossRef] [PubMed]
32. Hibbs, M.L.; Tarlinton, D.M.; Armes, J.; Grail, D.; Hodgson, G.; Maglitto, R.; Stacker, S.A.; Dunn, A.R. Multiple defects in the immune system of Lyn-deficient mice, culminating in autoimmune disease. *Cell* **1995**, *83*, 301–311. [CrossRef]
33. Ban, T.; Sato, G.R.; Nishiyama, A.; Akiyama, A.; Takasuna, M.; Umehara, M.; Suzuki, S.; Ichino, M.; Matsunaga, S.; Kimura, A.; et al. Lyn Kinase Suppresses the Transcriptional Activity of IRF5 in the TLR-MyD88 Pathway to Restrain the Development of Autoimmunity. *Immunity* **2016**, *45*, 319–332. [CrossRef]
34. Park, J.S.; Yang, S.; Hwang, S.H.; Choi, J.; Kwok, S.K.; Kong, Y.Y.; Youn, J.; Cho, M.L.; Park, S.H. B Cell-Specific Deletion of CR6-Interacting Factor 1 Drives Lupus-like Autoimmunity by Activation of Interleukin-17, Interleukin-6, and Pathogenic Follicular Helper T Cells in a Mouse Model. *Arthritis Rheumatol.* **2022**, *74*, 1211–1222. [CrossRef] [PubMed]
35. Lietke, D.S. *CRIF1 and Its Function in Anti-Viral Immunity*; Ludwig Maximilian University of Munich: Munich, Germany, 2017.
36. Lee, K.; Park, J.; Tanno, H.; Georgiou, G.; Diamond, B.; Kim, S.J. Peripheral T cell activation, not thymic selection, expands the T follicular helper repertoire in a lupus-prone murine model. *Proc. Natl. Acad. Sci. USA* **2023**, *120*, e2309780120. [CrossRef] [PubMed]
37. Kim, S.J.; Schatzle, S.; Ahmed, S.S.; Haap, W.; Jang, S.H.; Gregersen, P.K.; Georgiou, G.; Diamond, B. Increased cathepsin S in Prdm1(-/-) dendritic cells alters the T(FH) cell repertoire and contributes to lupus. *Nat. Immunol.* **2017**, *18*, 1016–1024. [CrossRef]
38. Kim, V.; Lee, K.; Tian, H.; Jang, S.H.; Diamond, B.; Kim, S.J. IL-17-producing follicular Th cells enhance plasma cell differentiation in lupus-prone mice. *JCI Insight* **2022**, *7*, e157332. [CrossRef]
39. Ko, Y.A.; Chan, Y.H.; Liu, C.H.; Liang, J.J.; Chuang, T.H.; Hsueh, Y.P.; Lin, Y.L.; Lin, K.I. Blimp-1-Mediated Pathway Promotes Type I IFN Production in Plasmacytoid Dendritic Cells by Targeting to Interleukin-1 Receptor-Associated Kinase M. *Front. Immunol.* **2018**, *9*, 1828. [CrossRef]
40. Reuschle, Q.; Van Heddegem, L.; Bosteels, V.; Moncan, M.; Depauw, S.; Wadier, N.; Marechal, S.; De Nolf, C.; Delgado, V.; Messai, Y.; et al. Loss of function of XBP1 splicing activity of IRE1alpha favors B cell tolerance breakdown. *J. Autoimmun.* **2024**, *142*, 103152. [CrossRef]
41. Murga, M.; Fernandez-Capetillo, O.; Field, S.J.; Moreno, B.; Borlado, L.R.; Fujiwara, Y.; Balomenos, D.; Vicario, A.; Carrera, A.C.; Orkin, S.H.; et al. Mutation of E2F2 in mice causes enhanced T lymphocyte proliferation, leading to the development of autoimmunity. *Immunity* **2001**, *15*, 959–970. [CrossRef]
42. Marin-Vidalled, M.J.; Bolivar, A.; Zubiaga, A.; Lopez-Hoyos, M. The combined effect of BCL-2 over-expression and E2F2 deficiency induces an autoimmune syndrome in non-susceptible mouse strain C57BL/6. *Autoimmunity* **2010**, *43*, 111–120. [CrossRef] [PubMed]
43. Wang, S.; Wang, L.; Wu, C.; Sun, S.; Pan, J.H. E2F2 directly regulates the STAT1 and PI3K/AKT/NF-kappaB pathways to exacerbate the inflammatory phenotype in rheumatoid arthritis synovial fibroblasts and mouse embryonic fibroblasts. *Arthritis Res. Ther.* **2018**, *20*, 225. [CrossRef] [PubMed]
44. Akizuki, S.; Ishigaki, K.; Kochi, Y.; Law, S.M.; Matsuo, K.; Ohmura, K.; Suzuki, A.; Nakayama, M.; Iizuka, Y.; Koseki, H.; et al. PLD4 is a genetic determinant to systemic lupus erythematosus and involved in murine autoimmune phenotypes. *Ann. Rheum. Dis.* **2019**, *78*, 509–518. [CrossRef] [PubMed]
45. Gavin, A.L.; Blane, T.R.; Thinnes, T.C.; Gerlt, E.; Marshak-Rothstein, A.; Huang, D.; Nemazee, D. Disease in the Pld4thss/thss Model of Murine Lupus Requires TLR9. *Immunohorizons* **2023**, *7*, 577–586. [CrossRef] [PubMed]
46. Gavin, A.L.; Huang, D.; Huber, C.; Martensson, A.; Tardif, V.; Skog, P.D.; Blane, T.R.; Thinnes, T.C.; Osborn, K.; Chong, H.S.; et al. PLD3 and PLD4 are single-stranded acid exonucleases that regulate endosomal nucleic-acid sensing. *Nat. Immunol.* **2018**, *19*, 942–953. [CrossRef]

47. Yu, P.; Constien, R.; Dear, N.; Katan, M.; Hanke, P.; Bunney, T.D.; Kunder, S.; Quintanilla-Martinez, L.; Huffstadt, U.; Schroder, A.; et al. Autoimmunity and inflammation due to a gain-of-function mutation in phospholipase C gamma 2 that specifically increases external Ca2+ entry. *Immunity* **2005**, *22*, 451–465. [CrossRef]
48. Becker-Herman, S.; Meyer-Bahlburg, A.; Schwartz, M.A.; Jackson, S.W.; Hudkins, K.L.; Liu, C.; Sather, B.D.; Khim, S.; Liggitt, D.; Song, W.; et al. WASp-deficient B cells play a critical, cell-intrinsic role in triggering autoimmunity. *J. Exp. Med.* **2011**, *208*, 2033–2042. [CrossRef]
49. Jackson, S.W.; Scharping, N.E.; Kolhatkar, N.S.; Khim, S.; Schwartz, M.A.; Li, Q.-Z.; Hudkins, K.L.; Alpers, C.E.; Liggitt, D.; Rawlings, D.J. Opposing Impact of B Cell–Intrinsic TLR7 and TLR9 Signals on Autoantibody Repertoire and Systemic Inflammation. *J. Immunol.* **2014**, *192*, 4525–4532. [CrossRef]
50. Jiang, Y.; Xiang, Y.; Lin, C.; Zhang, W.; Yang, Z.; Xiang, L.; Xiao, Y.; Chen, L.; Ran, Q.; Li, Z. Multifunctions of CRIF1 in cancers and mitochondrial dysfunction. *Front. Oncol.* **2022**, *12*, 1009948. [CrossRef]
51. Nadeau, S.; Martins, G.A. Conserved and Unique Functions of Blimp1 in Immune Cells. *Front. Immunol.* **2021**, *12*, 805260. [CrossRef]
52. Brodie, E.J.; Infantino, S.; Low, M.S.Y.; Tarlinton, D.M. Lyn, Lupus, and (B) Lymphocytes, a Lesson on the Critical Balance of Kinase Signaling in Immunity. *Front. Immunol.* **2018**, *9*, 401. [CrossRef]
53. Jackson, J.T.; Mulazzani, E.; Nutt, S.L.; Masters, S.L. The role of PLCgamma2 in immunological disorders, cancer, and neurodegeneration. *J. Biol. Chem.* **2021**, *297*, 100905. [CrossRef]
54. Rey-Suarez, I.; Wheatley, B.A.; Koo, P.; Bhanja, A.; Shu, Z.; Mochrie, S.; Song, W.; Shroff, H.; Upadhyaya, A. WASP family proteins regulate the mobility of the B cell receptor during signaling activation. *Nat. Commun.* **2020**, *11*, 439. [CrossRef] [PubMed]
55. Junjappa, R.P.; Patil, P.; Bhattarai, K.R.; Kim, H.R.; Chae, H.J. IRE1alpha Implications in Endoplasmic Reticulum Stress-Mediated Development and Pathogenesis of Autoimmune Diseases. *Front. Immunol.* **2018**, *9*, 1289. [CrossRef]
56. Park, S.M.; Kang, T.I.; So, J.S. Roles of XBP1s in Transcriptional Regulation of Target Genes. *Biomedicines* **2021**, *9*, 791. [CrossRef]
57. Freitas, E.C.; de Oliveira, M.S.; Monticielo, O.A. Pristane-induced lupus: Considerations on this experimental model. *Clin. Rheumatol.* **2017**, *36*, 2403–2414. [CrossRef]
58. Satoh, M.; Richards, H.B.; Shaheen, V.M.; Yoshida, H.; Shaw, M.; Naim, J.O.; Wooley, P.H.; Reeves, W.H. Widespread susceptibility among inbred mouse strains to the induction of lupus autoantibodies by pristane. *Clin. Exp. Immunol.* **2000**, *121*, 399–405. [CrossRef]
59. Bender, A.T.; Wu, Y.; Cao, Q.; Ding, Y.; Oestreicher, J.; Genest, M.; Akare, S.; Ishizaka, S.T.; Mackey, M.F. Assessment of the translational value of mouse lupus models using clinically relevant biomarkers. *Transl. Res.* **2014**, *163*, 515–532. [CrossRef]
60. Postal, M.; Vivaldo, J.F.; Fernandez-Ruiz, R.; Paredes, J.L.; Appenzeller, S.; Niewold, T.B. Type I interferon in the pathogenesis of systemic lupus erythematosus. *Curr. Opin. Immunol.* **2020**, *67*, 87–94. [CrossRef]
61. Savarese, E.; Steinberg, C.; Pawar, R.D.; Reindl, W.; Akira, S.; Anders, H.J.; Krug, A. Requirement of Toll-like receptor 7 for pristane-induced production of autoantibodies and development of murine lupus nephritis. *Arthritis Rheum.* **2008**, *58*, 1107–1115. [CrossRef]
62. Urbonaviciute, V.; Starke, C.; Pirschel, W.; Pohle, S.; Frey, S.; Daniel, C.; Amann, K.; Schett, G.; Herrmann, M.; Voll, R.E. Toll-like receptor 2 is required for autoantibody production and development of renal disease in pristane-induced lupus. *Arthritis Rheum.* **2013**, *65*, 1612–1623. [CrossRef]
63. Summers, S.A.; Hoi, A.; Steinmetz, O.M.; O'Sullivan, K.M.; Ooi, J.D.; Odobasic, D.; Akira, S.; Kitching, A.R.; Holdsworth, S.R. TLR9 and TLR4 are required for the development of autoimmunity and lupus nephritis in pristane nephropathy. *J. Autoimmun.* **2010**, *35*, 291–298. [CrossRef] [PubMed]
64. Bossaller, L.; Christ, A.; Pelka, K.; Nündel, K.; Chiang, P.I.; Pang, C.; Mishra, N.; Busto, P.; Bonegio, R.G.; Schmidt, R.E.; et al. TLR9 Deficiency Leads to Accelerated Renal Disease and Myeloid Lineage Abnormalities in Pristane-Induced Murine Lupus. *J. Immunol.* **2016**, *197*, 1044–1053. [CrossRef] [PubMed]
65. Giordano, D.; Kuley, R.; Draves, K.E.; Elkon, K.B.; Giltiay, N.V.; Clark, E.A. B cell-activating factor (BAFF) from dendritic cells, monocytes and neutrophils is required for B cell maturation and autoantibody production in SLE-like autoimmune disease. *Front. Immunol.* **2023**, *14*, 1050528. [CrossRef] [PubMed]
66. Yoo, E.J.; Oh, K.H.; Piao, H.; Kang, H.J.; Jeong, G.W.; Park, H.; Lee, C.J.; Ryu, H.; Yang, S.H.; Kim, M.G.; et al. Macrophage transcription factor TonEBP promotes systemic lupus erythematosus and kidney injury via damage-induced signaling pathways. *Kidney Int.* **2023**, *104*, 163–180. [CrossRef] [PubMed]
67. Miyagawa, F.; Tagaya, Y.; Ozato, K.; Asada, H. Essential Requirement for IFN Regulatory Factor 7 in Autoantibody Production but Not Development of Nephritis in Murine Lupus. *J. Immunol.* **2016**, *197*, 2167–2176. [CrossRef] [PubMed]
68. Motwani, M.; McGowan, J.; Antonovitch, J.; Gao, K.M.; Jiang, Z.; Sharma, S.; Baltus, G.A.; Nickerson, K.M.; Marshak-Rothstein, A.; Fitzgerald, K.A. cGAS-STING Pathway Does Not Promote Autoimmunity in Murine Models of SLE. *Front. Immunol.* **2021**, *12*, 605930. [CrossRef]
69. Corzo, C.A.; Varfolomeev, E.; Setiadi, A.F.; Francis, R.; Klabunde, S.; Senger, K.; Sujatha-Bhaskar, S.; Drobnick, J.; Do, S.; Suto, E.; et al. The kinase IRAK4 promotes endosomal TLR and immune complex signaling in B cells and plasmacytoid dendritic cells. *Sci. Signal.* **2020**, *13*, eaaz1053. [CrossRef]

70. Lin, W.; Seshasayee, D.; Lee, W.P.; Caplazi, P.; McVay, S.; Suto, E.; Nguyen, A.; Lin, Z.; Sun, Y.; DeForge, L.; et al. Dual B cell immunotherapy is superior to individual anti-CD20 depletion or BAFF blockade in murine models of spontaneous or accelerated lupus. *Arthritis Rheumatol.* **2015**, *67*, 215–224. [CrossRef]
71. Gardet, A.; Chou, W.C.; Reynolds, T.L.; Velez, D.B.; Fu, K.; Czerkowicz, J.M.; Bajko, J.; Ranger, A.M.; Allaire, N.; Kerns, H.M.; et al. Pristane-Accelerated Autoimmune Disease in (SWR X NZB) F1 Mice Leads to Prominent Tubulointerstitial Inflammation and Human Lupus Nephritis-Like Fibrosis. *PLoS ONE* **2016**, *11*, e0164423. [CrossRef]
72. Satoh, M.; Weintraub, J.P.; Yoshida, H.; Shaheen, V.M.; Richards, H.B.; Shaw, M.; Reeves, W.H. Fas and Fas ligand mutations inhibit autoantibody production in pristane-induced lupus. *J. Immunol.* **2000**, *165*, 1036–1043. [CrossRef] [PubMed]
73. Yokogawa, M.; Takaishi, M.; Nakajima, K.; Kamijima, R.; Fujimoto, C.; Kataoka, S.; Terada, Y.; Sano, S. Epicutaneous application of toll-like receptor 7 agonists leads to systemic autoimmunity in wild-type mice: A new model of systemic Lupus erythematosus. *Arthritis Rheumatol.* **2014**, *66*, 694–706. [CrossRef] [PubMed]
74. Gleichmann, E.; Gleichmann, H. Pathogenesis of graft-versus-host reactions (GVHR) and GVH-like diseases. *J. Invest. Dermatol.* **1985**, *85*, 115s–120s. [CrossRef] [PubMed]
75. Srinivasan, M.; Flynn, R.; Price, A.; Ranger, A.; Browning, J.L.; Taylor, P.A.; Ritz, J.; Antin, J.H.; Murphy, W.J.; Luznik, L.; et al. Donor B-cell alloantibody deposition and germinal center formation are required for the development of murine chronic GVHD and bronchiolitis obliterans. *Blood* **2012**, *119*, 1570–1580. [CrossRef] [PubMed]
76. Bracken, S.J.; Suthers, A.N.; DiCioccio, R.A.; Su, H.; Anand, S.; Poe, J.C.; Jia, W.; Visentin, J.; Basher, F.; Jordan, C.Z.; et al. Heightened TLR7 signaling primes BCR-activated B cells in chronic graft-versus-host disease for effector functions. *Blood Adv.* **2024**, *8*, 667–680. [CrossRef] [PubMed]
77. Garimella, M.G.; He, C.; Chen, G.; Li, Q.Z.; Huang, X.; Karlsson, M.C.I. The B cell response to both protein and nucleic acid antigens displayed on apoptotic cells are dependent on endosomal pattern recognition receptors. *J. Autoimmun.* **2021**, *117*, 102582. [CrossRef] [PubMed]
78. Hayakawa, K.; Fujishiro, M.; Yoshida, Y.; Kataoka, Y.; Sakuma, S.; Nishi, T.; Ikeda, K.; Morimoto, S.; Takamori, K.; Sekigawa, I. Exposure of female NZBWF1 mice to imiquimod-induced lupus nephritis at an early age via a unique mechanism that differed from spontaneous onset. *Clin. Exp. Immunol.* **2022**, *208*, 33–46. [CrossRef] [PubMed]
79. Ma, L.; Terrell, M.; Brown, J.; Castellanos Garcia, A.; Elshikha, A.; Morel, L. TLR7/TLR8 activation and susceptibility genes synergize to breach gut barrier in a mouse model of lupus. *Front. Immunol.* **2023**, *14*, 1187145. [CrossRef] [PubMed]
80. Liu, Z.; Bethunaickan, R.; Huang, W.; Ramanujam, M.; Madaio, M.P.; Davidson, A. IFN-alpha confers resistance of systemic lupus erythematosus nephritis to therapy in NZB/W F1 mice. *J. Immunol.* **2011**, *187*, 1506–1513. [CrossRef]
81. Pollard, K.M.; Escalante, G.M.; Huang, H.; Haraldsson, K.M.; Hultman, P.; Christy, J.M.; Pawar, R.D.; Mayeux, J.M.; Gonzalez-Quintial, R.; Baccala, R.; et al. Induction of Systemic Autoimmunity by a Xenobiotic Requires Endosomal TLR Trafficking and Signaling from the Late Endosome and Endolysosome but Not Type I IFN. *J. Immunol.* **2017**, *199*, 3739–3747. [CrossRef]
82. Gill, R.F.; Mathieu, P.A.; Lash, L.H.; Rosenspire, A.J. Naturally occurring autoimmune disease in (NZB X NZW) F1 mice is correlated with suppression of MZ B cell development due to aberrant B Cell Receptor (BCR) signaling, which is exacerbated by exposure to inorganic mercury. *Toxicol. Sci.* **2023**, *197*, 211–221. [CrossRef] [PubMed]
83. Favor, O.K.; Chauhan, P.S.; Pourmand, E.; Edwards, A.M.; Wagner, J.G.; Lewandowski, R.P.; Heine, L.K.; Harkema, J.R.; Lee, K.S.S.; Pestka, J.J. Lipidome modulation by dietary omega-3 polyunsaturated fatty acid supplementation or selective soluble epoxide hydrolase inhibition suppresses rough LPS-accelerated glomerulonephritis in lupus-prone mice. *Front. Immunol.* **2023**, *14*, 1124910. [CrossRef] [PubMed]
84. Hasegawa, K.; Hayashi, T. Synthetic CpG oligodeoxynucleotides accelerate the development of lupus nephritis during preactive phase in NZB x NZWF1 mice. *Lupus* **2003**, *12*, 838–845. [CrossRef] [PubMed]
85. Chen, J.; Liao, S.; Zhou, H.; Yang, L.; Guo, F.; Chen, S.; Li, A.; Pan, Q.; Yang, C.; Liu, H.F.; et al. Humanized Mouse Models of Systemic Lupus Erythematosus: Opportunities and Challenges. *Front. Immunol.* **2021**, *12*, 816956. [CrossRef] [PubMed]
86. Maria, N.I.; Papoin, J.; Raparia, C.; Sun, Z.; Josselsohn, R.; Lu, A.; Katerji, H.; Syeda, M.M.; Polsky, D.; Paulson, R.; et al. Human TLR8 induces inflammatory bone marrow erythromyeloblastic islands and anemia in SLE-prone mice. *Life Sci. Alliance* **2023**, *6*, e202302241. [CrossRef] [PubMed]
87. Cakan, E.; Ai Kioon, M.D.; Garcia-Carmona, Y.; Glauzy, S.; Oliver, D.; Yamakawa, N.; Vega Loza, A.; Du, Y.; Schickel, J.N.; Boeckers, J.M.; et al. TLR9 ligand sequestration by chemokine CXCL4 negatively affects central B cell tolerance. *J. Exp. Med.* **2023**, *220*, e20230944. [CrossRef] [PubMed]
88. Schaper, F.; de Leeuw, K.; Horst, G.; Maas, F.; Bootsma, H.; Heeringa, P.; Limburg, P.C.; Westra, J. Autoantibodies to box A of high mobility group box 1 in systemic lupus erythematosus. *Clin. Exp. Immunol.* **2017**, *188*, 412–419. [CrossRef]
89. Abdulahad, D.A.; Westra, J.; Bijzet, J.; Limburg, P.C.; Kallenberg, C.G.; Bijl, M. High mobility group box 1 (HMGB1) and anti-HMGB1 antibodies and their relation to disease characteristics in systemic lupus erythematosus. *Arthritis Res. Ther.* **2011**, *13*, R71. [CrossRef]
90. Wirestam, L.; Schierbeck, H.; Skogh, T.; Gunnarsson, I.; Ottosson, L.; Erlandsson-Harris, H.; Wetterö, J.; Sjowall, C. Antibodies against High Mobility Group Box protein-1 (HMGB1) versus other anti-nuclear antibody fine-specificities and disease activity in systemic lupus erythematosus. *Arthritis Res. Ther.* **2015**, *17*, 338. [CrossRef]

91. Tanaka, A.; Ito, T.; Kibata, K.; Inagaki-Katashiba, N.; Amuro, H.; Nishizawa, T.; Son, Y.; Ozaki, Y.; Nomura, S. Serum high-mobility group box 1 is correlated with interferon-alpha and may predict disease activity in patients with systemic lupus erythematosus. *Lupus* **2019**, *28*, 1120–1127. [CrossRef]
92. Urbonaviciute, V.; Furnrohr, B.G.; Meister, S.; Munoz, L.; Heyder, P.; De Marchis, F.; Bianchi, M.E.; Kirschning, C.; Wagner, H.; Manfredi, A.A.; et al. Induction of inflammatory and immune responses by HMGB1-nucleosome complexes: Implications for the pathogenesis of SLE. *J. Exp. Med.* **2008**, *205*, 3007–3018. [CrossRef]
93. Das, N.; Dewan, V.; Grace, P.M.; Gunn, R.J.; Tamura, R.; Tzarum, N.; Watkins, L.R.; Wilson, I.A.; Yin, H. HMGB1 Activates Proinflammatory Signaling via TLR5 Leading to Allodynia. *Cell Rep.* **2016**, *17*, 1128–1140. [CrossRef]
94. Ma, K.; Li, J.; Wang, X.; Lin, X.; Du, W.; Yang, X.; Mou, F.; Fang, Y.; Zhao, Y.; Hong, X.; et al. TLR4(+)CXCR4(+) plasma cells drive nephritis development in systemic lupus erythematosus. *Ann. Rheum. Dis.* **2018**, *77*, 1498–1506. [CrossRef]
95. Li, S.J.; Ruan, D.D.; Wu, W.Z.; Wu, M.; Wu, Q.Y.; Wang, H.L.; Ji, Y.Y.; Zhang, Y.P.; Lin, X.F.; Fang, Z.T.; et al. Potential regulatory role of the Nrf2/HMGB1/TLR4/NF-kappaB signaling pathway in lupus nephritis. *Pediatr. Rheumatol. Online J.* **2023**, *21*, 130. [CrossRef]
96. Huang, Q.; Shen, S.; Qu, H.; Huang, Y.; Wu, D.; Jiang, H.; Yuan, C. Expression of HMGB1 and TLR4 in neuropsychiatric systemic lupus erythematosus patients with seizure disorders. *Ann. Transl. Med.* **2020**, *8*, 9. [CrossRef]
97. Elloumi, N.; Tahri, S.; Fakhfakh, R.; Abida, O.; Mahfoudh, N.; Hachicha, H.; Marzouk, S.; Bahloul, Z.; Masmoudi, H. Role of innate immune receptors TLR4 and TLR2 polymorphisms in systemic lupus erythematosus susceptibility. *Ann. Hum. Genet.* **2022**, *86*, 137–144. [CrossRef]
98. Lee, Y.H.; Lee, H.S.; Choi, S.J.; Ji, J.D.; Song, G.G. Associations between TLR polymorphisms and systemic lupus erythematosus: A systematic review and meta-analysis. *Clin. Exp. Rheumatol.* **2012**, *30*, 262–265.
99. Sanchez, E.; Orozco, G.; Lopez-Nevot, M.A.; Jimenez-Alonso, J.; Martin, J. Polymorphisms of toll-like receptor 2 and 4 genes in rheumatoid arthritis and systemic lupus erythematosus. *Tissue Antigens* **2004**, *63*, 54–57. [CrossRef]
100. Alajoleen, R.M.; Oakland, D.N.; Estaleen, R.; Shakeri, A.; Lu, R.; Appiah, M.; Sun, S.; Neumann, J.; Kawauchi, S.; Cecere, T.E.; et al. Tlr5 deficiency exacerbates lupus-like disease in the MRL/lpr mouse model. *Front. Immunol.* **2024**, *15*, 1359534. [CrossRef]
101. Patole, P.S.; Pawar, R.D.; Lech, M.; Zecher, D.; Schmidt, H.; Segerer, S.; Ellwart, A.; Henger, A.; Kretzler, M.; Anders, H.J. Expression and regulation of Toll-like receptors in lupus-like immune complex glomerulonephritis of MRL-Fas(lpr) mice. *Nephrol. Dial. Transpl.* **2006**, *21*, 3062–3073. [CrossRef]
102. Elloumi, N.; Fakhfakh, R.; Abida, O.; Ayadi, L.; Marzouk, S.; Hachicha, H.; Fourati, M.; Bahloul, Z.; Mhiri, M.N.; Kammoun, K.; et al. Relevant genetic polymorphisms and kidney expression of Toll-like receptor (TLR)-5 and TLR-9 in lupus nephritis. *Clin. Exp. Immunol.* **2017**, *190*, 328–339. [CrossRef]
103. Rupasree, Y.; Naushad, S.M.; Varshaa, R.; Mahalakshmi, G.S.; Kumaraswami, K.; Rajasekhar, L.; Kutala, V.K. Application of Various Statistical Models to Explore Gene-Gene Interactions in Folate, Xenobiotic, Toll-Like Receptor and STAT4 Pathways that Modulate Susceptibility to Systemic Lupus Erythematosus. *Mol. Diagn. Ther.* **2016**, *20*, 83–95. [CrossRef]
104. Hou, Y.; Wang, L.; Luo, C.; Tang, W.; Dai, R.; An, Y.; Tang, X. Clinical characteristics of early-onset paediatric systemic lupus erythematosus in a single centre in China. *Rheumatology* **2023**, *62*, 3373–3381. [CrossRef]
105. Oldenburg, M.; Kruger, A.; Ferstl, R.; Kaufmann, A.; Nees, G.; Sigmund, A.; Bathke, B.; Lauterbach, H.; Suter, M.; Dreher, S.; et al. TLR13 recognizes bacterial 23S rRNA devoid of erythromycin resistance-forming modification. *Science* **2012**, *337*, 1111–1115. [CrossRef]
106. Li, X.D.; Chen, Z.J. Sequence specific detection of bacterial 23S ribosomal RNA by TLR13. *Elife* **2012**, *1*, e00102. [CrossRef]
107. Lee, S.M.; Yip, T.F.; Yan, S.; Jin, D.Y.; Wei, H.L.; Guo, R.T.; Peiris, J.S.M. Recognition of Double-Stranded RNA and Regulation of Interferon Pathway by Toll-Like Receptor 10. *Front. Immunol.* **2018**, *9*, 516. [CrossRef]
108. Rodrigues, C.R.; Balachandran, Y.; Aulakh, G.K.; Singh, B. TLR10: An intriguing Toll-like receptor with many unanswered questions. *J. Innate Immun.* **2024**, *16*, 96–104. [CrossRef]
109. Caielli, S.; Wan, Z.; Pascual, V. Systemic Lupus Erythematosus Pathogenesis: Interferon and Beyond. *Annu. Rev. Immunol.* **2023**, *41*, 533–560. [CrossRef]
110. Scherlinger, M.; Guillotin, V.; Truchetet, M.E.; Contin-Bordes, C.; Sisirak, V.; Duffau, P.; Lazaro, E.; Richez, C.; Blanco, P. Systemic lupus erythematosus and systemic sclerosis: All roads lead to platelets. *Autoimmun. Rev.* **2018**, *17*, 625–635. [CrossRef]
111. Robert, M.; Scherlinger, M. Platelets are a major player and represent a therapeutic opportunity in systemic lupus erythematosus. *Jt. Bone Spine* **2024**, *91*, 105622. [CrossRef]
112. Linge, P.; Fortin, P.R.; Lood, C.; Bengtsson, A.A.; Boilard, E. The non-haemostatic role of platelets in systemic lupus erythematosus. *Nat. Rev. Rheumatol.* **2018**, *14*, 195–213. [CrossRef] [PubMed]
113. Scherlinger, M.; Richez, C.; Tsokos, G.C.; Boilard, E.; Blanco, P. The role of platelets in immune-mediated inflammatory diseases. *Nat. Rev. Immunol.* **2023**, *23*, 495–510. [CrossRef] [PubMed]
114. Baroni Pietto, M.C.; Glembotsky, A.C.; Lev, P.R.; Marin Oyarzun, C.R.; De Luca, G.; Gomez, G.; Collado, M.V.; Charo, N.; Cellucci, A.S.; Heller, P.G.; et al. Toll-like receptor expression and functional behavior in platelets from patients with systemic lupus erythematosus. *Immunobiology* **2024**, *229*, 152782. [CrossRef]
115. Hornung, V.; Rothenfusser, S.; Britsch, S.; Krug, A.; Jahrsdöfer, B.; Giese, T.; Endres, S.; Hartmann, G. Quantitative Expression of Toll-Like Receptor 1–10 mRNA in Cellular Subsets of Human Peripheral Blood Mononuclear Cells and Sensitivity to CpG Oligodeoxynucleotides1. *J. Immunol.* **2002**, *168*, 4531–4537. [CrossRef]

116. Demaria, O.; Pagni, P.P.; Traub, S.; de Gassart, A.; Branzk, N.; Murphy, A.J.; Valenzuela, D.M.; Yancopoulos, G.D.; Flavell, R.A.; Alexopoulou, L. TLR8 deficiency leads to autoimmunity in mice. *J. Clin. Investig.* **2010**, *120*, 3651–3662. [CrossRef] [PubMed]
117. Tilstra, J.S.; John, S.; Gordon, R.A.; Leibler, C.; Kashgarian, M.; Bastacky, S.; Nickerson, K.M.; Shlomchik, M.J. B cell-intrinsic TLR9 expression is protective in murine lupus. *J. Clin. Investig.* **2020**, *130*, 3172–3187. [CrossRef] [PubMed]
118. Heil, F.; Hemmi, H.; Hochrein, H.; Ampenberger, F.; Kirschning, C.; Akira, S.; Lipford, G.; Wagner, H.; Bauer, S. Species-Specific Recognition of Single-Stranded RNA via Toll-like Receptor 7 and 8. *Science* **2004**, *303*, 1526–1529. [CrossRef] [PubMed]
119. Peng, S.L. Signaling in B cells via Toll-like receptors. *Curr. Opin. Immunol.* **2005**, *17*, 230–236. [CrossRef]
120. Wen, L.; Zhang, B.; Wu, X.; Liu, R.; Fan, H.; Han, L.; Zhang, Z.; Ma, X.; Chu, C.-Q.; Shi, X. Toll-like receptors 7 and 9 regulate the proliferation and differentiation of B cells in systemic lupus erythematosus. *Front. Immunol.* **2023**, *14*, 1093208. [CrossRef]
121. Rubin, S.J.S.; Bloom, M.S.; Robinson, W.H. B cell checkpoints in autoimmune rheumatic diseases. *Nat. Rev. Rheumatol.* **2019**, *15*, 303–315. [CrossRef]
122. Leadbetter, E.A.; Rifkin, I.R.; Hohlbaum, A.M.; Beaudette, B.C.; Shlomchik, M.J.; Marshak-Rothstein, A. Chromatin–IgG complexes activate B cells by dual engagement of IgM and Toll-like receptors. *Nature* **2002**, *416*, 603–607. [CrossRef] [PubMed]
123. Viglianti, G.A.; Lau, C.M.; Hanley, T.M.; Miko, B.A.; Shlomchik, M.J.; Marshak-Rothstein, A. Activation of Autoreactive B Cells by CpG dsDNA. *Immunity* **2003**, *19*, 837–847. [CrossRef] [PubMed]
124. Christensen, S.R.; Shupe, J.; Nickerson, K.; Kashgarian, M.; Flavell, R.A.; Shlomchik, M.J. Toll-like Receptor 7 and TLR9 Dictate Autoantibody Specificity and Have Opposing Inflammatory and Regulatory Roles in a Murine Model of Lupus. *Immunity* **2006**, *25*, 417–428. [CrossRef]
125. Lau, C.M.; Broughton, C.; Tabor, A.S.; Akira, S.; Flavell, R.A.; Mamula, M.J.; Christensen, S.R.; Shlomchik, M.J.; Viglianti, G.A.; Rifkin, I.R.; et al. RNA-associated autoantigens activate B cells by combined B cell antigen receptor/Toll-like receptor 7 engagement. *J. Exp. Med.* **2005**, *202*, 1171–1177. [CrossRef] [PubMed]
126. Lin, L.; Gerth, A.J.; Peng, S.L. CpG DNA redirects class-switching towards 'Th1-like' Ig isotype production via TLR9 and MyD88. *Eur. J. Immunol.* **2004**, *34*, 1483–1487. [CrossRef] [PubMed]
127. He, B.; Qiao, X.; Cerutti, A. CpG DNA Induces IgG Class Switch DNA Recombination by Activating Human B Cells through an Innate Pathway That Requires TLR9 and Cooperates with IL-101. *J. Immunol.* **2004**, *173*, 4479–4491. [CrossRef] [PubMed]
128. Ehlers, M.; Fukuyama, H.; McGaha, T.L.; Aderem, A.; Ravetch, J.V. TLR9/MyD88 signaling is required for class switching to pathogenic IgG2a and 2b autoantibodies in SLE. *J. Exp. Med.* **2006**, *203*, 553–561. [CrossRef]
129. Eckl-Dorna, J.; Batista, F.D. BCR-mediated uptake of antigen linked to TLR9 ligand stimulates B-cell proliferation and antigen-specific plasma cell formation. *Blood* **2009**, *113*, 3969–3977. [CrossRef] [PubMed]
130. Rivera, C.E.; Zhou, Y.; Chupp, D.P.; Yan, H.; Fisher, A.D.; Simon, R.; Zan, H.; Xu, Z.; Casali, P. Intrinsic B cell TLR-BCR linked coengagement induces class-switched, hypermutated, neutralizing antibody responses in absence of T cells. *Sci. Adv.* **2023**, *9*, eade8928. [CrossRef]
131. Christensen, S.R.; Kashgarian, M.; Alexopoulou, L.; Flavell, R.A.; Akira, S.; Shlomchik, M.J. Toll-like receptor 9 controls anti-DNA autoantibody production in murine lupus. *J. Exp. Med.* **2005**, *202*, 321–331. [CrossRef]
132. Rahman, A.H.; Eisenberg, R.A. The role of toll-like receptors in systemic lupus erythematosus. *Springer Semin. Immunopathol.* **2006**, *28*, 131–143. [CrossRef]
133. Yi, A.-K.; Chang, M.; Peckham, D.W.; Krieg, A.M.; Ashman, R.F. CpG Oligodeoxyribonucleotides Rescue Mature Spleen B Cells from Spontaneous Apoptosis and Promote Cell Cycle Entry1. *J. Immunol.* **1998**, *160*, 5898–5906. [CrossRef] [PubMed]
134. Han, S.-S.; Chung, S.-T.; Robertson, D.A.; Chelvarajan, R.L.; Bondada, S. CpG oligodeoxynucleotides rescue BKS-2 immature B cell lymphoma from anti-IgM-mediated growth inhibition by up-regulation of egr-1. *Int. Immunol.* **1999**, *11*, 871–879. [CrossRef]
135. Nickerson, K.M.; Christensen, S.R.; Shupe, J.; Kashgarian, M.; Kim, D.; Elkon, K.; Shlomchik, M.J. TLR9 Regulates TLR7- and MyD88-Dependent Autoantibody Production and Disease in a Murine Model of Lupus. *J. Immunol.* **2010**, *184*, 1840–1848. [CrossRef] [PubMed]
136. Teichmann, L.L.; Schenten, D.; Medzhitov, R.; Kashgarian, M.; Shlomchik, M.J. Signals via the adaptor MyD88 in B cells and DCs make distinct and synergistic contributions to immune activation and tissue damage in lupus. *Immunity* **2013**, *38*, 528–540. [CrossRef]
137. Tilstra, J.S.; Kim, M.; Gordon, R.A.; Leibler, C.; Cosgrove, H.A.; Bastacky, S.; Nickerson, K.M.; Shlomchik, M.J. B cell–intrinsic Myd88 regulates disease progression in murine lupus. *J. Exp. Med.* **2023**, *220*, e20230263. [CrossRef]
138. Hwang, S.-H.; Lee, H.; Yamamoto, M.; Jones, L.A.; Dayalan, J.; Hopkins, R.; Zhou, X.J.; Yarovinsky, F.; Connolly, J.E.; Curotto de Lafaille, M.A.; et al. B Cell TLR7 Expression Drives Anti-RNA Autoantibody Production and Exacerbates Disease in Systemic Lupus Erythematosus–Prone Mice. *J. Immunol.* **2012**, *189*, 5786–5796. [CrossRef]
139. Satterthwaite, A.B. TLR7 Signaling in Lupus B Cells: New Insights into Synergizing Factors and Downstream Signals. *Curr. Rheumatol. Rep.* **2021**, *23*, 80. [CrossRef] [PubMed]
140. Desnues, B.; Macedo, A.B.; Roussel-Queval, A.; Bonnardel, J.; Henri, S.; Demaria, O.; Alexopoulou, L. TLR8 on dendritic cells and TLR9 on B cells restrain TLR7-mediated spontaneous autoimmunity in C57BL/6 mice. *Proc. Natl. Acad. Sci. USA* **2014**, *111*, 1497–1502. [CrossRef]
141. Scofield, R.H.; Bruner, G.R.; Namjou, B.; Kimberly, R.P.; Ramsey-Goldman, R.; Petri, M.; Reveille, J.D.; Alarcón, G.S.; Vilá, L.M.; Reid, J.; et al. Klinefelter's syndrome (47,XXY) in male systemic lupus erythematosus patients: Support for the notion of a gene-dose effect from the X chromosome. *Arthritis Rheum.* **2008**, *58*, 2511–2517. [CrossRef]

142. Souyris, M.; Cenac, C.; Azar, P.; Daviaud, D.; Canivet, A.; Grunenwald, S.; Pienkowski, C.; Chaumeil, J.; Mejía, J.E.; Guéry, J.-C. TLR7 escapes X chromosome inactivation in immune cells. *Sci. Immunol.* **2018**, *3*, eaap8855. [CrossRef] [PubMed]
143. Youness, A.; Cenac, C.; Faz-López, B.; Grunenwald, S.; Barrat, F.J.; Chaumeil, J.; Mejía, J.E.; Guéry, J.-C. TLR8 escapes X chromosome inactivation in human monocytes and CD4+ T cells. *Biol. Sex. Differ.* **2023**, *14*, 60. [CrossRef]
144. Wang, T.; Marken, J.; Chen, J.; Tran, V.B.; Li, Q.-Z.; Li, M.; Cerosaletti, K.; Elkon, K.B.; Zeng, X.; Giltiay, N.V. High TLR7 Expression Drives the Expansion of CD19+CD24hiCD38hi Transitional B Cells and Autoantibody Production in SLE Patients. *Front. Immunol.* **2019**, *10*, 01243. [CrossRef] [PubMed]
145. Deng, Y.; Zhao, J.; Sakurai, D.; Kaufman, K.M.; Edberg, J.C.; Kimberly, R.P.; Kamen, D.L.; Gilkeson, G.S.; Jacob, C.O.; Scofield, R.H.; et al. MicroRNA-3148 Modulates Allelic Expression of Toll-Like Receptor 7 Variant Associated with Systemic Lupus Erythematosus. *PLOS Genet.* **2013**, *9*, e1003336. [CrossRef]
146. Shen, N.; Fu, Q.; Deng, Y.; Qian, X.; Zhao, J.; Kaufman, K.M.; Wu, Y.L.; Yu, C.Y.; Tang, Y.; Chen, J.-Y.; et al. Sex-specific association of X-linked Toll-like receptor 7 (TLR7) with male systemic lupus erythematosus. *Proc. Natl. Acad. Sci. USA* **2010**, *107*, 15838–15843. [CrossRef] [PubMed]
147. Wang, C.-M.; Chang, S.-W.; Wu, Y.-J.J.; Lin, J.-C.; Ho, H.-H.; Chou, T.-C.; Yang, B.; Wu, J.; Chen, J.-Y. Genetic variations in Toll-like receptors (TLRs 3/7/8) are associated with systemic lupus erythematosus in a Taiwanese population. *Sci. Rep.* **2014**, *4*, 3792. [CrossRef]
148. Brown, G.J.; Cañete, P.F.; Wang, H.; Medhavy, A.; Bones, J.; Roco, J.A.; He, Y.; Qin, Y.; Cappello, J.; Ellyard, J.I.; et al. TLR7 gain-of-function genetic variation causes human lupus. *Nature* **2022**, *605*, 349–356. [CrossRef] [PubMed]
149. Nickerson, K.M.; Wang, Y.; Bastacky, S.; Shlomchik, M.J. Toll-like receptor 9 suppresses lupus disease in Fas-sufficient MRL Mice. *PLoS ONE* **2017**, *12*, e0173471. [CrossRef] [PubMed]
150. Lartigue, A.; Courville, P.; Auquit, I.; François, A.; Arnoult, C.; Tron, F.; Gilbert, D.; Musette, P. Role of TLR9 in Anti-Nucleosome and Anti-DNA Antibody Production in lpr Mutation-Induced Murine Lupus1. *J. Immunol.* **2006**, *177*, 1349–1354. [CrossRef]
151. Santiago-Raber, M.L.; Dunand-Sauthier, I.; Wu, T.; Li, Q.Z.; Uematsu, S.; Akira, S.; Reith, W.; Mohan, C.; Kotzin, B.L.; Izui, S. Critical role of TLR7 in the acceleration of systemic lupus erythematosus in TLR9-deficient mice. *J. Autoimmun.* **2010**, *34*, 339–348. [CrossRef]
152. Stoehr, A.D.; Schoen, C.T.; Mertes, M.M.M.; Eiglmeier, S.; Holecska, V.; Lorenz, A.K.; Schommartz, T.; Schoen, A.-L.; Hess, C.; Winkler, A.; et al. TLR9 in Peritoneal B-1b Cells Is Essential for Production of Protective Self-Reactive IgM To Control Th17 Cells and Severe Autoimmunity. *J. Immunol.* **2011**, *187*, 2953–2965. [CrossRef] [PubMed]
153. Yu, P.; Wellmann, U.; Kunder, S.; Quintanilla-Martinez, L.; Jennen, L.; Dear, N.; Amann, K.; Bauer, S.; Winkler, T.H.; Wagner, H. Toll-like receptor 9-independent aggravation of glomerulonephritis in a novel model of SLE. *Int. Immunol.* **2006**, *18*, 1211–1219. [CrossRef] [PubMed]
154. Cosgrove, H.A.; Gingras, S.; Kim, M.; Bastacky, S.; Tilstra, J.S.; Shlomchik, M.J. B cell-intrinsic TLR7 expression drives severe lupus in TLR9-deficient mice. *JCI Insight* **2023**, *8*, e172219. [CrossRef] [PubMed]
155. Celhar, T.; Yasuga, H.; Lee, H.Y.; Zharkova, O.; Tripathi, S.; Thornhill, S.I.; Lu, H.K.; Au, B.; Lim, L.H.K.; Thamboo, T.P.; et al. Toll-Like Receptor 9 Deficiency Breaks Tolerance to RNA-Associated Antigens and Up-Regulates Toll-Like Receptor 7 Protein in Sle1 Mice. *Arthritis Rheumatol.* **2018**, *70*, 1597–1609. [CrossRef] [PubMed]
156. Fukui, R.; Saitoh, S.-I.; Kanno, A.; Onji, M.; Shibata, T.; Ito, A.; Onji, M.; Matsumoto, M.; Akira, S.; Yoshida, N.; et al. Unc93B1 Restricts Systemic Lethal Inflammation by Orchestrating Toll-like Receptor 7 and 9 Trafficking. *Immunity* **2011**, *35*, 69–81. [CrossRef] [PubMed]
157. Huh, J.W.; Shibata, T.; Hwang, M.; Kwon, E.H.; Jang, M.S.; Fukui, R.; Kanno, A.; Jung, D.J.; Jang, M.H.; Miyake, K.; et al. UNC93B1 is essential for the plasma membrane localization and signaling of Toll-like receptor 5. *Proc. Natl. Acad. Sci. USA* **2014**, *111*, 7072–7077. [CrossRef] [PubMed]
158. Kim, Y.-M.; Brinkmann, M.M.; Paquet, M.-E.; Ploegh, H.L. UNC93B1 delivers nucleotide-sensing toll-like receptors to endolysosomes. *Nature* **2008**, *452*, 234–238. [CrossRef]
159. Fukui, R.; Saitoh, S.; Matsumoto, F.; Kozuka-Hata, H.; Oyama, M.; Tabeta, K.; Beutler, B.; Miyake, K. Unc93B1 biases Toll-like receptor responses to nucleic acid in dendritic cells toward DNA- but against RNA-sensing. *J. Exp. Med.* **2009**, *206*, 1339–1350. [CrossRef] [PubMed]
160. Leibler, C.; John, S.; Elsner, R.A.; Thomas, K.B.; Smita, S.; Joachim, S.; Levack, R.C.; Callahan, D.J.; Gordon, R.A.; Bastacky, S.; et al. Genetic dissection of TLR9 reveals complex regulatory and cryptic proinflammatory roles in mouse lupus. *Nat. Immunol.* **2022**, *23*, 1457–1469. [CrossRef]
161. Hanna Kazazian, N.; Wang, Y.; Roussel-Queval, A.; Marcadet, L.; Chasson, L.; Laprie, C.; Desnues, B.; Charaix, J.; Irla, M.; Alexopoulou, L. Lupus Autoimmunity and Metabolic Parameters Are Exacerbated Upon High Fat Diet-Induced Obesity Due to TLR7 Signaling. *Front. Immunol.* **2019**, *10*, 02015. [CrossRef]
162. Fejtkova, M.; Sukova, M.; Hlozkova, K.; Skvarova Kramarzova, K.; Rackova, M.; Jakubec, D.; Bakardjieva, M.; Bloomfield, M.; Klocperk, A.; Parackova, Z.; et al. TLR8/TLR7 dysregulation due to a novel TLR8 mutation causes severe autoimmune hemolytic anemia and autoinflammation in identical twins. *Am. J. Hematol.* **2022**, *97*, 338–351. [CrossRef] [PubMed]
163. Lind, N.A.; Rael, V.E.; Pestal, K.; Liu, B.; Barton, G.M. Regulation of the nucleic acid-sensing Toll-like receptors. *Nat. Rev. Immunol.* **2022**, *22*, 224–235. [CrossRef] [PubMed]

164. Song, H.-S.; Park, S.; Huh, J.-W.; Lee, Y.-R.; Jung, D.-J.; Yang, C.; Kim, S.H.; Kim, H.M.; Kim, Y.-M. N-glycosylation of UNC93B1 at a Specific Asparagine Residue Is Required for TLR9 Signaling. *Front. Immunol.* **2022**, *13*, 875083. [CrossRef] [PubMed]
165. Majer, O.; Liu, B.; Woo, B.J.; Kreuk, L.S.M.; Van Dis, E.; Barton, G.M. Release from UNC93B1 reinforces the compartmentalized activation of select TLRs. *Nature* **2019**, *575*, 371–374. [CrossRef] [PubMed]
166. Ni, H.; Wang, Y.; Yao, K.; Wang, L.; Huang, J.; Xiao, Y.; Chen, H.; Liu, B.; Yang, C.Y.; Zhao, J. Cyclical palmitoylation regulates TLR9 signalling and systemic autoimmunity in mice. *Nat. Commun.* **2024**, *15*, 1. [CrossRef]
167. Majer, O.; Liu, B.; Kreuk, L.S.M.; Krogan, N.; Barton, G.M. UNC93B1 recruits syntenin-1 to dampen TLR7 signalling and prevent autoimmunity. *Nature* **2019**, *575*, 366–370. [CrossRef]
168. Mishra, H.; Schlack-Leigers, C.; Lim, E.L.; Thieck, O.; Magg, T.; Raedler, J.; Wolf, C.; Klein, C.; Ewers, H.; Lee-Kirsch, M.A.; et al. Disrupted degradative sorting of TLR7 is associated with human lupus. *Sci. Immunol.* **2024**, *9*, eadi9575. [CrossRef] [PubMed]
169. Wolf, C.; Lim, E.L.; Mokhtari, M.; Kind, B.; Odainic, A.; Lara-Villacanas, E.; Koss, S.; Mages, S.; Menzel, K.; Engel, K.; et al. UNC93B1 variants underlie TLR7-dependent autoimmunity. *Sci. Immunol.* **2024**, *9*, eadi9769. [CrossRef]
170. Sato, R.; Shibata, T.; Tanaka, Y.; Kato, C.; Yamaguchi, K.; Furukawa, Y.; Shimizu, E.; Yamaguchi, R.; Imoto, S.; Miyano, S.; et al. Requirement of glycosylation machinery in TLR responses revealed by CRISPR/Cas9 screening. *Int. Immunol.* **2017**, *29*, 347–355. [CrossRef]
171. Sun, J.; Duffy, K.E.; Ranjith-Kumar, C.T.; Xiong, J.; Lamb, R.J.; Santos, J.; Masarapu, H.; Cunningham, M.; Holzenburg, A.; Sarisky, R.T.; et al. Structural and Functional Analyses of the Human Toll-like Receptor 3: ROLE OF GLYCOSYLATION*. *J. Biol. Chem.* **2006**, *281*, 11144–11151. [CrossRef]
172. Amith, S.R.; Jayanth, P.; Franchuk, S.; Siddiqui, S.; Seyrantepe, V.; Gee, K.; Basta, S.; Beyaert, R.; Pshezhetsky, A.V.; Szewczuk, M.R. Dependence of pathogen molecule-induced Toll-like receptor activation and cell function on Neu1 sialidase. *Glycoconj. J.* **2009**, *26*, 1197–1212. [CrossRef] [PubMed]
173. Ramos-Martínez, I.; Ramos-Martínez, E.; Cerbón, M.; Pérez-Torres, A.; Pérez-Campos Mayoral, L.; Hernández-Huerta, M.T.; Martínez-Cruz, M.; Pérez-Santiago, A.D.; Sánchez-Medina, M.A.; García-Montalvo, I.A.; et al. The Role of B Cell and T Cell Glycosylation in Systemic Lupus Erythematosus. *Int. J. Mol. Sci.* **2023**, *24*, 863. [CrossRef] [PubMed]
174. Cancro, M.P. Age-Associated B Cells. *Annu. Rev. Immunol.* **2020**, *38*, 315–340. [CrossRef] [PubMed]
175. Mouat, I.C.; Goldberg, E.; Horwitz, M.S. Age-associated B cells in autoimmune diseases. *Cell. Mol. Life Sci.* **2022**, *79*, 402. [CrossRef]
176. Jenks, S.A.; Cashman, K.S.; Zumaquero, E.; Marigorta, U.M.; Patel, A.V.; Wang, X.; Tomar, D.; Woodruff, M.C.; Simon, Z.; Bugrovsky, R.; et al. Distinct Effector B Cells Induced by Unregulated Toll-like Receptor 7 Contribute to Pathogenic Responses in Systemic Lupus Erythematosus. *Immunity* **2018**, *49*, 725–739.e726. [CrossRef] [PubMed]
177. Wang, S.; Wang, J.; Kumar, V.; Karnell, J.L.; Naiman, B.; Gross, P.S.; Rahman, S.; Zerrouki, K.; Hanna, R.; Morehouse, C.; et al. IL-21 drives expansion and plasma cell differentiation of autoreactive CD11chiT-bet+ B cells in SLE. *Nat. Commun.* **2018**, *9*, 1758. [CrossRef] [PubMed]
178. Rubtsov, A.V.; Rubtsova, K.; Fischer, A.; Meehan, R.T.; Gillis, J.Z.; Kappler, J.W.; Marrack, P. Toll-like receptor 7 (TLR7)–driven accumulation of a novel CD11c+ B-cell population is important for the development of autoimmunity. *Blood* **2011**, *118*, 1305–1315. [CrossRef]
179. Aranburu, A.; Höök, N.; Gerasimcik, N.; Corleis, B.; Ren, W.; Camponeschi, A.; Carlsten, H.; Grimsholm, O.; Mårtensson, I.-L. Age-associated B cells expanded in autoimmune mice are memory cells sharing H-CDR3-selected repertoires. *Eur. J. Immunol.* **2018**, *48*, 509–521. [CrossRef] [PubMed]
180. Dai, D.; Gu, S.; Han, X.; Ding, H.; Jiang, Y.; Zhang, X.; Yao, C.; Hong, S.; Zhang, J.; Shen, Y.; et al. The transcription factor ZEB2 drives the formation of age-associated B cells. *Science* **2024**, *383*, 413–421. [CrossRef]
181. Naradikian, M.S.; Myles, A.; Beiting, D.P.; Roberts, K.J.; Dawson, L.; Herati, R.S.; Bengsch, B.; Linderman, S.L.; Stelekati, E.; Spolski, R.; et al. Cutting Edge: IL-4, IL-21, and IFN-γ Interact To Govern T-bet and CD11c Expression in TLR-Activated B Cells. *J. Immunol.* **2016**, *197*, 1023–1028. [CrossRef]
182. Nickerson, K.M.; Smita, S.; Hoehn, K.B.; Marinov, A.D.; Thomas, K.B.; Kos, J.T.; Yang, Y.; Bastacky, S.I.; Watson, C.T.; Kleinstein, S.H.; et al. Age-associated B cells are heterogeneous and dynamic drivers of autoimmunity in mice. *J. Exp. Med.* **2023**, *220*, e20221346. [CrossRef]
183. Peng, S.L.; Szabo, S.J.; Glimcher, L.H. T-bet regulates IgG class switching and pathogenic autoantibody production. *Proc. Natl. Acad. Sci. USA* **2002**, *99*, 5545–5550. [CrossRef] [PubMed]
184. Woldemeskel, B.A.; Dykema, A.G.; Garliss, C.C.; Cherfils, S.; Smith, K.N.; Blankson, J.N. CD4+ T cells from COVID-19 mRNA vaccine recipients recognize a conserved epitope present in diverse coronaviruses. *J. Clin. Investig.* **2022**, *132*, e156083. [CrossRef] [PubMed]
185. Yasaka, K.; Yamazaki, T.; Sato, H.; Shirai, T.; Cho, M.; Ishida, K.; Ito, K.; Tanaka, T.; Ogasawara, K.; Harigae, H.; et al. Phospholipase D4 as a signature of toll-like receptor 7 or 9 signaling is expressed on blastic T-bet + B cells in systemic lupus erythematosus. *Arthritis Res. Ther.* **2023**, *25*, 200. [CrossRef] [PubMed]
186. Kalliolias, G.D.; Basdra, E.K.; Papavassiliou, A.G. Targeting TLR Signaling Cascades in Systemic Lupus Erythematosus and Rheumatoid Arthritis: An Update. *Biomedicines* **2024**, *12*, 138. [CrossRef] [PubMed]
187. Patinote, C.; Karroum, N.B.; Moarbess, G.; Cirnat, N.; Kassab, I.; Bonnet, P.A.; Deleuze-Masquéfa, C. Agonist and antagonist ligands of toll-like receptors 7 and 8: Ingenious tools for therapeutic purposes. *Eur. J. Med. Chem.* **2020**, *193*, 112238. [CrossRef]

188. Cenac, C.; Ducatez, M.F.; Guéry, J.-C. Hydroxychloroquine inhibits proteolytic processing of endogenous TLR7 protein in human primary plasmacytoid dendritic cells. *Eur. J. Immunol.* **2022**, *52*, 54–61. [CrossRef]
189. Ewald, S.E.; Lee, B.L.; Lau, L.; Wickliffe, K.E.; Shi, G.-P.; Chapman, H.A.; Barton, G.M. The ectodomain of Toll-like receptor 9 is cleaved to generate a functional receptor. *Nature* **2008**, *456*, 658–662. [CrossRef]
190. Schrezenmeier, E.; Dörner, T. Mechanisms of action of hydroxychloroquine and chloroquine: Implications for rheumatology. *Nat. Rev. Rheumatol.* **2020**, *16*, 155–166. [CrossRef]
191. Guiducci, C.; Gong, M.; Xu, Z.; Gill, M.; Chaussabel, D.; Meeker, T.; Chan, J.H.; Wright, T.; Punaro, M.; Bolland, S.; et al. TLR recognition of self nucleic acids hampers glucocorticoid activity in lupus. *Nature* **2010**, *465*, 937–941. [CrossRef]
192. Deshmukh, A.; Pereira, A.; Geraci, N.; Tzvetkov, E.; Przetak, M.; Catalina, M.D.; Morand, E.F.; Bender, A.T.; Vaidyanathan, B. Preclinical Evidence for the Glucocorticoid-Sparing Potential of a Dual Toll-Like Receptor 7/8 Inhibitor in Autoimmune Diseases. *J. Pharmacol. Exp. Ther.* **2024**, *388*, 751–764. [CrossRef]
193. Shisha, T.; Posch, M.G.; Lehmann, J.; Feifel, R.; Junt, T.; Hawtin, S.; Schuemann, J.; Avrameas, A.; Danekula, R.; Misiolek, P.; et al. First-in-Human Study of the Safety, Pharmacokinetics, and Pharmacodynamics of MHV370, a Dual Inhibitor of Toll-Like Receptors 7 and 8, in Healthy Adults. *Eur. J. Drug Metab. Pharmacokinet.* **2023**, *48*, 553–566. [CrossRef] [PubMed]
194. Hawtin, S.; André, C.; Collignon-Zipfel, G.; Appenzeller, S.; Bannert, B.; Baumgartner, L.; Beck, D.; Betschart, C.; Boulay, T.; Brunner, H.I.; et al. Preclinical characterization of the Toll-like receptor 7/8 antagonist MHV370 for lupus therapy. *Cell Rep. Med.* **2023**, *4*, 101036. [CrossRef] [PubMed]
195. Tojo, S.; Zhang, Z.; Matsui, H.; Tahara, M.; Ikeguchi, M.; Kochi, M.; Kamada, M.; Shigematsu, H.; Tsutsumi, A.; Adachi, N.; et al. Structural analysis reveals TLR7 dynamics underlying antagonism. *Nat. Commun.* **2020**, *11*, 5204. [CrossRef]
196. Ishizaka, S.T.; Hawkins, L.; Chen, Q.; Tago, F.; Yagi, T.; Sakaniwa, K.; Zhang, Z.; Shimizu, T.; Shirato, M. A novel Toll-like receptor 7/8-specific antagonist E6742 ameliorates clinically relevant disease parameters in murine models of lupus. *Eur. J. Pharmacol.* **2023**, *957*, 175962. [CrossRef] [PubMed]
197. Murakami, Y.; Fukui, R.; Tanaka, R.; Motoi, Y.; Kanno, A.; Sato, R.; Yamaguchi, K.; Amano, H.; Furukawa, Y.; Suzuki, H.; et al. Anti-TLR7 Antibody Protects Against Lupus Nephritis in NZBWF1 Mice by Targeting B Cells and Patrolling Monocytes. *Front. Immunol.* **2021**, *12*, 777197. [CrossRef]
198. Achek, A.; Kwon, H.K.; Patra, M.C.; Shah, M.; Hong, R.; Lee, W.H.; Baek, W.Y.; Choi, Y.S.; Kim, G.Y.; Pham, T.L.H.; et al. A peptide derived from the core beta-sheet region of TIRAP decoys TLR4 and reduces inflammatory and autoimmune symptoms in murine models. *EBioMedicine* **2020**, *52*, 102645. [CrossRef] [PubMed]
199. Moroni, G.; Frontini, G.; Ponticelli, C. When and How Is It Possible to Stop Therapy in Patients with Lupus Nephritis: A Narrative Review. *Clin. J. Am. Soc. Nephrol.* **2021**, *16*, 1909–1917. [CrossRef] [PubMed]
200. Le Naour, J.; Kroemer, G. Trial watch: Toll-like receptor ligands in cancer therapy. *OncoImmunology* **2023**, *12*, 2180237. [CrossRef]
201. Srinivasa, A.; Tosounidou, S.; Gordon, C. Increased Incidence of Gastrointestinal Side Effects in Patients Taking Hydroxychloroquine: A Brand-related Issue? *J. Rheumatol.* **2017**, *44*, 398. [CrossRef]
202. Shang, L.; Wang, L.; Shi, X.; Wang, N.; Zhao, L.; Wang, J.; Liu, C. HMGB1 was negatively regulated by HSF1 and mediated the TLR4/MyD88/NF-kappaB signal pathway in asthma. *Life Sci.* **2020**, *241*, 117120. [CrossRef] [PubMed]
203. Xue, J.; Suarez, J.S.; Minaai, M.; Li, S.; Gaudino, G.; Pass, H.I.; Carbone, M.; Yang, H. HMGB1 as a therapeutic target in disease. *J. Cell Physiol.* **2021**, *236*, 3406–3419. [CrossRef] [PubMed]

Disclaimer/Publisher's Note: The statements, opinions and data contained in all publications are solely those of the individual author(s) and contributor(s) and not of MDPI and/or the editor(s). MDPI and/or the editor(s) disclaim responsibility for any injury to people or property resulting from any ideas, methods, instructions or products referred to in the content.

Review

Interplay between the Chaperone System and Gut Microbiota Dysbiosis in Systemic Lupus Erythematosus Pathogenesis: Is Molecular Mimicry the Missing Link between Those Two Factors?

Alessandra Maria Vitale [1,*,†], Letizia Paladino [1,†], Celeste Caruso Bavisotto [1,2], Rosario Barone [1,*], Francesca Rappa [1], Everly Conway de Macario [2,3], Francesco Cappello [1,2], Alberto J. L. Macario [2,3] and Antonella Marino Gammazza [1]

1 Department of Biomedicine, Neurosciences and Advanced Diagnostics (BiND), University of Palermo, 90127 Palermo, Italy; letizia.paladino@unipa.it (L.P.); celeste.carusobavisotto@unipa.it (C.C.B.); francesca.rappa@unipa.it (F.R.); francesco.cappello@unipa.it (F.C.); antonella.marinogammazza@unipa.it (A.M.G.)
2 Euro-Mediterranean Institute of Science and Technology (IEMEST), 90139 Palermo, Italy; econwaydemacario@som.umaryland.edu (E.C.d.M.); ajlmacario@som.umaryland.edu (A.J.L.M.)
3 Department of Microbiology and Immunology, School of Medicine, University of Maryland at Baltimore-Institute of Marine and Environmental Technology (IMET), Baltimore, MD 21202, USA
* Correspondence: alessandramaria.vitale@unipa.it (A.M.V.); rosario.barone@unipa.it (R.B.)
† These authors contributed equally.

Abstract: Systemic lupus erythematosus (SLE) is a multifactorial autoimmune disease characterized by self-immune tolerance breakdown and the production of autoantibodies, causing the deposition of immune complexes and triggering inflammation and immune-mediated damage. SLE pathogenesis involves genetic predisposition and a combination of environmental factors. Clinical manifestations are variable, making an early diagnosis challenging. Heat shock proteins (Hsps), belonging to the chaperone system, interact with the immune system, acting as pro-inflammatory factors, autoantigens, as well as immune tolerance promoters. Increased levels of some Hsps and the production of autoantibodies against them are correlated with SLE onset and progression. The production of these autoantibodies has been attributed to molecular mimicry, occurring upon viral and bacterial infections, since they are evolutionary highly conserved. Gut microbiota dysbiosis has been associated with the occurrence and severity of SLE. Numerous findings suggest that proteins and metabolites of commensal bacteria can mimic autoantigens, inducing autoimmunity, because of molecular mimicry. Here, we propose that shared epitopes between human Hsps and those of gut commensal bacteria cause the production of anti-Hsp autoantibodies that cross-react with human molecules, contributing to SLE pathogenesis. Thus, the involvement of the chaperone system, gut microbiota dysbiosis, and molecular mimicry in SLE ought to be coordinately studied.

Keywords: systemic lupus erythematosus; chaperone system; gut microbiota; leaky gut; autoimmunity; molecular mimicry; chaperonopathy; chaperonotherapy

1. Introduction

The chaperone system (CS) is composed of molecular chaperones, some of which are heat shock proteins (Hsps), co-chaperones, chaperone co-factors, and chaperone interactors and receptors [1]. The canonical functions of the CS are directed to the maintenance of protein homeostasis and, for these functions, it interacts with the ubiquitin-proteasome system (UPS) and with the chaperone-mediated autophagy (CMA) machinery [2–4]. Chaperones perform their canonical functions not alone, as monomers, but in teams, which are oligomers made up of identical subunits, e.g., Hsp60, or constituted of non-identical but similar subunits, e.g., CCT [5–7]. Furthermore, the teams interact between themselves and form functional networks, e.g., Hsp70/DnaK-Hsp40/DnaJ-Prefoldin [8,9].

In the last few years, increasing evidence has pointed out the "other side of the coin" of the CS. In fact, when abnormal in structure/function/location/concentration, its members may become etiopathogenetic factors, causing diseases known as the chaperonopathies [10–12].

The involvement of Hsps in autoimmunity has been investigated for many years, and autoimmune diseases (ADs) can be classified into the group of chaperonopathies by mistake or collaborationism, i.e., acquired chaperonopathies in which a chaperone functions to favor the pathogenic mechanism and leads to disease [5,10–15]. However, their role is still under investigation. They may either promote immune cell activation and pro-inflammatory cytokine production and act as autoantigens eliciting autoantibodies, or perform a pro-immune tolerance restoring activity [16,17]. Depending on the role, Hsps have been proposed for the development of novel therapeutic strategies (positive or negative chaperonotherapy) [18–20]. Among the ADs in which the CS members, especially the Hsps, are believed to play a role is systemic lupus erythematosus (SLE) [21]. SLE is a chronic, multisystemic autoimmune/inflammatory disease affecting almost every organ and tissue of the body, with multiple clinical manifestations ranging from milder symptoms, such as skin rashes or non-erosive arthritis, to more serious and potentially life-threatening complications mostly affecting the kidney and the central nervous system [22–25]. SLE can affect persons of all ages and ethnic groups and both sexes. However, more than 90% of newly diagnosed cases are women in their childbearing years, with a female-to-male ratio of 9–10:1 [26]. On the contrary, men are diagnosed at a more advanced age and often show a more severe phenotype, with an overall higher risk for progression into SLE complications such as lupus nephritis (LN) and end-stage renal disease (ESRD) [26,27].

A distinctive hallmark of SLE is the breakdown of self-tolerance and the production of various autoantibodies, including antinuclear antibodies (ANAs) [28]. The interaction between autoantibodies and self-antigens produces immune complexes, which occur in circulation or localize in multiple tissues, triggering inflammation and complement activation causing immune-mediated organ damage [29]. SLE etiopathogenesis and molecular mechanisms remain largely unknown. However, numerous findings suggest a genetic predisposition to SLE development acting together with a combination of immunological, endocrine, and environmental factors [30–33].

In the last few years, the role of the gut microbiota has been investigated in the etiopathogenesis of SLE and other ADs. A normal/healthy gut microbiota contributes to the development of a functioning immune system [34]. On the contrary, gut microbiota alteration (dysbiosis) can result in the breakdown of immune tolerance, the over-activation of T cells, and the production of pro-inflammatory cytokines. All these events, in turn, can activate autoimmune responses, leading to the development of ADs [34]. Numerous findings suggest that the reason for this relationship may reside in the bacterial metabolites/products translocation from the intestinal lumen into the circulation because of increased intestinal permeability [35].

Here, we provide an overview of the involvement of the CS and gut microbiota dysbiosis in SLE pathogenesis, suggesting molecular mimicry as a potential link between them. A detailed understanding of the relationship between these three factors will likely contribute to the identification of novel promising biomarkers and therapeutic targets.

2. The Chaperone System and SLE

The role of the CS in SLE etiopathogenesis is multifaceted and not yet fully understood. Three conditions have elicited particular interest: (i) Hsps' overexpression; (ii) the production of anti-Hsp autoantibodies, and (iii) Hsps' presence on the surface of peripheral blood mononuclear cells (PBMCs), which correlates with high disease activity [36,37].

Higher levels of Hsp90 were found in PBMCs of patients with active SLE compared to patients with inactive disease, age- and sex-matched healthy controls, or patients who suffered from rheumatoid arthritis [38,39]. Similarly, Hsp70 levels were found to be elevated in PBMCs from SLE patients compared with those from healthy age- and sex-matched volunteers [38]. However, there was no correlation between the two Hsps, and only Hsp90 levels positively correlated with disease activity and onset [40]. The early increased levels of Hsp90 in some SLE patients is primarily dependent upon the enhanced transcription of the *HSP90β* gene, suggesting the activation of a specific gene program underlying the pathogenic mechanism of the disease [40–42]. On the contrary, the later elevation of Hsp70 levels is attributed to a stress response against the ongoing disease process [40,42]. Similarly to Hsp70, Hsp27 levels are also associated with disease activity. Both Hsp70 and Hsp27 levels were investigated in the renal tissue of patients with different forms of LN (diffuse proliferative, focal proliferative, and membranous) and were found within the cytoplasm of tubular epithelial cells of all patients [40]. A significant positive correlation was found between Hsp27 levels and disease severity in patients with diffuse proliferative nephritis [43].

PBMCs (lymphocytes and monocytes) from SLE patients not only had elevated intracellular levels of Hsp90, but also elevated levels on their surface, suggesting its role as an autoantigen leading to the production of autoantibodies [44,45]. Autoantibodies (IgM and IgG) against Hsp90 were found in the sera from a significant proportion of patients with SLE, both adults and children, compared to healthy controls [46–48]. Adults carrying higher antibody levels were more likely to have renal disease following an intense deposition of the protein in subepithelial, subendothelial, and mesangial areas of the glomeruli [47,49].

Higher levels of Hsp90 and anti-Hsp90 autoantibodies in the sera from SLE patients were also associated with higher levels of IL6 [50]. Both IL6 and IL10 have been found to be higher in SLE patients and positively correlated with disease activity and complications [51–53]. Both cytokines induce the transcription of the *HSP90β* gene in cultured PBMCs [54,55]. Elevation of these cytokines in SLE patients may induce an increase in Hsp90 levels, both intracellularly and on the surface of cells, which, in turn, leads to autoantibody production [55,56]. These results suggest that Hsp90 contributes to disease onset and progression, and to the establishment of inflammation. Therefore, targeting Hsp90 to diminish its levels may be a promising therapeutic treatment to delay disease progression [57]. For instance, in an SLE mouse model, it was observed that chemical treatment targeting the surface translocation of gp96 diminished and alleviated SLE-associated manifestations, like glomerulonephritis, proteinuria, and levels of antinuclear and DNA antibodies. All of this was accompanied by a reduction in the maturation of dendritic cells (DCs) and antigen-presenting cells, and by the activation of B and T cells [58]. The administration of a DNA vaccine encoding Hsp90 induced tolerogenic immune responses, with a reduction in anti-dsDNA autoantibody production, that limited SLE manifestations (e.g., renal disease) and extended the survival in lupus-prone mice [59]. Similar outcomes were obtained using a DNA vaccine encoding Hsp70 [60].

All these results suggest that chaperonotherapy may be effective, namely, a treatment strategy consisting of inhibiting/eliminating (negative chaperonotherapy) or boosting/replacing (positive chaperonotherapy) the pathogenic chaperone. For instance, it has been reported that the small heat shock protein (sHsp), alpha-B crystallin (HSPB5; CRYAB), attenuates the severity and disease progression of LN in lupus-prone mice (positive chaperonopathy) [18,61].

3. The Gut Microbiota in SLE

The gut microbiota is a complex population composed of a large number of commensal microorganisms (some estimates reach 100 trillion) residing in the gastrointestinal tract, which has co-evolved with its host and provides benefits to it in multiple ways, including digestion, the production of nutrients, and detoxification, ensuring a complex and mutual beneficial relationship [62]. The gut microbiota plays a key role in the biology and homeostasis of cells of the innate and adaptive immune system. Therefore, an imbalance in the quantity and/or quality of its composition, including a loss of beneficial bacteria, an excessive growth of potentially harmful bacteria, or a loss of overall bacterial diversity, i.e., dysbiosis, may trigger autoimmunity [34,63–65]. Dysbiosis has been primarily associated with inflammatory bowel diseases (IBDs), such as Crohn's disease (CD) and ulcerative colitis (UC) [66]. Several studies have demonstrated the association between an imbalance of the gut microbiota and the etiopathogenesis of extra-intestinal diseases, including autoimmune diseases such as SLE [67–70].

The dynamics of the gut microbiota has been investigated in a murine lupus-prone model, and differences in the composition and overall diversity were found compared to healthy controls [71]. The gut microbiota was different in males as compared to females, with an over-representation of *Lachnospiraceae* in females that was associated with an earlier onset and more severe manifestation of SLE [71,72]. This was taken as evidence that sex affects the disease course, likely because of the control exerted by sex hormones in the regulation of the immune system. The use of probiotic lactobacilli and retinoic acid as dietary supplements improved symptoms, suggesting that this type of treatment could be efficacious in relieving inflammatory flares in lupus patients [71].

In a mouse LN model, the lack of *Lactobacillus* occurred before (not after) disease onset, suggesting its involvement in disease pathogenesis, and conversely, restoration of the *Lactobacillus* population enhanced the gut mucosal barrier, suppressed gut inflammation, and attenuated LN, prolonging mice survival [73]. However, *Lactobacillus* played an opposite role in studies performed with different lupus mouse models. For instance, the gut microbiota changed before and after disease onset in lupus-prone mice, with an increase in specific genera during disease progression [74]. A positive correlation between the abundance of *Lactobacillus* species and poorer renal function and higher-level systemic autoimmunity was observed.

The association between gut microbiota dysbiosis and SLE pathogenesis has a genetic basis, since fecal microbiome transplantation from SLE mice induced significant changes in immune cell distribution and overall changes in their genetic profiles, with an upregulation of certain lupus susceptibility genes [75]. Similarly, in humans, clear differences in the composition and richness of the gut microbiota were also observed between SLE patients and healthy controls, and numerous findings have suggested that gut microbiota dysbiosis is one of the mechanisms underlying SLE pathogenesis (Figure 1) [76–83].

A human healthy gut microbiota primarily consists of the phyla Firmicutes, Bacteroidetes, Actinobacteria, Proteobacteria, Fusobacteria, and Verrucomicrobia, with Firmicutes and Bacteroidetes being the most abundant [84–87]. The Firmicutes/Bacteroidetes ratio is altered in various disorders [88,89] and is affected by the diet [90]. In SLE patients, marked dysbiosis was observed, with a significant decrease in the Firmicutes/Bacteroidetes ratio as compared with healthy controls (HCs) [76–78,83], and with the enrichment of the phylum Proteobacteria [74,77,80,82]. The reduced Firmicutes/Bacteroidetes ratio in SLE patients was correlated with lymphocyte activation and Th17 differentiation from naïve CD4(+) lymphocytes, favoring inflammatory mechanisms [78]. Conversely, the enrichment of the gut microbiota with bacterial strains belonging to the Firmicutes phylum reduced the IL-17/IFNγ balance and prevented the over-activation of CD4$^+$ lymphocytes. This suggests that supplementation with probiotics containing Treg-inducer strains able to restore the Treg/Th17/Th1 balance would be a beneficial treatment for SLE patients [78]. An imbalance of pro-inflammatory and anti-inflammatory T cells in SLE patients was observed that was correlated to changes in the intestinal microbial population [82].

Differences in gut microbiota dysbiosis were observed in SLE patients with active disease compared to those with inactive disease. For instance, an abundance of the genera *Streptococcus*, *Campylobacter*, and *Veillonella* and a decrease in the genus *Bifidobacterium* were observed [79]. Other authors have reported increased *Desulfovibrio piger*, *Bacteroides thetaiotaomicron*, and *Ruminococcus gnavus* species and decreased Bacilli class and *Ruminococcaceae* and *Lactobacillaceae* families in active SLE patients compared to inactive SLE patients [83]. However, one study found no significant differences in the *Firmicutes/Bacteroidetes* ratio between SLE patients and healthy controls [74], confirming the high variability in the human gut microbiota already observed in mouse models and the impossibility to outline a universally valid profile that would distinguish SLE patients from healthy controls.

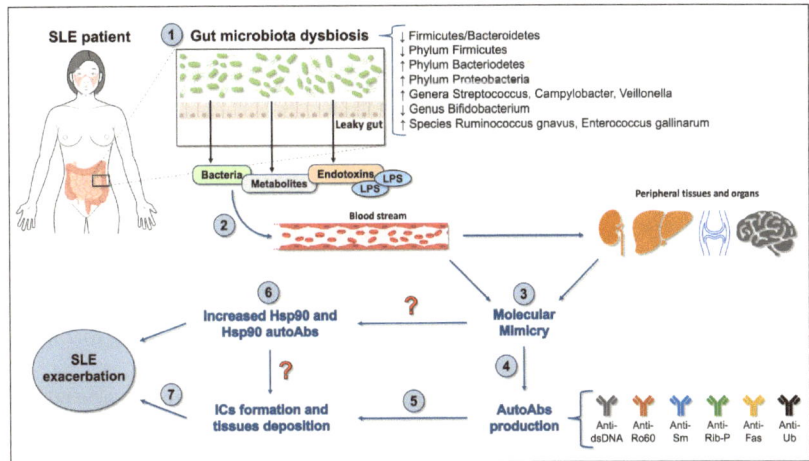

Figure 1. An overview of the role of the gut microbiota in SLE. Gut microbiota dysbiosis in SLE patients shows a significant reduction in both the richness and diversity of the gut microbiota, including a lower Firmicutes/Bacteroidetes ratio (1). Gut microbiota dysbiosis may cause an increase in intestinal permeability (leaky gut) and favor the translocation of pathogens and their products/metabolites from the intestinal lumen to the systemic circulation and thereby to other organs (2), resulting in inflammation and antigenic cross-reactivity via the mechanism of molecular mimicry (3). The translocation of the gut commensal autoantigen-mimicking peptides induces the production of autoantibodies, such as anti-Ro60, anti-Sm, anti-dsDNA, anti-Rib-P, anti-Fas, and anti-Ub, as shown (4). These antibodies cross-react with self-antigens, forming immune complexes that deposit in peripheral tissues (5), exacerbating SLE conditions (7). This event could explain the increase in the Hsp and anti-Hsp antibody levels observed both in the circulation and in the peripheral tissues of SLE patients (6). Abbreviations: AutoAbs, autoantibodies; Anti-dsDNA, anti-double-stranded DNA; Anti-Fas, Anti- FS-7-associated surface antigen; Anti-Rib-P, anti-ribosomal-P; Anti-Ro60, RNA-binding 60 kDa Ro; Anti-Sm, anti-Smith; AntiUb, anti-ubiquitin; LPS, lipopolysaccharide; SLE, systemic lupus erythematosus.

4. Molecular Mimicry, Hsps, and Gut Microbiota Dysbiosis in SLE

The breakdown of self-tolerance plays a critical role in the occurrence and development of SLE, leading to the production of autoantibodies and the formation of cytotoxic immune complexes triggering immune and inflammatory responses [28]. All these events are common among different autoimmune conditions and may be triggered by an infection via the molecular mimicry mechanism [91]. The term molecular mimicry describes the sharing of antigens between a parasite and its host, which facilitates the evasion of the host's immune response and the establishment of immunological tolerance [92]. In recent years, the phenomenon was often associated with autoimmunity. Amino acid sequence or structural similarities between foreign antigens and self-antigens may favor the activation of autoreactive T or B cells, resulting in autoimmune responses in some susceptible individuals [93]. The hypothesis of post-infection pathogenic events caused by molecular mimicry has been proposed to explain SLE etiopathogenesis, and various pathogens have been identified as possible culprits [94–98].

The evolutionary conservation of Hsps in prokaryotes and eukaryotes suggests the involvement of a molecular mimicry mechanism in the production of anti-Hsp autoantibodies in a variety of autoreactive disorders, including SLE [99,100]. For instance, high cross-reactivity was reported between isolated SLE IgGs and Hsp70 and other intracellular proteins from *Mycobacterium tuberculosis* [101]. The sera from SLE patients contain IgGs that bind to Hsp60 present on the surface of epithelial cells, favoring phosphatidylserine exposure and cell apoptosis [102]. Also, proteins and metabolites of commensal bacteria of the gut can mimic autoantigens and induce autoimmunity through molecular mimicry [35]. The impairment of the barrier function of the intestinal epithelium, which augments intestinal permeability (leaky gut), may favor the translocation of bacteria and bacterial components, such as lipopolysaccharides (LPSs) and endotoxins, from the intestinal lumen to the systemic circulation which thereby reach other organs [103]. These bacterial components, in turn, may act as cross-reactive autoantigens and trigger autoimmune responses in hosts carrying high-risk human leukocyte antigen (HLA) genes [35,103]. For instance, numerous findings have suggested that gut commensal microbes may mimic retinal antigen(s), favoring the production of autoreactive T cells, triggering autoimmune uveitis [104]. In synovia and PBMCs from patients affected by rheumatoid arthritis, two autoantigens, N-acetylglucosamine-6-sulfatase and filamin A, targeted by T and B cells have been found [105]. Both antigens show high sequence homology with epitopes of some gut commensals, suggesting that immunological triggers at mucosal sites, such as the gut microbiota, may promote autoimmunity that affects joints, likely via the molecular mimicry mechanism [100]. A microbial peptide shared by several major classes of bacteria including *Escherichia coli*, which is one of the most common commensal bacteria of the human gut microbiota, can induce multiple sclerosis (MS)-like disease in humanized mice by cross-reacting with a T cell receptor that recognizes a peptide from myelin basic protein acting as candidate MS autoantigen [106]. Similarly, a peptide from *E. coli* has been demonstrated to induce autoimmune pancreatitis, likely by mimicking some self-antigens [107].

Increasing evidence suggests that a leaky gut is present in some, if not all, SLE patients, allowing pathogens and their products/metabolites to leak out from the gut lumen and penetrate the blood stream, reaching other organs and triggering inflammation and autoimmunity through the mechanism of molecular mimicry (Figure 1) [108]. The earliest anti-nuclear autoantibodies detected in SLE patients target the RNA-binding 60 kDa Ro protein and their production may be driven by Ro60 orthologs produced by commensal bacteria from different niches in genetic susceptible individuals through aberrant cross-reactive immune responses [109]. This hypothesis is supported by the observation that colonization of germ-free mice with *Bacteroides thetaiotaomicron* containing Ro60 ortholog caused T and B cell responses against human Ro60 and glomerular immune complex deposition [109]. The gut of SLE patients has an overall higher representation of *Ruminococcus gnavus* [83]. Anti-dsDNA autoantibodies cross-react with antigens from a *Ruminococcus gnavus* strain, contributing to the immune pathogenesis of LN, which suggests the possibility of developing a biomarker assay with diagnostic and prognostic value to assess the risk of LN [110]. In the sera from SLE patients, a significant positive correlation between higher titers of anti-*Enterococcus gallinarum* IgGs and the presence of autoantibodies, including anti-Ribosomal P (anti-Rib-P), anti-dsDNA, and anti-Smith (anti-Sm) autoantibodies, has been observed [111]. Moreover, *E. gallinarum* was detected in liver biopsies from lupus and autoimmune hepatitis patients, demonstrating that a gut pathobiont can translocate and promote autoimmunity in genetically predisposed hosts [112]. In a cohort of untreated SLE patients, numerous autoantigen-mimicking microbial peptides have been identified [81]. A peptide-mimicking human Fas antigen from *Akkermansia muciniphila* was found to bind to the IgGs produced by memory B cells from a subgroup of SLE patients, but not those from healthy controls [81]. *Bacteroides fragilis* is a Gram-negative obligate anaerobic bacterium of the normal human gut microbiota. *B. fragilis* ubiquitin (BfUb) shares 63% identity and more than 99% structural similarity with human ubiquitin (hUb) [113]. It has been reported that the sera from patients suffering from various ADs, including SLE and RA, contain higher levels of antibodies to BfUb compared to healthy volunteers, suggesting that molecular mimicry of hUb by BfUb could be a trigger for autoimmunity [113].

To date, no definitive data exist in the literature proving that the autoimmune response against endogenous Hsps in SLE patients may be caused by dysbiosis of the gut microbiota, accompanied by leaky gut, mediated by a molecular mimicry mechanism. However, this hypothesis is plausible because of the high similarity between human and bacterial Hsps. Moreover, numerous findings have demonstrated that the cross-reactivity between human and gut microbial Hsps is involved in the development of other autoimmune conditions. For example, IgG autoantibodies against human mitochondrial Hsp60 were significantly higher in the sera of patients with rheumatic autoimmune diseases, including SLE, than in healthy controls, and it was suggested that the antibodies were produced because GroEL, the *E. coli* Hsp60, shares immunogenic–antigenic epitopes with the mitochondrial chaperonin [114,115]. Microorganisms isolated from the jejunal mucosa of individuals affected by Kawasaki disease produce large amounts of Hsp60 and elicit the production of endogenous Hsp60 [116]. In turn, both bacterial and human Hsp60 molecules induce the activation of the immune system, triggering an inflammatory response against blood vessels typical of the disease [116]. It has been suggested that T cells specific to gut bacterial Hsps could cross-react against endogenous Hsps overexpressed in retinal ganglion cells and axons from glaucomatous mice and human glaucoma patients in response to elevated intraocular pressure, leading to progressive neurodegeneration in the eye [117].

A similar cross-reactivity mechanism between bacterial and human Hsps could cause the production of the autoantibodies against Hsp90 and Hsp70 found in SLE patients. The two chaperones occur both in bacteria and in humans with a high sequence similarity and are known to be immunogenic [118,119].

5. Conclusions and Future Perspectives

The SLE clinical manifestations can vary widely from individual to individual, ranging from milder symptoms to more severe and life-threatening ones. Because of this heterogeneity in phenotypes and clinical manifestations, which often mimic those of other conditions, and the lack of clear and robust diagnostic criteria, the diagnosis of SLE is still challenging, and the consequent diagnostic delay often prevents the timely choice of appropriate treatment, worsening both short- and long-term outcomes [120–122]. Therefore, identification of novel, strong, and unique biomarkers for early and accurate diagnosis could improve disease management and lead to personalized therapeutic interventions with tolerable side effects and curative results. To identify these biomarkers, knowledge of the factors involved in SLE pathogenesis is necessary.

Autoantibodies circulating in body fluids or forming immune complexes in peripheral tissues have been used as valuable diagnostic and prognostic biomarkers in SLE for predicting pathogenic pathways and for guiding therapeutic treatments [123,124]. Therefore, in recent years, several efforts have been made to improve the detection of autoantibodies. Synthetic peptides mimicking post-translationally modified autoantigens have been successfully used for the development of specific in vitro diagnostic/prognostic assays of autoimmune diseases, including SLE [125]. Moreover, the use of post-translationally modified peptides has allowed identification of autoantibodies associated with the most severe phenotypes [126].

Another way to make progress in this area is to research the immune mechanisms underlying the SLE pathogenesis. Here, we offer an overview of the involvement of two apparently independent and not interconnected factors in SLE etiopathogenesis, i.e., the CS and gut microbiota dysbiosis. Molecular mimicry could be the link between these two factors, whose pathogenicity in SLE is currently under scrutiny. Therefore, a comparison of primary and higher-order structures of components of the CS in human and gut microbes, which for instance may be facilitated by in silico analysis [127], could allow us to further elucidate the role of molecular mimicry in SLE. In this way, it may be possible to obtain new insights into disease pathogenesis and to develop novel and more efficacious therapeutic interventions that, for instance, could be based on the inhibition of the activity of the pathogenic Hsp(s) (negative chaperonotherapy).

Author Contributions: A.M.V., F.C. and A.M.G.: conceptualization; A.M.V., L.P., C.C.B., R.B., F.R. and A.M.G.: writing—original draft preparation; A.M.V., E.C.d.M., F.C.; A.J.L.M. and A.M.G.: writing—review and editing; A.M.V. and L.P.: figure preparation and editing; F.C and A.M.G.: supervision. All authors have read and agreed to the published version of the manuscript.

Funding: This research received no external funding.

Conflicts of Interest: The authors declare no conflicts of interest.

References

1. Macario, A.J.L.; Conway de Macario, E. Chaperone proteins and chaperonopathies. In *Stress: Physiology, Biochemistry, and Pathology. Handbook of Stress Series*; Fink, G., Ed.; Elsevier/Academic Press: Cambridge, MA, USA, 2019; Volume 3, Chapter 12; pp. 135–152.
2. Carlisle, C.; Prill, K.; Pilgrim, D. Chaperones and the proteasome system: Regulating the construction and demolition of striated muscle. *Int. J. Mol. Sci.* **2017**, *19*, 32. [CrossRef] [PubMed]
3. Kocaturk, N.M.; Gozuacik, D. Crosstalk between mammalian autophagy and the ubiquitin-proteasome system. *Front. Cell. Dev. Biol.* **2018**, *6*, 128. [CrossRef] [PubMed]
4. Margulis, B.; Tsimokha, A.; Zubova, S.; Guzhova, I. Molecular chaperones and proteolytic machineries regulate protein homeostasis in aging cells. *Cells* **2020**, *9*, 1308. [CrossRef] [PubMed]
5. Macario, A.J.L.; Conway de Macario, E.; Cappello, F. *The Chaperonopathies. Diseases with Defective Molecular Chaperones*; Springer: Dordrecht, The Netherlands, 2013.
6. Willison, K.R. The structure and evolution of eukaryotic chaperonin-containing TCP-1 and its mechanism that folds actin into a protein spring. *Biochem. J.* **2018**, *475*, 3009–3034. [CrossRef] [PubMed]
7. Dahiya, V.; Buchner, J. Functional principles and regulation of molecular chaperones. *Adv. Protein Chem. Struct. Biol.* **2019**, *114*, 1–60. [PubMed]
8. Gestaut, D.; Roh, S.H.; Ma, B.; Pintilie, G.; Joachimiak, L.A.; Leitner, A.; Walzthoeni, T.; Aebersold, R.; Chiu, W.; Frydman, J. The chaperonin TRiC/CCT associates with prefoldin through a conserved electrostatic interface essential for cellular proteostasis. *Cell* **2019**, *177*, 751–765.e15. [CrossRef] [PubMed]
9. Havalová, H.; Ondrovičová, G.; Keresztesová, B.; Bauer, J.A.; Pevala, V.; Kutejová, E.; Kunová, N. Mitochondrial HSP70 chaperone system-the influence of post-translational modifications and involvement in human diseases. *Int. J. Mol. Sci.* **2021**, *22*, 8077. [CrossRef] [PubMed]
10. Macario, A.J.L.; Conway de Macario, E. Sick chaperones, cellular stress, and disease. *N. Engl. J. Med.* **2005**, *353*, 1489–1501. [CrossRef] [PubMed]
11. David, S.; Vitale, A.M.; Fucarino, A.; Scalia, F.; Vergilio, G.; Conway de Macario, E.; Macario, A.J.L.; Caruso Bavisotto, C.; Pitruzzella, A. The challenging riddle about the janus-type role of Hsp60 and related extracellular vesicles and miRNAs in carcinogenesis and the promises of its solution. *Appl. Sci.* **2021**, *11*, 1175. [CrossRef]
12. Paladino, L.; Vitale, A.M.; Santonocito, R.; Pitruzzella, A.; Cipolla, C.; Graceffa, G.; Bucchieri, F.; Conway de Macario, E.; Macario, A.J.L.; Rappa, F. Molecular Chaperones and Thyroid Cancer. *Int. J. Mol. Sci.* **2021**, *22*, 4196. [CrossRef]
13. Gaston, J.S. Are heat shock proteins involved in autoimmunity? *Int. J. Clin. Lab. Res.* **1992**, *22*, 90–94. [CrossRef] [PubMed]
14. Kaufmann, S.H. Heat shock proteins and autoimmunity: A critical appraisal. *Int. Arch. Allergy Immunol.* **1994**, *103*, 317–322. [CrossRef] [PubMed]
15. Rajaiah, R.; Moudgil, K.D. Heat-shock proteins can promote as well as regulate autoimmunity. *Autoimmun. Rev.* **2009**, *8*, 388–393. [CrossRef] [PubMed]
16. van Eden, W.; Jansen, M.A.A.; Ludwig, I.; van Kooten, P.; van der Zee, R.; Broere, F. The enigma of heat shock proteins in immune tolerance. *Front. Immunol.* **2017**, *8*, 1599. [CrossRef] [PubMed]
17. Androvitsanea, A.; Stylianou, K.; Drosataki, E.; Petrakis, I. The pathophysiological role of heat shock response in autoimmunity: A literature review. *Cells* **2021**, *10*, 2626. [CrossRef]
18. Cappello, F.; Marino Gammazza, A.; Palumbo Piccionello, A.; Campanella, C.; Pace, A.; Conway de Macario, E.; Macario, A.J.L. Hsp60 chaperonopathies and chaperonotherapy: Targets and agents. *Expert Opin. Ther. Targets* **2014**, *18*, 185–208. [CrossRef] [PubMed]
19. Tukaj, S.; Kaminski, M. Heat shock proteins in the therapy of autoimmune diseases: Too simple to be true? *Cell Stress Chaperones* **2019**, *24*, 475–479. [CrossRef]
20. Zummo, L.; Vitale, A.M.; Caruso Bavisotto, C.; De Curtis, M.; Garbelli, R.; Giallonardo, A.T.; Di Bonaventura, C.; Fanella, M.; Conway de Macario, E.; Cappello, F.; et al. Molecular chaperones and miRNAs in epilepsy: Pathogenic implications and therapeutic prospects. *Int. J. Mol. Sci.* **2021**, *22*, 8601. [CrossRef] [PubMed]
21. Latchman, D.S.; Isenberg, D.A. The role of Hsp90 in SLE. *Autoimmunity* **1994**, *19*, 211–218. [CrossRef]
22. Kuper, B.C.; Failla, S. Systemic lupus erythematosus: A multisystem autoimmune disorder. *Nurs. Clin. N. Am.* **2000**, *35*, 253–265. [CrossRef]
23. Rahman, A.; Isenberg, D.A. Systemic lupus erythematosus. *N. Engl. J. Med.* **2008**, *358*, 929–939. [CrossRef] [PubMed]
24. Cojocaru, M.; Cojocaru, I.M.; Silosi, I.; Vrabie, C.D. Manifestations of systemic lupus erythematosus. *Maedica* **2011**, *6*, 330–336. [PubMed]
25. Doria, A.; Iaccarino, L.; Ghirardello, A.; Zampieri, S.; Arienti, S.; Sarzi-Puttini, P.; Atzeni, F.; Piccoli, A.; Todesco, S. Long-term prognosis and causes of death in systemic lupus erythematosus. *Am. J. Med.* **2006**, *119*, 700–706. [CrossRef] [PubMed]

26. Ramírez Sepúlveda, J.I.; Bolin, K.; Mofors, J.; Leonard, D.; Svenungsson, E.; Jönsen, A.; Bengtsson, C.; DISSECT Consortium; Nordmark, G.; Rantapää Dahlqvist, S.; et al. Sex differences in clinical presentation of systemic lupus erythematosus. *Biol. Sex Differ.* **2019**, *10*, 60. [CrossRef]
27. Wolf, B.; Blaschke, C.R.K.; Mungaray, S.; Weselman, B.T.; Stefanenko, M.; Fedoriuk, M.; Bai, H.; Rodgers, J.; Palygin, O.; Drake, R.R.; et al. Metabolic markers and association of biological sex in lupus nephritis. *Int. J. Mol. Sci.* **2023**, *24*, 16490. [CrossRef] [PubMed]
28. Woods, M.; Zou, Y.R.; Davidson, A. Defects in germinal center selection in SLE. *Front. Immunol.* **2015**, *6*, 425. [CrossRef] [PubMed]
29. Herrmann, M.; Voll, R.E.; Kalden, J.R. Etiopathogenesis of systemic lupus erythematosus. *Immunol. Today* **2000**, *21*, 424–426. [CrossRef] [PubMed]
30. Ramos, P.S.; Brown, E.E.; Kimberly, R.P.; Langefeld, C.D. Genetic factors predisposing to systemic lupus erythematosus and lupus nephritis. *Semin. Nephrol.* **2010**, *30*, 164–176. [CrossRef] [PubMed]
31. Kamen, D.L. Environmental influences on systemic lupus erythematosus expression. *Rheum. Dis. Clin. N. Am.* **2014**, *40*, 401–412. [CrossRef]
32. Pan, L.; Lu, M.P.; Wang, J.H.; Xu, M.; Yang, S.R. Immunological pathogenesis and treatment of systemic lupus erythematosus. *World J. Pediatr.* **2020**, *16*, 19–30. [CrossRef]
33. Woo, J.M.P.; Parks, C.G.; Jacobsen, S.; Costenbader, K.H.; Bernatsky, S. The role of environmental exposures and gene-environment interactions in the etiology of systemic lupus erythematosus. *J. Intern. Med.* **2022**, *291*, 755–778. [CrossRef] [PubMed]
34. Wu, H.J.; Wu, E. The role of gut microbiota in immune homeostasis and autoimmunity. *Gut Microbes.* **2012**, *3*, 4–14. [CrossRef] [PubMed]
35. Garabatos, N.; Santamaria, P. Gut microbial antigenic mimicry in autoimmunity. *Front. Immunol.* **2022**, *13*, 873607. [CrossRef] [PubMed]
36. Dhillon, V.; Latchman, D.; Isenberg, D. Heat shock proteins and systemic lupus erythematosus. *Lupus* **1991**, *1*, 3–8. [CrossRef] [PubMed]
37. Stephanou, A.; Latchman, D.S.; Isenberg, D.A. The regulation of heat shock proteins and their role in systemic lupus erythematosus. *Semin. Arthritis Rheum.* **1998**, *28*, 155–162. [CrossRef]
38. Deguchi, Y.; Negoro, S.; Kishimoto, S. Heat-shock protein synthesis by human peripheral mononuclear cells from SLE patients. *Biochem. Biophys. Res. Commun.* **1987**, *148*, 1063–1068. [CrossRef]
39. Norton, P.M.; Isenberg, D.A.; Latchman, D.S. Elevated levels of the 90 kd heat shock protein in a proportion of SLE patients with active disease. *J. Autoimmun.* **1989**, *2*, 187–195. [CrossRef] [PubMed]
40. Dhillon, V.B.; McCallum, S.; Norton, P.; Twomey, B.M.; Erkeller-Yuksel, F.; Lydyard, P.; Isenberg, D.A.; Latchman, D.S. Differential heat shock protein overexpression and its clinical relevance in systemic lupus erythematosus. *Ann. Rheum. Dis.* **1993**, *52*, 436–442. [CrossRef] [PubMed]
41. Twomey, B.M.; Dhillon, V.B.; McCallum, S.; Isenberg, D.A.; Latchman, D.S. Elevated levels of the 90 kD heat shock protein in patients with systemic lupus erythematosus are dependent upon enhanced transcription of the hsp90 beta gene. *J. Autoimmun.* **1993**, *6*, 495–506. [CrossRef]
42. Faulds, G.B.; Isenberg, D.A.; Latchman, D.S. The tissue specific elevation in synthesis of the 90 kDa heat shock protein precedes the onset of disease in lupus prone MRL/lpr mice. *J. Rheumatol.* **1994**, *21*, 234–238.
43. Tsagalis, G.C.; Nikolopoulou, N.; Sotsiou, F.; Hadjiconstantinou, V. The expression of heat shock proteins 27 and 70 in lupus nephritis. *Hosp. Chron.* **2006**, *1*, 125–129.
44. Minota, S.; Winfield, J.B. IgG anti-lymphocyte antibodies in systemic lupus erythematosus react with surface molecules shared by peripheral T cells and a primitive T cell line. *J. Immunol.* **1987**, *138*, 1750–1756. [CrossRef] [PubMed]
45. Erkeller-Yüksel, F.M.; Isenberg, D.A.; Dhillon, V.B.; Latchman, D.S.; Lydyard, P.M. Surface expression of heat shock protein 90 by blood mononuclear cells from patients with systemic lupus erythematosus. *J. Autoimmun.* **1992**, *5*, 803–814. [CrossRef] [PubMed]
46. Minota, S.; Koyasu, S.; Yahara, I.; Winfield, J. Autoantibodies to the heat-shock protein Hsp90 in systemic lupus erythematosus. *J. Clin. Investig.* **1988**, *81*, 106–109. [CrossRef] [PubMed]
47. Conroy, S.E.; Faulds, G.B.; Williams, W.; Latchman, D.S.; Isenberg, D.A. Detection of autoantibodies to the 90 kDa heat shock protein in systemic lupus erythematosus and other autoimmune diseases. *Br. J. Rheumatol.* **1994**, *33*, 923–926. [CrossRef] [PubMed]
48. Conroy, S.E.; Tucker, L.; Latchman, D.S.; Isenberg, D.A. Incidence of anti Hsp 90 and 70 antibodies in children with SLE, juvenile dermatomyositis and juvenile chronic arthritis. *Clin. Exp. Rheumatol.* **1996**, *14*, 99–104. [PubMed]
49. Kenderov, A.; Minkova, V.; Mihailova, D.; Giltiay, N.; Kyurkchiev, S.; Kehayov, I.; Kazatchkine, M.; Kaveri, S.; Pashov, A. Lupus-specific kidney deposits of HSP90 are associated with altered IgG idiotypic interactions of anti-HSP90 autoantibodies. *Clin. Exp. Immunol.* **2002**, *129*, 169–176. [CrossRef] [PubMed]
50. Ripley, B.J.; Isenberg, D.A.; Latchman, D.S. Elevated levels of the 90 kDa heat shock protein (Hsp90) in SLE correlate with levels of IL-6 and autoantibodies to hsp90. *J. Autoimmun.* **2001**, *17*, 341–346. [CrossRef]
51. Linker-Israeli, M.; Deans, R.J.; Wallace, D.J.; Prehn, J.; Ozeri-Chen, T.; Klinenberg, J.R. Elevated levels of endogenous IL-6 in systemic lupus erythematosus. A putative role in pathogenesis. *J. Immunol.* **1991**, *147*, 117–123. [CrossRef]
52. Park, Y.B.; Lee, S.K.; Kim, D.S.; Lee, J.; Lee, C.H.; Song, C.H. Elevated interleukin-10 levels correlated with disease activity in systemic lupus erythematosus. *Clin. Exp. Rheumatol.* **1998**, *16*, 283–288.

53. Mercader-Salvans, J.; García-González, M.; Gómez-Bernal, F.; Quevedo-Abeledo, J.C.; de Vera-González, A.; González-Delgado, A.; López-Mejías, R.; Martín-González, C.; González-Gay, M.Á.; Ferraz-Amaro, I. Relationship between Disease Characteristics and Circulating Interleukin 6 in a Well-characterized cohort of patients with systemic lupus erythematosus. *Int J. Mol. Sci.* **2023**, *24*, 14006. [CrossRef] [PubMed]
54. Stephanou, A.; Amin, V.; Isenberg, D.A.; Akira, S.; Kishimoto, T.; Latchman, D.S. Interleukin 6 activates heat-shock protein 90β gene expression. *Biochem. J.* **1997**, *321*, 103–106. [CrossRef] [PubMed]
55. Ripley, B.J.; Stephanou, A.; Isenberg, D.A.; Latchman, D.S. Interleukin-10 activates heat-shock protein 90β gene expression. *Immunology* **1999**, *97*, 226–231. [CrossRef] [PubMed]
56. Stephanou, A.; Conroy, S.; Isenberg, D.A.; Maione, D.; Poli, V.; Ciliberto, G.; Latchman, D.S. Elevation of IL-6 in transgenic mice results in increased levels of the 90 kDa heat shock protein (Hsp90) and the production of anti-Hsp90 antibodies. *J. Autoimmun.* **1998**, *11*, 249–253. [CrossRef] [PubMed]
57. Shukla, H.D.; Pitha, P.M. Role of Hsp90 in systemic lupus erythematosus and its clinical relevance. *Autoimmune Dis.* **2012**, *2012*, 728605. [CrossRef] [PubMed]
58. Han, J.M.; Kwon, N.H.; Lee, J.Y.; Jeong, S.J.; Jung, H.J.; Kim, H.R.; Li, Z.; Kim, S. Identification of gp96 as a novel target for treatment of autoimmune disease in mice. *PLoS ONE* **2010**, *5*, e9792. [CrossRef] [PubMed]
59. Liu, A.; Shi, F.D.; Cohen, I.R.; Castaldo, G.; Matarese, G.; Quintana, F.J.; La Cava, A. DNA vaccine encoding heat shock protein 90 protects from murine lupus. *Arthritis Res. Ther.* **2020**, *22*, 152. [CrossRef] [PubMed]
60. Liu, A.; Ferretti, C.; Shi, F.D.; Cohen, I.R.; Quintana, F.J.; La Cava, A. DNA vaccination with Hsp70 protects against systemic lupus erythematosus in (NZB × NZW)F1 mice. *Arthritis Rheumatol.* **2020**, *72*, 997–1002. [CrossRef]
61. Berg, S.I.T.; Knapp, J.; Braunstein, M.; Shirriff, C. The small heat shock protein HSPB5 attenuates the severity of lupus nephritis in lupus-prone mice. *Autoimmunity* **2022**, *55*, 192–202. [CrossRef]
62. Thursby, E.; Juge, N. Introduction to the human gut microbiota. *Biochem. J.* **2017**, *474*, 1823–1836. [CrossRef]
63. Hill, D.A.; Artis, D. Intestinal bacteria and the regulation of immune cell homeostasis. *Annu. Rev. Immunol.* **2010**, *28*, 623–667. [CrossRef] [PubMed]
64. Haverson, K.; Rehakova, Z.; Sinkora, J.; Sver, L.; Bailey, M. Immune development in jejunal mucosa after colonization with selected commensal gut bacteria: A study in germ-free pigs. *Vet. Immunol. Immunopathol.* **2007**, *119*, 243–253. [CrossRef] [PubMed]
65. Yoo, J.Y.; Groer, M.; Dutra, S.V.O.; Sarkar, A.; McSkimming, D.I. Gut microbiota and immune system interactions. *Microorganisms* **2020**, *8*, 1587, https://doi.org/10.3390/microorganisms8101587;Erratum in *Microorganisms* **2020**, *8*, 2046. [CrossRef] [PubMed]
66. Santana, P.T.; Rosas, S.L.B.; Ribeiro, B.E.; Marinho, Y.; de Souza, H.S.P. Dysbiosis in inflammatory bowel disease: Pathogenic role and potential therapeutic targets. *Int. J. Mol. Sci.* **2022**, *23*, 3464. [CrossRef] [PubMed]
67. Intili, G.; Paladino, L.; Rappa, F.; Alberti, G.; Plicato, A.; Calabrò, F.; Fucarino, A.; Cappello, F.; Bucchieri, F.; Tomasello, G.; et al. From dysbiosis to neurodegenerative diseases through different communication pathways: An overview. *Biology* **2023**, *12*, 195. [CrossRef] [PubMed]
68. Xu, H.; Liu, M.; Cao, J.; Li, X.; Fan, D.; Xia, Y.; Lu, X.; Li, J.; Ju, D.; Zhao, H. The dynamic interplay between the gut microbiota and autoimmune diseases. *J. Immunol. Res.* **2019**, *2019*, 7546047. [CrossRef] [PubMed]
69. Kim, J.W.; Kwok, S.K.; Choe, J.Y.; Park, S.H. Recent advances in our understanding of the link between the intestinal microbiota and systemic lupus erythematosus. *Int. J. Mol. Sci.* **2019**, *20*, 4871. [CrossRef]
70. Miyauchi, E.; Shimokawa, C.; Steimle, A.; Desai, M.S.; Ohno, H. The impact of the gut microbiome on extra-intestinal autoimmune diseases. *Nat. Rev. Immunol.* **2023**, *23*, 9–23. [CrossRef]
71. Zhang, H.; Liao, X.; Sparks, J.B.; Luo, X.M. Dynamics of gut microbiota in autoimmune lupus. *Appl. Environ. Microbiol.* **2014**, *80*, 7551–7560. [CrossRef]
72. Gomez, A.; Luckey, D.; Taneja, V. The gut microbiome in autoimmunity: Sex matters. *Clin. Immunol.* **2015**, *159*, 154–162. [CrossRef]
73. Mu, Q.; Zhang, H.; Liao, X.; Lin, K.; Liu, H.; Edwards, M.R.; Ahmed, S.A.; Yuan, R.; Li, L.; Cecere, T.E.; et al. Control of lupus nephritis by changes of gut microbiota. *Microbiome* **2017**, *5*, 73. [CrossRef]
74. Luo, X.M.; Edwards, M.R.; Mu, Q.; Yu, Y.; Vieson, M.D.; Reilly, C.M.; Ahmed, S.A.; Bankole, A.A. Gut microbiota in human systemic lupus erythematosus and a mouse model of lupus. *Appl. Environ. Microbiol.* **2018**, *84*, e02288-17. [CrossRef]
75. Ma, Y.; Xu, X.; Li, M.; Cai, J.; Wei, Q.; Niu, H. Gut microbiota promote the inflammatory response in the pathogenesis of systemic lupus erythematosus. *Mol. Med.* **2019**, *25*, 35. [CrossRef]
76. Hevia, A.; Milani, C.; López, P.; Cuervo, A.; Arboleya, S.; Duranti, S.; Turroni, F.; González, S.; Suárez, A.; Gueimonde, M.; et al. Intestinal dysbiosis associated with systemic lupus erythematosus. *mBio* **2014**, *5*, e01548-14. [CrossRef] [PubMed]
77. He, Z.; Shao, T.; Li, H.; Xie, Z.; Wen, C. Alterations of the gut microbiome in Chinese patients with systemic lupus erythematosus. *Gut Pathog.* **2016**, *8*, 64. [CrossRef] [PubMed]
78. López, P.; de Paz, B.; Rodríguez-Carrio, J.; Hevia, A.; Sánchez, B.; Margolles, A.; Suárez, A. Th17 responses and natural IgM antibodies are related to gut microbiota composition in systemic lupus erythematosus patients. *Sci. Rep.* **2016**, *6*, 24072. [CrossRef]
79. Li, Y.; Wang, H.F.; Li, X.; Li, H.X.; Zhang, Q.; Zhou, H.W.; He, Y.; Li, P.; Fu, C.; Zhang, X.H.; et al. Disordered intestinal microbes are associated with the activity of Systemic Lupus Erythematosus. *Clin. Sci.* **2019**, *133*, 821–838. [CrossRef]
80. Wei, F.; Xu, H.; Yan, C.; Rong, C.; Liu, B.; Zhou, H. Changes of intestinal flora in patients with systemic lupus erythematosus in northeast China. *PLoS ONE* **2019**, *14*, e0213063. [CrossRef] [PubMed]

81. Chen, B.D.; Jia, X.M.; Xu, J.Y.; Zhao, L.D.; Ji, J.Y.; Wu, B.X.; Ma, Y.; Li, H.; Zuo, X.X.; Pan, W.Y.; et al. An autoimmunogenic and proinflammatory profile defined by the gut microbiota of patients with untreated systemic lupus erythematosus. *Arthritis Rheumatol.* **2021**, *73*, 232–243. [CrossRef]
82. Zhang, S.X.; Wang, J.; Chen, J.W.; Zhang, M.X.; Zhang, Y.F.; Hu, F.Y.; Lv, Z.Q.; Gao, C.; Li, Y.F.; Li, X.F. The level of peripheral regulatory T cells is linked to changes in gut commensal microflora in patients with systemic lupus erythematosus. *Ann. Rheum. Dis.* **2021**, *80*, e177. [CrossRef]
83. Toumi, E.; Goutorbe, B.; Plauzolles, A.; Bonnet, M.; Mezouar, S.; Militello, M.; Mege, J.L.; Chiche, L.; Halfon, P. Gut microbiota in systemic lupus erythematosus patients and lupus mouse model: A cross species comparative analysis for biomarker discovery. *Front. Immunol.* **2022**, *13*, 943241. [CrossRef] [PubMed]
84. Eckburg, P.B.; Bik, E.M.; Bernstein, C.N.; Purdom, E.; Dethlefsen, L.; Sargent, M.; Gill, S.R.; Nelson, K.E.; Relman, D.A. Diversity of the human intestinal microbial flora. *Science* **2005**, *308*, 1635–1638. [CrossRef] [PubMed]
85. Rinninella, E.; Raoul, P.; Cintoni, M.; Franceschi, F.; Miggiano, G.A.D.; Gasbarrini, A.; Mele, M.C. What is the healthy gut microbiota composition? A changing ecosystem across age, environment, diet, and diseases. *Microorganisms* **2019**, *7*, 14. [CrossRef] [PubMed]
86. Human Microbiome Project Consortium. Structure, function and diversity of the healthy human microbiome. *Nature* **2012**, *486*, 207–214. [CrossRef] [PubMed]
87. Qin, J.; Li, R.; Raes, J.; Arumugam, M.; Burgdorf, K.S.; Manichanh, C.; Nielsen, T.; Pons, N.; Levenez, F.; Yamada, T.; et al. A human gut microbial gene catalogue established by metagenomic sequencing. *Nature* **2010**, *464*, 59–65. [CrossRef] [PubMed]
88. Larsen, N.; Vogensen, F.K.; van den Berg, F.W.; Nielsen, D.S.; Andreasen, A.S.; Pedersen, B.K.; Al-Soud, W.A.; Sørensen, S.J.; Hansen, L.H.; Jakobsen, M. Gut microbiota in human adults with type 2 diabetes differs from non-diabetic adults. *PLoS ONE* **2010**, *5*, e9085. [CrossRef] [PubMed]
89. Turnbaugh, P.J.; Ley, R.E.; Mahowald, M.A.; Magrini, V.; Mardis, E.R.; Gordon, J.I. An obesity-associated gut microbiome with increased capacity for energy harvest. *Nature* **2006**, *444*, 1027–1031. [CrossRef] [PubMed]
90. Wu, G.D.; Chen, J.; Hoffmann, C.; Bittinger, K.; Chen, Y.Y.; Keilbaugh, S.A.; Bewtra, M.; Knights, D.; Walters, W.A.; Knight, R.; et al. Linking long-term dietary patterns with gut microbial enterotypes. *Science* **2011**, *334*, 105–108. [CrossRef]
91. Wucherpfennig, K.W. Mechanisms for the induction of autoimmunity by infectious agents. *J. Clin. Investig.* **2001**, *108*, 1097–1104. [CrossRef]
92. Damian, R.T. Molecular mimicry: Antigen sharing by parasite and host and its consequences. *Am. Nat.* **1964**, *98*, 129–149. [CrossRef]
93. Rojas, M.; Restrepo-Jiménez, P.; Monsalve, D.M.; Pacheco, Y.; Acosta-Ampudia, Y.; Ramírez-Santana, C.; Leung, P.S.C.; Ansari, A.A.; Gershwin, M.E.; Anaya, J.M. Molecular mimicry and autoimmunity. *J. Autoimmun.* **2018**, *95*, 100–123. [CrossRef]
94. Sundar, K.; Jacques, S.; Gottlieb, P.; Villars, R.; Benito, M.E.; Taylor, D.K.; Spatz, L.A. Expression of the Epstein-Barr virus nuclear antigen-1 (EBNA-1) in the mouse can elicit the production of anti-dsDNA and anti-Sm antibodies. *J. Autoimmun.* **2004**, *23*, 127–140. [CrossRef] [PubMed]
95. Poole, B.D.; Scofield, R.H.; Harley, J.B.; James, J.A. Epstein-Barr virus and molecular mimicry in systemic lupus erythematosus. *Autoimmunity* **2006**, *39*, 63–70. [CrossRef]
96. Neo, J.Y.J.; Wee, S.Y.K.; Bonne, I.; Tay, S.H.; Raida, M.; Jovanovic, V.; Fairhurst, A.M.; Lu, J.; Hanson, B.J.; MacAry, P.A. Characterisation of a human antibody that potentially links cytomegalovirus infection with systemic lupus erythematosus. *Sci. Rep.* **2019**, *9*, 9998. [CrossRef] [PubMed]
97. Hsieh, A.H.; Kuo, C.F.; Chou, I.J.; Tseng, W.Y.; Chen, Y.F.; Yu, K.H.; Luo, S.F. Human cytomegalovirus pp65 peptide-induced autoantibodies cross-reacts with TAF9 protein and induces lupus-like autoimmunity in BALB/c mice. *Sci. Rep.* **2020**, *10*, 9662. [CrossRef] [PubMed]
98. Emiliani, Y.; Muzi, G.; Sánchez, A.; Sánchez, J.; Munera, M. Prediction of molecular mimicry between proteins from *Trypanosoma* sp. and human antigens associated with systemic lupus erythematosus. *Microb. Pathog.* **2022**, *172*, 105760. [CrossRef] [PubMed]
99. Zügel, U.; Kaufmann, S.H. Immune response against heat shock proteins in infectious diseases. *Immunobiology* **1999**, *201*, 22–35. [CrossRef] [PubMed]
100. Barone, R.; Marino Gammazza, A.; Paladino, L.; Pitruzzella, A.; Spinoso, G.; Salerno, M.; Sessa, F.; Pomara, C.; Cappello, F.; Rappa, F. Morphological alterations and stress protein variations in lung biopsies obtained from autopsies of COVID-19 subjects. *Cells* **2021**, *10*, 3136. [CrossRef] [PubMed]
101. Tasneem, S.; Islam, N.; Ali, R. Crossreactivity of SLE autoantibodies with 70 kDa heat shock proteins of *Mycobacterium tuberculosis*. *Microbiol. Immunol.* **2001**, *45*, 841–846. [CrossRef]
102. Dieudé, M.; Senécal, J.L.; Raymond, Y. Induction of endothelial cell apoptosis by heat-shock protein 60-reactive antibodies from anti-endothelial cell autoantibody-positive systemic lupus erythematosus patients. *Arthritis Rheum.* **2004**, *50*, 3221–3231. [CrossRef]
103. Mu, Q.; Kirby, J.; Reilly, C.M.; Luo, X.M. Leaky gut as a danger signal for autoimmune diseases. *Front. Immunol.* **2017**, *8*, 598. [CrossRef] [PubMed]
104. Fu, X.; Chen, Y.; Chen, D. The role of gut microbiome in autoimmune uveitis. *Ophthalmic Res.* **2021**, *64*, 168–177. [CrossRef] [PubMed]

105. Pianta, A.; Arvikar, S.L.; Strle, K.; Drouin, E.E.; Wang, Q.; Costello, C.E.; Steere, A.C. Two rheumatoid arthritis-specific autoantigens correlate microbial immunity with autoimmune responses in joints. *J. Clin. Investig.* **2017**, *127*, 2946–2956. [CrossRef] [PubMed]
106. Harkiolaki, M.; Holmes, S.L.; Svendsen, P.; Gregersen, J.W.; Jensen, L.T.; McMahon, R.; Friese, M.A.; van Boxel, G.; Etzensperger, R.; Tzartos, J.S.; et al. T cell-mediated autoimmune disease due to low-affinity crossreactivity to common microbial peptides. *Immunity* **2009**, *30*, 348–357, Erratum in *Immunity* **2009**, *30*, 610. [CrossRef]
107. Yanagisawa, N.; Haruta, I.; Shimizu, K.; Furukawa, T.; Higuchi, T.; Shibata, N.; Shiratori, K.; Yagi, J. Identification of commensal flora-associated antigen as a pathogenetic factor of autoimmune pancreatitis. *Pancreatology* **2014**, *14*, 100–106. [CrossRef] [PubMed]
108. Ma, L.; Morel, L. Loss of gut barrier integrity in lupus. *Front. Immunol.* **2022**, *13*, 919792. [CrossRef] [PubMed]
109. Greiling, T.M.; Dehner, C.; Chen, X.; Hughes, K.; Iñiguez, A.J.; Boccitto, M.; Ruiz, D.Z.; Renfroe, S.C.; Vieira, S.M.; Ruff, W.E.; et al. Commensal orthologs of the human autoantigen Ro60 as triggers of autoimmunity in lupus. *Sci. Transl. Med.* **2018**, *10*, eaan2306. [CrossRef] [PubMed]
110. Azzouz, D.; Omarbekova, A.; Heguy, A.; Schwudke, D.; Gisch, N.; Rovin, B.H.; Caricchio, R.; Buyon, J.P.; Alekseyenko, A.V.; Silverman, G.J.; et al. Lupus nephritis is linked to disease-activity associated expansions and immunity to a gut commensal. *Ann. Rheum. Dis.* **2019**, *78*, 947–956. [CrossRef]
111. Bagavant, H.; Araszkiewicz, A.M.; Ingram, J.K.; Cizio, K.; Merrill, J.T.; Arriens, C.; Guthridge, J.M.; James, J.A.; Deshmukh, U.S. Immune response to *Enterococcus gallinarum* in lupus patients is associated with a subset of lupus-associated autoantibodies. *Front. Immunol.* **2021**, *12*, 635072. [CrossRef]
112. Manfredo Vieira, S.; Hiltensperger, M.; Kumar, V.; Zegarra-Ruiz, D.; Dehner, C.; Khan, N.; Costa, F.R.C.; Tiniakou, E.; Greiling, T.; Ruff, W.; et al. Translocation of a gut pathobiont drives autoimmunity in mice and humans. *Science* **2018**, *359*, 1156–1161, https://doi.org/10.1126/science.aar7201;Erratum in *Science* **2018**, *360*, eaat9922. [CrossRef]
113. Stewart, L.; Edgar, J.D.M.; Blakely, G.; Patrick, S. Antigenic mimicry of ubiquitin by the gut bacterium *Bacteroides fragilis*: A potential link with autoimmune disease. *Clin. Exp. Immunol.* **2018**, *194*, 153–165. [CrossRef] [PubMed]
114. Handley, H.H.; Yu, J.; Yu, D.T.; Singh, B.; Gupta, R.S.; Vaughan, J.H. Autoantibodies to human heat shock protein (hsp)60 may be induced by Escherichia coli groEL. *Clin. Exp. Immunol.* **1996**, *103*, 429–435. [CrossRef] [PubMed]
115. Yokota, S.I.; Hirata, D.; Minota, S.; Higashiyama, T.; Kurimoto, M.; Yanagi, H.; Yura, T.; Kubota, H. Autoantibodies against chaperonin CCT in human sera with rheumatic autoimmune diseases: Comparison with antibodies against other Hsp60 family proteins. *Cell Stress Chaperones* **2000**, *5*, 337–346. [CrossRef] [PubMed]
116. Nagata, S.; Yamashiro, Y.; Ohtsuka, Y.; Shimizu, T.; Sakurai, Y.; Misawa, S.; Ito, T. Heat shock proteins and superantigenic properties of bacteria from the gastrointestinal tract of patients with Kawasaki disease. *Immunology* **2009**, *128*, 511–520. [CrossRef] [PubMed]
117. Chen, H.; Cho, K.S.; Vu, T.H.K.; Shen, C.H.; Kaur, M.; Chen, G.; Mathew, R.; McHam, M.L.; Fazelat, A.; Lashkari, K.; et al. Commensal microflora-induced T cell responses mediate progressive neurodegeneration in glaucoma. *Nat. Commun.* **2018**, *9*, 3209, Erratum in *Nat. Commun.* **2018**, *9*, 3914. [CrossRef] [PubMed]
118. Genest, O.; Wickner, S.; Doyle, S.M. Hsp90 and Hsp70 chaperones: Collaborators in protein remodeling. *J. Biol. Chem.* **2019**, *294*, 2109–2120. [CrossRef] [PubMed]
119. Tukaj, S.; Sitko, K. Heat Shock Protein 90 (Hsp90) and Hsp70 as potential therapeutic targets in autoimmune skin diseases. *Biomolecules* **2022**, *12*, 1153. [CrossRef] [PubMed]
120. Bruce, I.N.; Buie, J.; Bloch, L.; Bae, S.C.; Costenbader, K.; Levy, R.A.; Werth, V.P.; Marion, A.; Sangodkar, S.; Manzi, S. Lupus spectrum ambiguity has long-term negative implications for patients. *Lupus Sci. Med.* **2023**, *10*, e000856. [CrossRef] [PubMed]
121. Kuhn, A.; Bonsmann, G.; Anders, H.J.; Herzer, P.; Tenbrock, K.; Schneider, M. The diagnosis and treatment of systemic lupus erythematosus. *Dtsch. Ärzteblatt Int.* **2015**, *112*, 423–432. [CrossRef]
122. Kernder, A.; Richter, J.G.; Fischer-Betz, R.; Winkler-Rohlfing, B.; Brinks, R.; Aringer, M.; Schneider, M.; Chehab, G. Delayed diagnosis adversely affects outcome in systemic lupus erythematosus: Cross sectional analysis of the LuLa cohort. *Lupus* **2021**, *30*, 431–438. [CrossRef]
123. Yu, H.; Nagafuchi, Y.; Fujio, K. Clinical and Immunological Biomarkers for Systemic Lupus Erythematosus. *Biomolecules* **2021**, *11*, 928. [CrossRef] [PubMed]
124. Gómez-Bañuelos, E.; Fava, A.; Andrade, F. An update on autoantibodies in systemic lupus erythematosus. *Curr. Opin. Rheumatol.* **2023**, *35*, 61–67. [CrossRef] [PubMed]
125. Papini, A.M. The use of post-translationally modified peptides for detection of biomarkers of immune-mediated diseases. *J. Pept. Sci.* **2009**, *15*, 621–628. [CrossRef] [PubMed]
126. García-Moreno, C.; Gómara, M.J.; Castellanos-Moreira, R.; Sanmartí, R.; Haro, I. Peptides bearing multiple post-translational modifications as antigenic targets for severe rheumatoid arthritis patients. *Int. J. Mol. Sci.* **2021**, *22*, 13290. [CrossRef]
127. Vitale, A.M.; Conway de Macario, E.; Alessandro, R.; Cappello, F.; Macario, A.J.L.; Marino Gammazza, A. Missense mutations of human Hsp60: A computational analysis to unveil their pathological significance. *Front. Genet.* **2020**, *11*, 969. [CrossRef]

Disclaimer/Publisher's Note: The statements, opinions and data contained in all publications are solely those of the individual author(s) and contributor(s) and not of MDPI and/or the editor(s). MDPI and/or the editor(s) disclaim responsibility for any injury to people or property resulting from any ideas, methods, instructions or products referred to in the content.

Article

B Cell Kinetics upon Therapy Commencement for Active Extrarenal Systemic Lupus Erythematosus in Relation to Development of Renal Flares: Results from Three Phase III Clinical Trials of Belimumab

Ioannis Parodis [1,2,*], Alvaro Gomez [1], Julius Lindblom [1], Jun Weng Chow [1], Christopher Sjöwall [3], Savino Sciascia [4] and Mariele Gatto [5]

1. Division of Rheumatology, Department of Medicine Solna, Karolinska Institutet and Karolinska University Hospital, 17176 Stockholm, Sweden
2. Department of Rheumatology, Faculty of Medicine and Health, Örebro University, 70281 Örebro, Sweden
3. Division of Inflammation and Infection, Department of Biomedical and Clinical Sciences, Linköping University, 58183 Linköping, Sweden
4. Center of Research of Immunopathology and Rare Diseases and Nephrology and Dialysis, Department of Clinical and Biological Sciences, University of Turin, 10124 Turin, Italy
5. Unit of Rheumatology, Department of Medicine, University of Padua, 35040 Padua, Italy
* Correspondence: ioannis.parodis@ki.se; Tel.: +46-722-321-322

Abstract: Renal flares constitute major determinants of poor prognosis in people living with systemic lupus erythematosus (SLE). The aim of the present study was to investigate changes in B cell subsets in relation to renal flares upon initiation of standard therapy (ST) plus belimumab or placebo in patients with SLE. Using data from the BLISS-76, BLISS-SC, and BLISS Northeast Asia trials, we investigated associations of relative to baseline rapid (through week 8) and early (through week 24) percentage changes in circulating $CD19^+$ B cell subsets characterised through flow cytometry, anti-dsDNA antibodies, and complement levels with the occurrence of renal flares over one year. Patients who developed renal flares showed more prominent rapid decreases in $CD19^+CD20^+CD138^+$ short-lived plasma cells (−50.4% vs. −16.7%; $p = 0.019$) and $CD19^+CD20^-CD27^{bright}$ plasmablasts (−50.0% vs. −29.9%; $p = 0.020$) compared to non-flaring patients, followed by a subsequent return. Less prominent rapid reductions in $CD19^+CD27^-CD24^{bright}CD38^{bright}$ transitional B cells (−42.9% vs. −75.0%; $p = 0.038$) and $CD19^+CD20^-CD138^+$ peripheral long-lived plasma cells (−11.3% vs. −29.2%; $p = 0.019$) were seen in belimumab-treated—but not placebo-treated—patients who developed renal flares compared to belimumab-treated patients who did not. Rapid and early changes in anti-dsDNA or complement levels showed no clear association with renal flares. In summary, a rapid drop followed by a subsequent return in circulating short-lived plasma cells and plasmablasts upon treatment for active extra-renal SLE portended renal flares, indicating a need for therapeutic adjustments in patients showing such B cell patterns. Rapid decreases in transitional B cells and peripheral long-lived plasma cells upon belimumab therapy commencement may signify a greater protection against renal flares. B cell kinetics may prove useful in early drug evaluation.

Keywords: systemic lupus erythematosus; biomarkers; renal flares; B cells; plasma cells; B lymphocyte; belimumab; biologics

1. Introduction

Renal flares constitute major determinants of poor prognosis in patients with systemic lupus erythematosus (SLE) since they contribute to renal and overall organ damage accrual as well as to increased disease- and treatment-related morbidity and costs [1–4]. Renal flares are coupled with increases in proteinuria and/or serum creatinine levels as well as substantial nephron loss, eventually resulting in irreversible worsening of renal function [5,6]. Risk factors for renal flares in SLE include persistently active extrarenal disease, low complement levels, and positive anti-U1RNP and anti-dsDNA antibodies [7,8], yet patient monitoring is mainly based on fluctuations in proteinuria and serum creatinine, abnormalities in the urinary sediment, and changes in serological markers, which are often subject to inconsistencies owing to different assays and timings of sample collection [9–11].

Belimumab blocks the soluble counterpart of B cell activating factor (BAFF; also known as B lymphocyte stimulator, BLyS) and has been used for the treatment of SLE for over a decade [12]. It has shown ability to induce durable disease control and reduce the risk of disease flares, including renal flares, in clinical trials and several real-life observational studies [13–18], and after a recent phase III lupus nephritis (LN)-specific clinical trial [19], belimumab received approval from regulatory agencies for use as an add-on therapy in addition to standard immunosuppressive therapy (mycophenolate mofetil or low-dose intravenous cyclophosphamide) in patients with SLE and active renal involvement [20]. Still, some patients may develop renal flares during belimumab therapy, including de novo LN, as exemplified in a recent report [21], mandating identification of patient profiles with susceptibility to develop renal flares despite immunosuppressive therapy, including therapy with belimumab, as an urgent need towards determination of individualised therapeutic modifications required to prevent renal flares in the short term and kidney function loss over the longer term.

In this regard, identification of reproducible biological changes occurring soon after treatment initiation that are associated with renal flares could introduce a novel concept in surveillance upon commencement of a new therapy, early evaluation of its effectiveness, and evaluation of the need for treatment modification in selected patients. Hence, in this study, we aimed at investigating early changes in B cell and plasma cell subsets in relation to the development of renal flares during non-biological standard therapy (ST) plus belimumab or placebo within the frame of three phase III clinical trials of belimumab in SLE.

2. Results

2.1. Patient Characteristics

Demographics and clinical and serological data of the patients, including comparisons between patients who developed and patients who did not develop renal flares through week 52, are reported in Table 1. Patients who developed renal flares were younger at baseline (34.6 ± 11.6 years vs. 39.5 ± 11.9 years; $p = 0.001$). Higher proportions of patients among those who developed renal flares were on glucocorticoids at baseline (93.8% vs. 81.5%; $p = 0.012$) and were of Asian ancestry (42.2% vs. 14.7%; $p < 0.001$) compared to patients who did not develop renal flares, while lower proportions of patients among those who developed renal flares were White/Caucasian (35.9% vs. 63.5%; $p < 0.001$). A total of 633/1715 patients (36.9%) had a history of or current renal SLE at baseline (renal BILAG A–D), and 152 patients (8.9%) had active renal disease (renal BILAG A or B). A higher proportion of patients with renal BILAG A–B developed renal flares through week 52 compared to patients who did not (28.1% vs. 8.1%; $p < 0.001$). Detailed information about BILAG-based organ involvement at baseline is presented in Supplementary Table S1.

The corresponding results from comparisons between patients who developed renal flares through the end of follow-up—i.e., week 52 in BLISS-SC and BLISS-NEA but week 76 in BLISS-76—are presented in Supplementary Table S2. Table 2 shows baseline B cell and plasma cell counts as well as comparisons between patients who developed renal flares through week 52 and patients who did not. In Table 2, results are stratified by study to account for batch variations in cell analyses across studies, and the corresponding results for renal flares through the end of follow-up are detailed in Supplementary Table S3.

Table 1. Characteristics of patients who developed renal flares vs. patients who did not from baseline through week 52 in the pooled BLISS study population.

	All Patients n = 1715	Renal Flare n = 64	No Renal Flare n = 1651	p Value	OR	95% CI (OR)	RR	95% CI (RR)
Patient characteristics								
Age at baseline (years)	39.3 ± 11.9	34.6 ± 11.6	39.5 ± 11.9	**0.001**	N/A	N/A	N/A	N/A
Female sex	1608 (93.8%)	62 (96.9%)	1546 (93.6%)	0.294	2.11	0.51–8.73	2.06	0.51–8.32
Ancestry								
Asian	270 (15.7%)	27 (42.2%)	243 (14.7%)	<**0.001**	4.23	2.53–7.07	3.91	2.42–6.30
Black/African American	204 (11.9%)	8 (12.5%)	196 (11.9%)	0.879	1.10	0.52–2.35	1.10	0.53–2.27
Indigenous American *	170 (9.9%)	6 (9.4%)	164 (9.9%)	0.883	0.94	0.40–2.21	0.94	0.41–2.15
White/Caucasian	1071 (62.4%)	23 (35.9%)	1048 (63.5%)	<**0.001**	0.32	0.19–0.54	0.34	0.20–0.56
Clinical data								
SLE duration at baseline (years)	5.1 (1.6–10.6)	4.1 (1.1–10.0)	5.1 (1.6–10.6)	0.202	N/A	N/A	N/A	N/A
BILAG renal								
A	10 (0.6%)	2 (3.1%)	8 (0.5%)	0.051	6.63	1.38–31.85	5.50	1.55–19.46
B	142 (8.3%)	16 (25.0%)	126 (7.6%)	<**0.001**	4.03	2.23–7.31	3.69	2.15–6.33
C	383 (22.3%)	29 (45.3%)	354 (21.4%)	<**0.001**	3.04	1.83–5.04	2.88	1.79–4.65
D	98 (5.7%)	6 (9.4%)	92 (5.6%)	0.198	1.75	0.74–4.17	1.71	0.76–3.86
E	1082 (63.1%)	11 (17.2%)	1071 (64.9%)	<**0.001**	0.11	0.06–0.22	0.12	0.06–0.23
A–B	152 (8.9%)	18 (28.1%)	134 (8.1%)	<**0.001**	4.43	2.50–7.86	4.02	2.40–6.76
Treatment at baseline								
Glucocorticoids	1405 (81.9%)	60 (93.8%)	1345 (81.5%)	**0.012**	3.41	1.23–9.46	3.31	1.21–9.04
AMA [†]	1099 (64.1%)	36 (56.3%)	1063 (64.4%)	0.183	0.71	0.43–1.18	0.72	0.44–1.17
Immunosuppressants [‡]	882 (51.4%)	39 (60.9%)	843 (51.1%)	0.121	1.50	0.90–2.49	1.47	0.90–2.41
Azathioprine	336 (19.6%)	15 (23.4%)	321 (19.4%)	0.430	1.27	0.70–2.29	1.26	0.71–2.21
Methotrexate	248 (14.5%)	7 (10.9%)	241 (14.6%)	0.414	0.72	0.32–1.59	0.73	0.34–1.57
Mycophenolate mofetil or sodium	243 (14.2%)	12 (18.8%)	231 (14.0%)	0.284	1.42	0.75–2.70	1.39	0.76–2.56
Trial intervention								
Placebo	576 (33.6%)	26 (40.6%)	550 (33.3%)	0.224	1.37	0.82–2.28	1.35	0.83–2.21
Belimumab	1139 (66.4%)	38 (59.4%)	1101 (66.7%)	0.224	0.73	0.44–1.21	0.74	0.45–1.20
i.v. 1 mg/kg	271 (15.8%)	2 (3.1%)	269 (16.3%)	**0.005**	0.17	0.04–0.68	0.17	0.04–0.70
i.v. 10 mg/kg	312 (18.2%)	10 (15.6%)	302 (18.3%)	0.587	0.82	0.42–1.64	0.83	0.43–1.62
s.c. 200 mg	556 (32.4%)	26 (40.6%)	530 (32.1%)	0.153	1.45	0.87–2.41	1.43	0.88–2.32
Serological markers at baseline								
C3; mg/dL	95.0 (74.0–118.0)	75.0 (57.3–91.5)	96.0 (75.0–119.0)	<**0.001**	N/A	N/A	N/A	N/A
C4; mg/dL	15.0 (9.0–22.0)	11.0 (7.0–16.0)	15.0 (9.0–22.0)	<**0.001**	N/A	N/A	N/A	N/A
anti-dsDNA; IU/mL (all patients)	95.0 (29.0–288.0)	256.0 (97.5–632.0)	90.0 (29.0–275.3)	<**0.001**	N/A	N/A	N/A	N/A
anti-dsDNA; IU/mL (patients positive at baseline)	167.0 (89.0–497.3); n = 1172	279.0 (137.3–664.5); n = 56	163.5 (86.5–490.8); n = 1116	**0.003**	N/A	N/A	N/A	N/A

Data are presented as the number (percentage), mean ± standard deviation, or median (interquartile range), as appropriate. Additionally, odds ratio (OR) and the corresponding 95% confidence interval (CI), as well as risk ratio (RR) and the corresponding 95% CI, are indicated. In case of missing values, the total number of patients with available data is indicated. Percentages are derived using the total number of patients in the respective column as the denominator (i.e., all patients, patients who developed renal flares and patients who did not develop renal flares). P values were derived from non-parametrical Mann–Whitney U tests for continues variables and chi-squared (χ^2) or Fisher's exact tests for binomial variables, as appropriate. Statistically significant P values are in bold. * Alaska Native or American Indian from North, South, or Central America. [†] Hydroxychloroquine, chloroquine, mepacrine, mepacrine hydrochloride, or quinine sulfate. [‡] Azathioprine, cyclosporine, oral cyclophosphamide, leflunomide, methotrexate, mizoribine, mycophenolate sodium, or thalidomide. AMA: antimalarial agents; C3: complement component 3; C4: complement component 4; CI: confidence interval; i.v.: intravenous; N/A: not applicable; OR: odds ratio; RR: risk ratio; s.c.: subcutaneous; SLE: systemic lupus erythematosus; SRI-4: SLE Responder Index 4.

Table 2. B cell subset counts at baseline in patients who developed renal flares vs. patients who did not from baseline through week 52 in the BLISS-76, BLISS-SC, and BLISS Northeast Asia study populations.

B Cell Subsets	All Patients	Renal Flare	No Renal Flare	p Value
	BLISS-76			
	n = 819	n = 9	n = 810	
CD19$^+$CD20$^+$ ($\times 10^3$/mL)	91.5 (43.0–176.0); n = 756	95.5 (25.0–123.5); n = 8	91.0 (43.3–178.0); n = 748	0.386
CD19$^+$CD20$^+$CD27$^+$ ($\times 10^3$/mL)	14.0 (6.0–27.0); n = 756	13.5 (3.3–23.3); n = 8	14.0 (6.0–27.0); n = 748	0.456
CD19$^+$CD20$^+$CD69$^+$ (/mL)	2096.5 (938.3–4350.8); n = 744	2769.5 (708.3–9099.3); n = 736	2096.5 (938.3–4327.0); n = 736	0.531
CD19$^+$CD20$^+$CD27$^-$ ($\times 10^3$/mL)	75.0 (33.0–143.0); n = 756	77.5 (20.0–103.0); n = 8	75.0 (33.3–143.0); n = 748	0.479
CD19$^+$CD20$^+$CD138$^+$ (/mL)	819.0 (334.0–1811.5); n = 749	1127.0 (137.3–2752.5); n = 8	806.0 (335.–1807.5); n = 741	0.974
CD19$^+$CD20$^-$CD138$^+$ (/mL)	482.5 (211.0–1067.3); n = 748	589.5 (242.3–1740.0); n = 8	480.5 (211.0–1058.8); n = 740	0.464
CD19$^+$CD20$^-$CD27^{brt} (/mL)	299.0 (115.0–705.0); n = 747	365.0 (119.3–446.8); n = 8	298.0 (115.0–707.0); n = 739	0.838
CD19$^+$CD27^{brt}CD38^{brt} (/mL)	306.0 (116.0–701.8); n = 754	326.5 (159.0–402.8); n = 8	306.0 (115.8–706.0); n = 746	0.804
	BLISS-SC			
	n = 836	n = 47	n = 789	
CD19$^+$CD20$^+$ ($\times 10^3$/mL)	106.0 (56.0–196.0); n = 811	91.0 (41.3–270.5); n = 44	107.0 (57.0–194.0); n = 767	0.680
CD19$^+$CD20$^+$CD27$^+$ ($\times 10^3$/mL)	14.0 (7.0–29.0); n = 811	10.5 (5.3–28.8); n = 44	14.0 (7.0–29.0); n = 767	0.450
CD19$^+$CD20$^+$CD69$^+$ (/mL)	79.0 (33.0–199.0); n = 811	47.5 (23.5–137.3); n = 44	80.0 (34.0–202.0); n = 767	0.041
CD19$^+$CD20$^+$CD27$^-$ ($\times 10^3$/mL)	89.0 (43.0–167.0); n = 811	81.0 (24.8–239.8); n = 44	90.0 (43.0–166.0); n = 767	0.819
CD19$^+$CD20$^-$CD138$^+$ (/mL)	53.0 (20.0–127.0); n = 811	63.0 (23.3–152.8); n = 44	53.0 (20.0–126.0); n = 767	0.479
CD19$^+$CD20$^-$CD138$^+$ (/mL)	203.0 (67.0–505.0); n = 811	253.5 (46.3–698.8); n = 44	201.0 (68.0–501.0); n = 767	0.496
CD19$^+$CD20$^-$CD27^{brt} (/mL)	2000.0 (1000–4000.0); n = 811	2000.0 (1000.0–7000.0); n = 44	2000.0 (1000.0–4000.0); n = 767	0.060
CD19$^+$CD27^{brt}CD38^{brt} (/mL)	1732.0 (738.0–3926.0); n = 811	2442.0 (738.5–7416.3); n = 44	1714.0 (731.0–3793.0); n = 767	0.053
	BLISS Northeast Asia			
	n = 60	n = 8	n = 52	
CD19$^+$CD20$^+$ ($\times 10^3$/mL)	52.5 (22.8–96.8); n = 54	65.0 (12.0–80.0); n = 5	51.0 (25.5–105.0); n = 49	0.467
CD19$^+$CD20$^+$CD27$^+$ ($\times 10^3$/mL)	7.3 (3.7–10.6); n = 55	11.0 (3.3–19.1); n = 6	7.3 (3.5–10.5); n = 49	0.703
CD19$^+$CD20$^+$CD69$^+$ (/mL)	101.3 (45.9–183.0); n = 55	124.3 (77.0–170.2); n = 6	100.7 (45.6–185.4); n = 49	0.782
CD19$^+$CD20$^+$CD27$^-$ ($\times 10^3$/mL)	39.7 (18.6–87.5); n = 55	23.5 (5.6–58.2); n = 6	41.4 (19.8–98.4); n = 49	0.104
CD19$^+$CD20$^-$CD138$^+$ (/mL)	108.2 (58.1–258.1); n = 55	167.8 (113.0–599.3); n = 6	86.9 (54.0–218.7); n = 49	0.077
CD19$^+$CD20$^-$CD138$^+$ (/mL)	303.1 (174.5–668.8); n = 55	269.5 (49.7–467.4); n = 6	303.1 (176.7–698.3); n = 49	0.375
CD19$^+$CD20$^-$CD27^{brt} (/mL)	916.5 (262.8–2008.4); n = 55	1122.8 (315.0–1730.9); n = 6	904.3 (240.7–2446.1); n = 49	0.969
CD19$^+$CD27^{brt}CD38^{brt} (/mL)	934.9 (264.7–2095.6); n = 55	1161.5 (132.1–1867.2); n = 6	887.6 (274.6–2177.5); n = 49	0.969

Data are presented as medians (interquartile range) of absolute counts. In case of missing values, the total number of patients with available data is indicated. p values are derived from non-parametrical Mann–Whitney U tests. Statistically significant p values are in bold. brt: bright; SC: subcutaneous.

2.2. Associations with Renal Flares Occurring during Follow-Up

In the pooled datasets, 64/1715 patients (3.7%) developed at least one renal flare through week 52, and 69/1715 patients (4.0%) developed at least one renal flare through the end of the study period, i.e., including the follow-up period of week 52–76 in BLISS-76. Among patients who developed renal flares, the first renal flare through week 52 occurred after a mean time of 160.9 ± 102.9 days from baseline, and the first renal flare throughout the entire follow-up was documented after a mean time of 181.7 ± 124.5 days from baseline.

2.3. B Cell Changes

In the entire cohort (all treatment arms), patients who developed at least one renal flare through week 52 showed a more profound rapid decrease in $CD19^+CD20^+CD138^+$ short-lived plasma cells (−50.4% vs. −16.7%; $p = 0.019$) and $CD19^+CD20^-CD27^{bright}$ plasmablasts (−50.0% vs. −29.9%; $p = 0.020$) compared with patients who did not develop renal flares in logistic regression analysis after adjustment for potential confounders, as described in the Methods. In patients who developed renal flares, this initial drop in the aforementioned cell subsets was followed by a subsequent increase, while in patients who did not develop renal flares, these lymphocyte subsets continued the declining trend, as detailed in Supplementary Tables S4–S6. In contrast, patients who flared showed less prominent $CD19^+CD20^-CD138^+$ peripheral long-lived plasma cells through week 24 compared to patients who did not (−10.4% vs. −38.8%; $p = 0.028$).

Among patients who received add-on belimumab, patients who developed at least one renal flare showed a less profound rapid decrease from baseline through week 8 in $CD19^+CD20^-CD138^+$ peripheral long-lived plasma cells (−11.3% vs. −29.2%; $p = 0.019$) compared to patients who did not develop renal flares (Figure 1). Among patients who received standard therapy alone, no differences were seen in rapid or early changes in B cell or plasma cell subsets between patients who developed renal flares through week 52 and patients who did not.

Results from analysis in the entire cohort and analysis stratified by treatment arm for renal flares throughout the entire follow-up (baseline through week 52 in BLISS-SC and BLISS-NEA and through week 76 in BLISS-76) are detailed in Supplementary Tables S7–S9. Supplementary Tables S4–S9 also detail comparisons of changes in B cell and plasma cell subsets between patients who received ST plus belimumab and patients who received ST plus placebo.

In a subgroup analysis of the $CD19^+CD20^+CD27^-$ B cell subset in the BLISS-SC trial, a less prominent rapid decrease in $CD19^+CD27^-CD24^{bright}CD38^{bright}$ transitional B cells was seen in belimumab-treated patients who developed at least one renal flare through week 52 compared with belimumab-treated patients who did not (−42.9% vs. −75.0%; $p = 0.038$), as illustrated in Figure 2. In contrast, no differences were seen regarding rapid or early changes in transitional B cells between patients who developed renal flares and patients who did not among patients who were exposed to non-biological ST alone (Figure 2). Moreover, no differences were observed regarding changes in $CD19^+CD27^-CD24^{low}CD38^{low}$ naïve B cells between flaring and non-flaring patients. Detailed results from this analysis are presented in Supplementary Table S10.

2.4. Serological Markers

In the entire cohort (all treatment arms) patients who developed at least one renal flare through week 52 had higher baseline anti-dsDNA levels (median; IQR: 256.0; 97.5–632.0 IU/mL vs. 90.0; 29.0–275.3 IU/mL; $p < 0.001$) and lower C3 (median; IQR: 75.0; 57.3–91.5 mg/dL vs. 96.0; 75.0–119.0 mg/dL; $p < 0.001$) and C4 levels (median; IQR: 11.0; 7.0–16.0 mg/dL vs. 15.0; 9.0–22.0 mg/dL; $p < 0.001$) compared to patients who did not develop renal flares. Rapid and early changes of anti-dsDNA antibody levels, C3 levels, and C4 levels did not differ between patients who developed renal flares through week 52 and patients who did not. Similar patterns were seen in analysis stratified by treatment arms (Figure 3). The results are detailed in Supplementary Tables S4–S6, and the corresponding results for renal flares through week 76 are detailed in Supplementary Tables S7–S9. These tables also detail comparisons of changes in serological markers between patients who received ST plus belimumab and patients who received ST plus placebo.

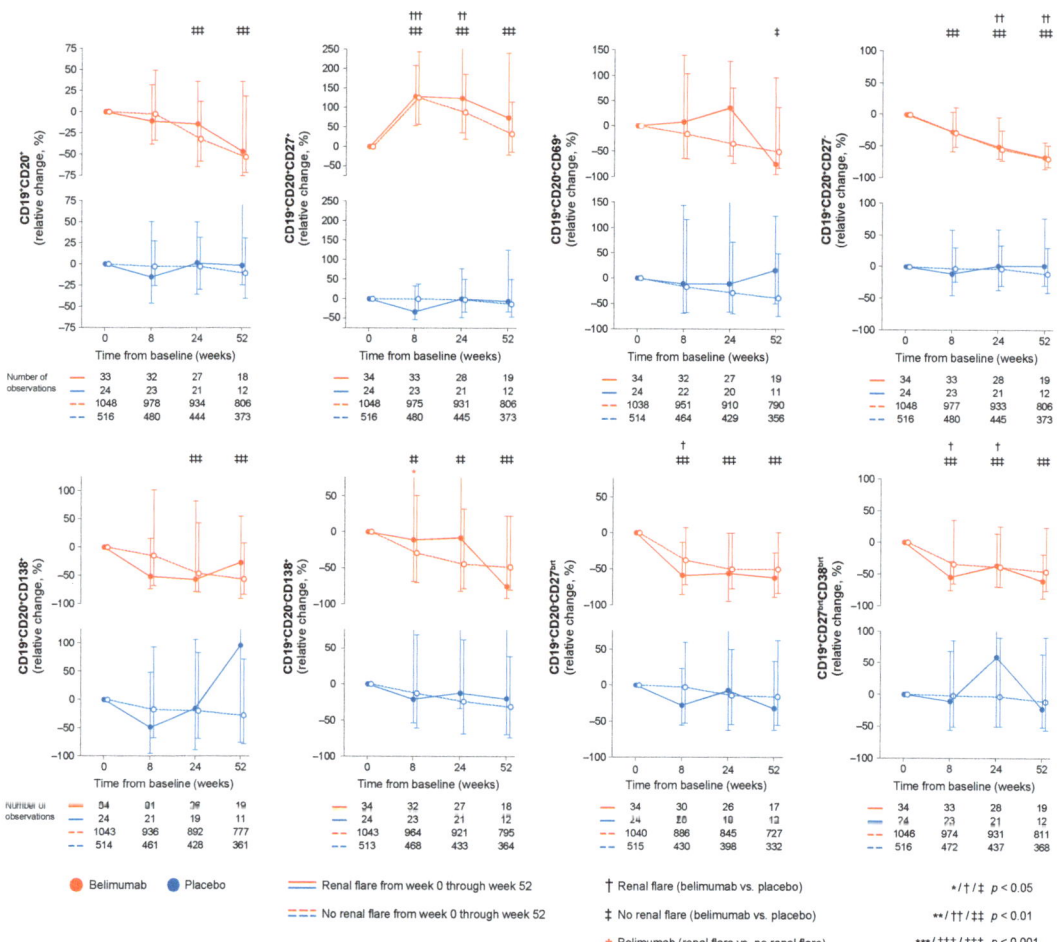

Figure 1. B cell alterations in relation to renal flares. The graphs delineate relative to baseline percentage changes in selected B cell and peripheral plasma cell subsets in patients who developed at least one renal flare during the study period (continuous lines) and patients who did not (dashed lines). Comparisons between patients who flared and patients who did not were conducted using multivariable logistic regression analysis to account for potential confounders and are illustrated for patients who received non-biological standard therapy plus belimumab (red lines) and patients who received non-biological standard therapy alone (blue lines). Comparisons between treatment arms were conducted using non-parametrical Mann–Whitney U tests. Whiskers indicate the interquartile range of distributions. The number of patients with available data at each time point is indicated for each patient subgroup.

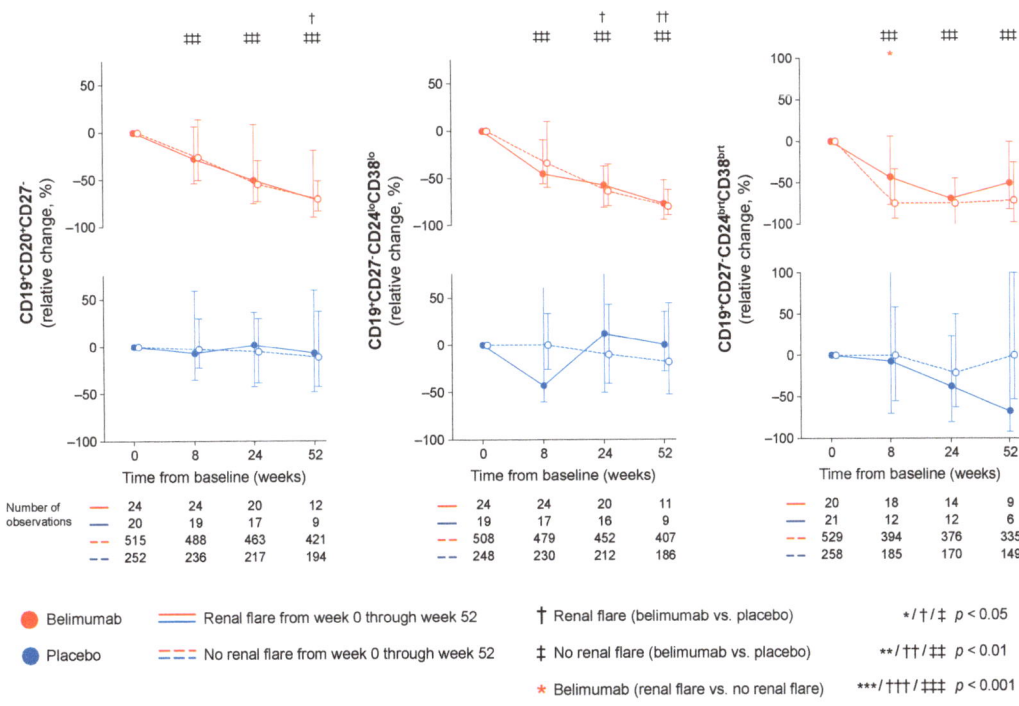

Figure 2. Transitional and naïve B cell alterations in relation to renal flares. The graphs delineate relative to baseline percentage changes in transitional and naïve B cell subsets in patients who developed at least one renal flare during the study period (continuous lines) and patients who did not (dashed lines) in a subanalysis of data from the BLISS-SC trial. Comparisons between patients who flared and patients who did not were conducted for patients with available data, stratified into patients who received non-biological standard therapy plus belimumab (red lines) and patients who received non-biological standard therapy alone (blue lines). P values are derived from non-parametric Mann–Whitney U tests. Whiskers indicate the interquartile range of distributions. The number of patients with available data at each time point is indicated for each patient subgroup.

2.5. Analyses in Relation to the First Documented Renal Flare

To further understand the observed kinetics of B cell and plasma cell subsets, anti-dsDNA antibody levels, and complement levels, we investigated absolute cell counts and anti-dsDNA, C3, and C4 levels in relation to the time of the first documented renal flare. More specifically, we compared the distributions of absolute cell counts and anti-dsDNA, C3, and C4 levels measured at the most adjacent timepoint before (median time: −7.9; IQR: −15.4–−4.1 weeks) and after (median time: 10.9; IQR: 3.9–12.7 weeks) the first renal flare. In this analysis, absolute $CD19^+CD20^+CD138^+$ short-lived plasma cell counts displayed a decrease between the last available measurement prior to the first documented renal flare (median: 422.5 cells/mL; IQR: 274.5–567.9 cells/mL) and the first available measurement after the renal fare (median: 183.0 cells/mL; IQR: 130.4–301.0 cells/mL; $p = 0.035$). In contrast, C4 levels displayed an increase from the first available measurement prior to renal flare (median: 9.5 mg/dL; IQR: 7.0–13.8 mg/dL) to the first measurement after the renal flare (median: 12.5 mg/dL; IQR 7.3–18.0 mg/dL; $p = 0.011$). All other cell subsets, anti-dsDNA antibody levels, and C3 levels showed no statistically significant change before and after the first documented renal flare ($p > 0.05$ for all comparisons).

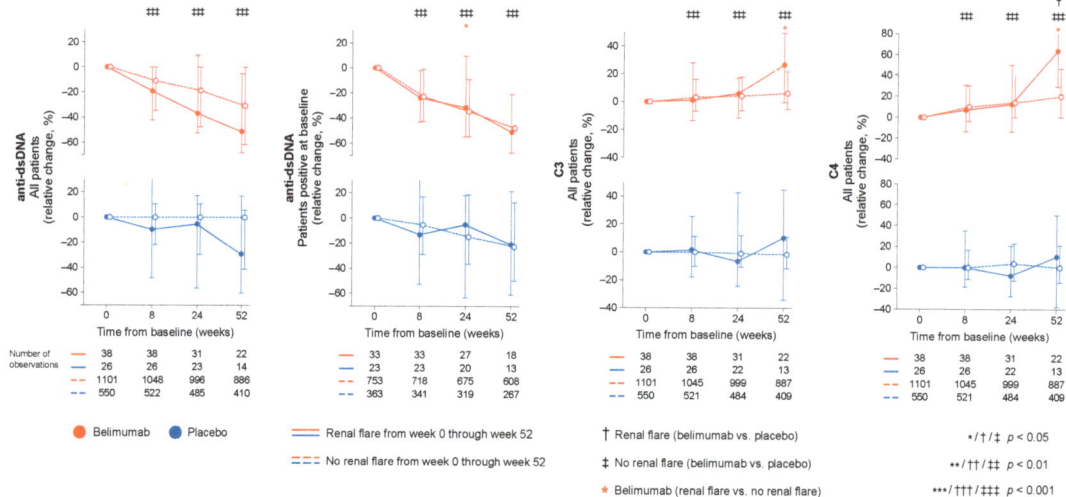

Figure 3. Changes in serological markers in relation to renal flares. The graphs delineate relative to baseline percentage changes in anti-dsDNA, C3, and C4 levels in patients who developed at least one renal flare during the study period (continuous lines) and patients who did not (dashed lines). Comparisons between patients who flared and patients who did not were conducted using multivariable logistic regression analysis to account for potential confounders and are illustrated for patients who received non-biological standard therapy plus belimumab (red lines) and patients who received non-biological standard therapy alone (blue lines). For anti-dsDNA levels, a separate analysis for patients with positive anti-dsDNA levels ($\geq$30 IU/mL) at baseline is also demonstrated. Comparisons between treatment arms were conducted using non-parametrical Mann–Whitney U tests. Whiskers indicate the interquartile range of distributions. The number of patients with available data at each time point is indicated for each patient subgroup. Anti-dsDNA: anti-double-stranded DNA antibodies; C3: complement component 3; C4: complement component 4.

3. Discussion

In this study, we investigated alterations across different circulating B cell subsets upon treatment for active SLE and their association with occurrence of renal flares. We showed that a course in short-lived plasma cells and plasmablasts characterised by a rapid decrease followed by a subsequent return was associated with the occurrence of renal flares; this pattern may thus signify a need for treatment modifications in selected patients. While this drop–return pattern was seen both in patients treated with add-on belimumab and patients treated with non-biological ST alone, the drop in plasmablasts was more prominent in belimumab-treated patients irrespective of the development of renal flares. It is worth noting that belimumab was herein shown to induce declining trends in plasma cell subsets early on upon treatment initiation, while in previous research, data on the effect of belimumab on plasma cells have been conflicting [22–24]. This may be due to the large study population in the present work and the resulting power amplification in statistical calculations as well as the detailed characterisation of peripheral plasma cells into different subsets. A similar pattern of an initial drop and subsequent return in memory B cells discriminated patients on non-biological ST who flared from those who did not flare in unadjusted analysis, which, however, did not reach statistical significance after adjustment for confounders. In contrast, circulating memory B cells showed a rapid increase upon belimumab treatment regardless of the occurrence of renal flares. This increase in circulating memory B cells occurring short time after commencement of belimumab therapy has been described in previous research [22–24] and has been speculated to be related to a secondary defect in their trafficking receptors [25]. Albeit not unexpected in light of its mode of action, belimumab was shown to induce a rapid and sustained decline in transitional B cells, which was less prominent in belimumab-treated patients who developed renal flares. This finding is novel and suggests that transitional B cell kinetics may be an early indicator of successful treatment with belimumab, with pronounced rapid reductions signifying a better protection against renal flares. Lastly, while high levels of anti-dsDNA antibodies and low levels of C3 and C4 at baseline were associated with renal flare development, rapid or early changes in these traditional serological markers were not.

While renal flares constitute a major contributing factor of poor long-term prognosis in patients with SLE [26–28], traditional biomarkers do not satisfactorily predict their occurrence [10], especially when evaluating the likelihood of renal flare-up upon commencing therapy for active SLE. In conformity with the above, early changes in anti-dsDNA or complement levels did not discriminate between patients who developed renal flares and patients who did not in the present study. Moreover, while several studies have shown that attainment of low proteinuria levels at one year of therapy for lupus nephritis is coupled with a better long-term renal prognosis, failure to attain this target was not clearly predictive of poor outcome [27,29,30], and another study found no clear association between proteinuria levels at one year of therapy and subsequent renal flares [31]. In contrast, this latter study revealed that active glomerular inflammatory lesions in per-protocol repeat kidney biopsies after the initial phase of therapy were predictive of subsequent renal flares [31]. Although direct examination of the kidney biopsy is considered the gold standard for determination of therapeutic need, its invasiveness makes it inappropriate in several cases, especially when the purpose is to predict future events rather than confirmation of activity and justification of therapy upon clinical indications. Moreover, while several theories exist, the exact mechanisms underlying inflammatory kidney injury in patients with SLE are not fully elucidated, and it is still unclear whether immune activation preceding nephritis starts in the periphery or in situ [5].

Various functions of B cells have been implicated in the pathogenesis of LN, including the production of inflammatory mediators or potentially nephritogenic autoantibodies and cytotoxicity mediated by interactions with components of the complement system. Studies of murine lupus have shown that B cells infiltrating the kidney tissue secrete antibodies with various antigen specificities and contribute to in situ immune complex formation [32–34]. Also in human studies, germinal-centre-like structures and T and B cell aggregates in the kidney have been shown to promote in situ secretion of pathogenic antibodies and immune complexes [35,36]. Moreover, in response to evidence that B cell depletion prevents or delays the onset of glomerulonephritis in lupus-prone mice [37,38] and induces complete or partial clinical remission in patients with lupus nephritis [39–41], B cell modulation with the BAFF inhibiting monoclonal antibody belimumab was recently shown successful in a lupus-nephritis-specific phase III clinical trial [19] and received approval for the treatment of this lupus manifestation. Moreover, the B-cell-depleting agent obinutuzumab has entered a phase III protocol after promising results in a phase II trial [41]. It is, however, worth noting that where the ability of B cells to secrete antibodies is impeded, lupus-prone mice have also been shown to develop nephritis [42], implying that B cell functions other than antibody production, such as antigen presentation or cytokine production, may also contribute to inflammatory kidney injury. Altogether, investigation of biological events in the periphery that can be anticipated to reflect the inflammatory activity in the kidney preceding renal flares has merit, and we hypothesised that kinetics of peripheral B cell and plasma cell subsets might prove to be a useful surveillance tool in this regard.

A kinetics pattern of a rapid drop in short-lived plasma cells and plasmablasts with a subsequent return was associated with the development of renal flares, while patients who did not develop renal flares showed more gradual decreases. Interestingly, this drop–return pattern was prominent in patients who received non-biological ST alone while the returning trend in these cell subsets was less pronounced or absent among patients who received add-on belimumab. It is worth noting that belimumab was herein shown to induce declining trends in certain plasma cell subsets early on upon treatment initiation, in part contrasting previous conflicting data [22–24], potentially owing to the large study population and resulting power amplification in statistical calculations as well as the detailed characterisation of peripheral plasma cells into different subsets. Another point of striking interest was the rapid decrease in peripheral long-lived plasma cells in belimumab-treated patients who did not develop renal flares, which was more prominent than in belimumab-treated patients who flared. In contrast, no such discriminative ability was observed for long-lived plasma cell kinetics in patients who were on non-biological ST alone. While the origin of long-lived plasma cells found in the periphery is unclear, this finding is in an intuitive direction and may prove useful in the early evaluation of belimumab therapy, signifying a better response and thus a protection against renal flare development in patients showing rapid reductions.

A similar pattern of an initial drop and subsequent return in memory B cells was seen in patients on non-biological ST who developed renal flares, while circulating memory B cells showed a rapid increase upon belimumab treatment regardless of renal flare occurrence. This increase in circulating memory B cells seen short time after initiation of belimumab treatment has been described in previous research [22–24], and it has been speculated to be related to a secondary defect in their trafficking receptors [25]. Thus, it may be argued that gradual decreases in selected B cell subsets may signify a durable response to treatment in terms of protection against renal flares, while return trends may be indicative of a rebound B cell enrichment or relative enrichment of certain subsets within the B cell pool.

While the difference did not reach statistical significance after adjustments, changes in activated B cells displayed numerically prominent differential patterns within the belimumab-treated population, with patients who developed renal flares showing increasing trends and patients who did not flare showing declines. The separation trend was seen at week 8, yielding an absolute difference of 23.9%, but was more prominent in the comparison of week 24, yielding an absolute difference of 70.7%. Despite the lack of statistical significance, the direction of this observation is intuitive, with B cells carrying activation markers accumulating towards a renal flare and decreasing activated B cells signifying favourable response to belimumab and protection against renal flares, warranting further study of this B cell subset in relation to responses to belimumab therapy.

In a subgroup analysis aiming at a better characterisation of the naïve and transitional B cells, transitional B cells showed rapid and sustained reductions in belimumab-treated patients, which were more prominent in patients who did not develop renal flares. In contrast, patients treated with non-biological ST alone showed less prominent decreases in transitional B cells, which did not distinguish flaring from non-flaring patients. Based on its mode of action, belimumab is expected to impact transitional and naïve B cells [43,44], while the more prominent decline in transitional B cells in belimumab-treated patients who were protected against renal flares may be speculated to be due to an augmented BAFF effect on transitional B cells in an environment of declining numbers of naïve B cells. Supportive of the latter may also be considered the previously documented increase in BAFF levels upon exposure to belimumab therapy [17].

While high levels of anti-dsDNA antibodies and low levels of C3 and C4 at baseline signified patients at risk for renal flares during follow-up, their rapid and early kinetics in response to therapy were not found to have any predictive value. Lastly, the higher levels of C4 and lower levels of short-lived plasma cells measured after the first documented renal flare compared with the last available measurement prior to the flare may be due to an effect of the glucocorticoid and/or immunosuppressive rescue therapy given to treat the observed flare. It is important to underline that our findings are rather hypothesis-generating and not intended to suggest the substitution of traditional serological markers with B cell and peripheral plasma cell kinetics. They are rather intended to suggest the use of both in a complemental fashion while monitoring drug efficacy, especially belimumab or other B cell targeting therapies, to obtain a better insight into the biological drug response and facilitate early treatment evaluation based on evidence-based expectations for subsequent clinical outcomes.

It is important to acknowledge that this study included a selected SLE population mainly displaying musculoskeletal and mucocutaneous activity at baseline; in total, 36.9% of the study participants had current or past renal involvement at baseline. Together with the short follow-up time, this explains the overall low incidence of renal flares during the study period and limits the generalisability of the findings in real-world SLE populations of higher percentages of renal involvement [1,5]. On the other hand, the study encompassed a large number of patients that commenced therapy for active, autoantibody-positive extrarenal disease, who are expected to be at a certain risk for developing renal flares [7] and were followed up in a structured manner which allowed for the detection of patterns of lymphocyte alterations over time after treatment commencement.

While SLE populations more enriched in active renal disease might yield a higher renal flare rate, it is of clinical relevance to also investigate renal flare development in a population commencing therapy for active extrarenal disease for several reasons. Firstly, because treatment given for extrarenal disease is not necessarily protective against development of renal activity and understanding how to prevent this is warranted. Secondly, a proportion of the study participants had active renal SLE (8.9%), and many had a history of renal involvement, albeit quiescent (5.7%), or stable (22.3%) renal disease at baseline. Thirdly, cases of de novo lupus nephritis development after commencement of belimumab therapy in patients with no prior renal SLE have been reported [21,45]. Hence, especially in light of the recent approval of add-on belimumab for active lupus nephritis [19], it is important to understand which patient subgroups are protected against renal flares during belimumab therapy and which patients are not. In the present investigation, the proportion of individuals who developed renal flares differed from those who did not in favour of belimumab only within patients treated with the low dose of i.v. belimumab (1 mg/kg). While the approved dose of add-on i.v. belimumab is 10 mg/kg, this dose was tested in patients with active LN and high levels of proteinuria, resulting in an increased drug clearance [19]. Altogether, the dose of belimumab in SLE patients with low-grade or no proteinuria may still require investigation in relation to drug effects on B cells with regulatory properties, as previously postulated [21], and indirectly supported by the prominent reductions of IL-10 upon belimumab therapy commencement for active extrarenal SLE [46].

4. Materials and Methods

4.1. Study Population

We analysed prospectively collected longitudinal data from patients with active SLE who participated in three multicentre, randomised, double-blind, placebo-controlled trials comparing belimumab (administered intravenously or subcutaneously) with placebo—i.e., BLISS-76 (NCT00410384; n = 819) [47], BLISS-SC (NCT01484496; n = 836) [48], and BLISS Northeast Asia (NEA; NCT01345253; n = 60) [49]—in a post hoc manner. The study population (n = 1715) was selected based on the a priori flow cytometry analysis plan for each one of the BLISS trials and therefore based on the availability of data on B cell subset counts, selected serological markers, and clinical data needed to determine renal flares. In the BLISS programmes, belimumab or placebo was administered on top of ST, including antimalarial agents, glucocorticoids, immunosuppressive agents, or combinations thereof.

In terms of design, the three trials were similar. Briefly, all patients were required to have a Safety of Estrogens in Lupus Erythematosus National Assessment-Systemic Lupus Erythematosus Disease Activity Index (SELENA-SLEDAI) [50] score ≥ 6 (BLISS-76) or ≥ 8 (BLISS-SC and BLISS-NEA) and had to be autoantibody-positive (antinuclear antibody titres $\geq$1:80 and/or anti-double stranded (ds)DNA levels $\geq$30 IU/mL) at the screening visit. All patients had received stable dosages of ST for at least 30 days prior to baseline. For BLISS-76 and BLISS-NEA, belimumab or placebo were administered intravenously on days 0, 14, and 28, and every 4th week thereafter through week 48 (NEA) or week 72 (BLISS-76). In BLISS-SC, belimumab 200 mg or placebo was administered subcutaneously weekly through week 52, on top of non-biological ST. Progressive restrictions were imposed during the trial periods on concurrent immunosuppressive and antimalarial medications, as well as glucocorticoid intake. The primary endpoint in all trials was the proportion of responders at week 52, with response being determined using the composite SLE Responder Index (SRI)-4 [51]. The similar trial design and endpoints allowed pooling of the data to increase power during statistical analyses.

4.2. Clinical Definitions

Renal flare was defined as the occurrence of one or more of the following features on two or more consecutive visits during the study period: (i) a reproducible increase in 24 h urine protein equivalent levels to >1 g if the baseline value was <0.2 g, >2 g if the baseline value was 0.2 g to 1 g, or >2 times the baseline value if the baseline value was >1 g; (ii) a reproducible increase in serum creatinine by $\geq 20\%$ or ≥ 0.3 mg/dL, accompanied by proteinuria (equivalent to >1 g/24 h), haematuria (≥ 4 red blood cells per high power field) and/or red blood cell casts; (iii) treatment-emergent reproducible haematuria (≥ 11 to 20 red blood cells per high power field) or a reproducible increase in haematuria by 2 grades compared to baseline associated with 25% dysmorphic red blood cells, glomerular in origin, exclusive of menses, and accompanied by either an ≥ 0.8 g increase in 24 h proteinuria (or equivalent amount measured by other means, such as the urinary protein to creatinine ratio) or new red blood cell casts [18]. Occurrence of renal flare was determined every fourth week during the study period.

History of or current renal involvement was defined as a renal score of A–D in the classic British Isles Lupus Assessment Group Index (BILAG) [52], while no history of renal involvement was defined a renal classic BILAG E. Active renal SLE was defined as a renal classic BILAG A or B. Organ damage was determined with the Systemic Lupus International Collaborating Clinics (SLICC)/American College of Rheumatology (ACR) Damage Index (SDI) [53].

4.3. Determination of B Cell Subsets and Serological Markers

Peripheral B cell and plasma cell subsets were determined via flow cytometry, and the gating strategy for cell separation was employed within the frame of the BLISS study programmes [47–49]. Flow cytometry was performed on samples captured at weeks 8, 24, and 52 in BLISS-76 and BLISS-SC, and at weeks 8, 12, and 52 in BLISS-NEA. The cell subsets were classified into total peripheral $CD19^+CD20^+$ B cells, $CD19^+CD20^+CD69^+$ activated B cells, $CD19^+CD20^+CD27^-$ naïve B cells, $CD19^+CD20^+CD27^+$ memory B cells, $CD19^+CD20^-CD27^{bright}$ plasmablasts, $CD19^+CD20^+CD138^+$ short-lived plasma cells, $CD19^+CD20^-CD138^+$ long-lived plasma cells, and $CD19^+CD38^{bright}CD27^{bright}$ SLE-associated plasma cells based on previous works deriving from the BLISS trials and other literature [23,54–56]. In a subgroup analysis to better characterise the $CD19^+CD20^+CD27^-$ cell subset performed in the population from the BLISS-SC trial, which encompassed a more detailed gating strategy, $CD19^+CD27^-CD24^{bright}CD38^{bright}$ designated transitional B cells, and $CD19^+CD27^-CD24^{low}CD38^{low}$ designated a befitting naïve B cell subset [57]. Levels of anti-dsDNA, C3, and C4 were determined within the frame of the BLISS programmes [47–49] and were made available through the Clinical Study Data Request (CSDR) consortium.

We analysed changes in B cell subsets and serum levels of anti-dsDNA, C3, and C4 that occurred through weeks 8, 24, and 52 relative to baseline (i.e., treatment initiation). The changes in B cell subsets between baseline and week 12 in the 60 patients from the BLISS-NEA trial were pooled with changes in B cell subsets between baseline and week 24 in the rest of the study population and were thus collectively termed changes through week 24. Changes occurring through week 8 were deemed rapid, and changes occurring through week 24 were deemed early; further changes were referred to as delayed. We next investigated associations between changes in B cell or plasma cell subsets or changes in serological markers and renal flares occurring until week 52 in a first analysis; throughout the entire follow-up, i.e., through week 52, for BLISS-SC and BLISS-NEA; and through week 76 for BLISS-76 in a subsequent analysis.

4.4. Ethics

Data from the BLISS trials were made available by GlaxoSmithKline (Uxbridge, UK) through the CSDR consortium. The trial protocols were approved by regional ethics review boards for all participating centres and complied with the ethical principles of the Declaration of Helsinki. Written informed consent was obtained from all study participants prior to enrolment. The present study was approved by the Swedish Ethical Review Authority (reference: 2019-05498).

4.5. Statistical Analysis

Descriptive statistics are reported as means and standard deviations or medians and interquartile ranges for continuous variables, while frequencies and percentages are reported for categorical variables. For comparisons of patient characteristics between patients who developed renal flares and patients who did not, non-parametrical Mann–Whitney U tests were used for continues variables, and chi-squared (χ^2) or Fisher's exact tests were used for binomial variables as appropriate. Comparisons of distributions of relative to baseline changes between flaring and non-flaring patients were conducted using multivariable logistic regression models; apart from the main exposure under investigation (i.e., relative to baseline percentage changes through week 8, week 24, or week 52 in B cell subset counts or serum levels of serological markers), other covariates in the models included age, ethnicity, glucocorticoid use, and belimumab use. Adjustment for belimumab use was not applicable in models stratified by treatment arm. Results from the logistic regression analyses are presented as the coefficient, odds ratio (OR), 95% confidence interval (CI), and P value for the main exposure in the respective multivariable logistic regression model.

In subgroup analyses from the BLISS-SC for a more in-depth characterisation of naïve and transitional B cells, the corresponding comparisons were performed using non-parametrical Mann–Whitney U tests due to the lack of a sufficient number of events (renal flares) limiting us from performing multivariable logistic regression analysis. Taking the randomisation in the clinical trials into consideration, comparisons between treatment arms were derived from non-parametrical Mann–Whitney U tests. Comparisons of distributions of related (paired) samples before and after the occurrence of the first recorded renal flare were conducted using the non-parametrical Wilcoxon signed-rank test. p values below 0.05 were deemed statistically significant. All analyses were performed using the R version 4.01 software (R Foundation for Statistical Computing, Vienna, Austria). The GraphPad Prism software version 9 (La Jolla, CA, USA) was used for the preparation of graphs.

5. Conclusions

To summarise, we showed that changes in the circulating B cell compartment in patients undergoing immunosuppressive treatment for active extra-renal SLE may help identify patients at risk for impending development of a renal flare and might hence have a place in disease surveillance as a complement to traditional parameters. Our findings provide implications that B cell kinetics with ability to inform about imminent renal flares differ between patients treated with non-biological standard therapy and patients receiving add-on belimumab owing to the effects of BAFF inhibition on the B cell compartment; this renders identification of therapy-specific patterns of B cell alterations of particular importance. The most striking results from the present study suggested that prominent rapid decreases in transitional B cells and peripheral long-lived plasma cells may signify a more favourable response to belimumab therapy and protection against renal flares.

Supplementary Materials: The following supporting information can be downloaded at: https://www.mdpi.com/article/10.3390/ijms232213941/s1.

Author Contributions: Conceptualization, I.P. and M.G.; methodology, I.P., A.G., J.L., and M.G.; software, I.P., A.G., and J.L.; formal analysis, I.P., A.G., and J.L.; investigation, I.P., A.G., J.L., J.W.C., C.S., S.S., and M.G.; resources, I.P.; data curation, A.G., J.L., and J.W.C.; writing—original draft preparation, I.P. and M.G.; writing—review and editing, I.P., A.G., J.L., J.W.C., C.S., S.S., and M.G.; visualization, A.G.; supervision, I.P., C.S., S.S., and M.G.; project administration, I.P.; funding acquisition, I.P. All authors have read and agreed to the published version of the manuscript.

Funding: This research was funded by grants from the Swedish Rheumatism Association (R-969696), King Gustaf V's 80-year Foundation (FAI-2020-0741; FAI-2020-0663), Swedish Society of Medicine (SLS-974449), Nyckelfonden (OLL-974804); Professor Nanna Svartz Foundation (2020-00368), Ulla and Roland Gustafsson Foundation (2021-26), Region Stockholm (FoUI-955483), and Karolinska Institutet.

Institutional Review Board Statement: Data from the BLISS trials were made available by GlaxoSmithKline (Uxbridge, UK) through the CSDR consortium. The trial protocols were approved by regional ethics review boards for all participating centres and complied with the ethical principles of the Declaration of Helsinki. The present study was approved by the Swedish Ethical Review Authority (reference: 2019-05498).

Informed Consent Statement: Informed consent was obtained from all subjects involved in the BLISS clinical trials.

Data Availability Statement: Data are available upon request through the Clinical Study Data Request (CSDR) portal: https://www.clinicalstudydatarequest.com (accessed on 13 August 2022).

Acknowledgments: The authors would like to thank GlaxoSmithKline for providing data from the BLISS-76 (NCT00410384), BLISS-SC (NCT01484496), and BLISS-NEA (NCT01345253) trials through the CSDR consortium as well as all patients with SLE who participated in the trials.

Conflicts of Interest: IP has received research funding and/or honoraria from Amgen, AstraZeneca, Aurinia Pharmaceuticals, Elli Lilly and Company, Gilead Sciences, GlaxoSmithKline, Janssen Pharmaceuticals, Novartis, and F. Hoffmann-La Roche AG. The other authors declare that they have no conflicts of interest related to this work. The funders had no role in the design of the study, the analyses or interpretation of data, or the writing of the manuscript.

References

1. Gasparotto, M.; Gatto, M.; Binda, V.; Doria, A.; Moroni, G. Lupus nephritis: Clinical presentations and outcomes in the 21st century. *Rheumatology (Oxford)* **2020**, *59*, v39–v51. [CrossRef] [PubMed]
2. Moroni, G.; Vercelloni, P.G.; Quaglini, S.; Gatto, M.; Gianfreda, D.; Sacchi, L.; Raffiotta, F.; Zen, M.; Costantini, G.; Urban, M.L.; et al. Changing patterns in clinical-histological presentation and renal outcome over the last five decades in a cohort of 499 patients with lupus nephritis. *Ann. Rheum. Dis.* **2018**, *77*, 1318–1325. [CrossRef] [PubMed]
3. Ugarte-Gil, M.F.; Acevedo-Vásquez, E.; Alarcón, G.S.; Pastor-Asurza, C.A.; Alfaro-Lozano, J.L.; Cucho-Venegas, J.M.; Segami, M.I.; Wojdyla, D.; Soriano, E.R.; Drenkard, C.; et al. The number of flares patients experience impacts on damage accrual in systemic lupus erythematosus: Data from a multiethnic Latin American cohort. *Ann. Rheum. Dis.* **2015**, *74*, 1019–1023. [CrossRef]
4. Doria, A.; Amoura, Z.; Cervera, R.; Khamastha, M.A.; Schneider, M.; Richter, J.; Guillemin, F.; Kobelt, G.; Maurel, F.; Garofano, A.; et al. Annual direct medical cost of active systemic lupus erythematosus in five European countries. *Ann. Rheum. Dis.* **2014**, *73*, 154–160. [CrossRef]
5. Anders, H.J.; Saxena, R.; Zhao, M.H.; Parodis, I.; Salmon, J.E.; Mohan, C. Lupus nephritis. *Nat. Rev. Dis. Prim.* **2020**, *6*, 7. [CrossRef]
6. Isenberg, D.A.; Allen, E.; Farewell, V.; D'Cruz, D.; Alarcon, G.S.; Aranow, C.; Bruce, I.N.; Dooley, M.A.; Fortin, P.R.; Ginzler, E.M.; et al. An assessment of disease flare in patients with systemic lupus erythematosus: A comparison of BILAG 2004 and the flare version of SELENA. *Ann. Rheum. Dis.* **2011**, *70*, 54–59. [CrossRef]
7. Ligtenberg, G.; Arends, S.; Stegeman, C.A.; de Leeuw, K. Predictors of renal flares and long-term renal outcome in patients with lupus nephritis: Results from daily clinical practice. *Clin. Exp. Rheumatol.* **2021**, *40*, 33–38. [CrossRef]
8. Luís, M.S.F.; Bultink, I.E.M.; da Silva, J.A.P.; Voskuyl, A.E.; Inês, L.S. Early predictors of renal outcome in patients with proliferative lupus nephritis: A 36-month cohort study. *Rheumatology (Oxford)* **2021**, *60*, 5134–5141. [CrossRef]
9. Pisetsky, D.S.; Lipsky, P.E. New insights into the role of antinuclear antibodies in systemic lupus erythematosus. *Nat. Rev. Rheumatol.* **2020**, *16*, 565–579. [CrossRef]
10. Gensous, N.; Marti, A.; Barnetche, T.; Blanco, P.; Lazaro, E.; Seneschal, J.; Truchetet, M.E.; Duffau, P.; Richez, C. Predictive biological markers of systemic lupus erythematosus flares: A systematic literature review. *Arthritis. Res. Ther.* **2017**, *19*, 238. [CrossRef]

11. Enocsson, H.; Sjöwall, C.; Wirestam, L.; Dahle, C.; Kastbom, A.; Rönnelid, J.; Wetterö, J.; Skogh, T. Four Anti-dsDNA Antibody Assays in Relation to Systemic Lupus Erythematosus Disease Specificity and Activity. *J. Rheumatol.* **2015**, *42*, 817–825. [CrossRef] [PubMed]
12. Parodis, I.; Stockfelt, M.; Sjowall, C. B Cell Therapy in Systemic Lupus Erythematosus: From Rationale to Clinical Practice. *Front. Med.* **2020**, *7*, 316. [CrossRef] [PubMed]
13. Gatto, M.; Saccon, F.; Andreoli, L.; Bartoloni, E.; Benvenuti, F.; Bortoluzzi, A.; Bozzolo, E.; Brunetta, E.; Canti, V.; Cardinaletti, P.; et al. Durable renal response and safety with add-on belimumab in patients with lupus nephritis in real-life setting (BeRLiSS-LN). Results from a large, nationwide, multicentric cohort. *J. Autoimmun.* **2021**, *124*, 102729. [CrossRef] [PubMed]
14. Gatto, M.; Saccon, F.; Zen, M.; Regola, F.; Fredi, M.; Andreoli, L.; Tincani, A.; Urban, M.L.; Emmi, G.; Ceccarelli, F.; et al. Early Disease and Low Baseline Damage as Predictors of Response to Belimumab in Patients WITH Systemic Lupus Erythematosus in a Real-Life Setting. *Arthritis Rheumatol.* **2020**, *72*, 1314–1324. [CrossRef] [PubMed]
15. Sciascia, S.; Radin, M.; Yazdany, J.; Levy, R.A.; Roccatello, D.; Dall'Era, M.; Cuadrado, M.J. Efficacy of belimumab on renal outcomes in patients with systemic lupus erythematosus: A systematic review. *Autoimmun. Rev.* **2017**, *16*, 287–293. [CrossRef] [PubMed]
16. Iaccarino, L.; Bettio, S.; Reggia, R.; Zen, M.; Frassi, M.; Andreoli, L.; Gatto, M.; Piantoni, S.; Nalotto, L.; Franceschini, F.; et al. Effects of Belimumab on Flare Rate and Expected Damage Progression in Patients With Active Systemic Lupus Erythematosus. *Arthritis Care Res. (Hoboken)* **2017**, *69*, 115–123. [CrossRef] [PubMed]
17. Parodis, I.; Sjowall, C.; Jonsen, A.; Ramskold, D.; Zickert, A.; Frodlund, M.; Sohrabian, A.; Arnaud, L.; Ronnelid, J.; Malmstrom, V.; et al. Smoking and pre-existing organ damage reduce the efficacy of belimumab in systemic lupus erythematosus. *Autoimmun. Rev.* **2017**, *16*, 343–351. [CrossRef]
18. Dooley, M.A.; Houssiau, F.; Aranow, C.; D'Cruz, D.P.; Askanase, A.; Roth, D.A.; Zhong, Z.J.; Cooper, S.; Freimuth, W.W.; Ginzler, E.M.; et al. Effect of belimumab treatment on renal outcomes: Results from the phase 3 belimumab clinical trials in patients with SLE. *Lupus* **2013**, *22*, 63–72. [CrossRef]
19. Furie, R.; Rovin, B.H.; Houssiau, F.; Malvar, A.; Teng, Y.K.O.; Contreras, G.; Amoura, Z.; Yu, X.; Mok, C.C.; Santiago, M.B.; et al. Two-Year, Randomized, Controlled Trial of Belimumab in Lupus Nephritis. *N. Engl. J. Med.* **2020**, *383*, 1117–1128. [CrossRef]
20. Parodis, I.; Houssiau, F.A. From sequential to combination and personalised therapy in lupus nephritis: Moving towards a paradigm shift? *Ann. Rheum. Dis.* **2021**, *81*, 15–19. [CrossRef]
21. Parodis, I.; Vital, E.M.; Hassan, S.U.; Jonsen, A.; Bengtsson, A.A.; Eriksson, P.; Leonard, D.; Gunnarsson, I.; Ronnblom, L.; Sjowall, C. De novo lupus nephritis during treatment with belimumab. *Rheumatology (Oxford)* **2021**, *60*, 4348–4354. [CrossRef]
22. Jacobi, A.M.; Huang, W.; Wang, T.; Freimuth, W.; Sanz, I.; Furie, R.; Mackay, M.; Aranow, C.; Diamond, B.; Davidson, A. Effect of long-term belimumab treatment on B cells in systemic lupus erythematosus: Extension of a phase II, double-blind, placebo-controlled, dose-ranging study. *Arthritis Rheum.* **2010**, *62*, 201–210. [CrossRef] [PubMed]
23. Stohl, W.; Hiepe, F.; Latinis, K.M.; Thomas, M.; Scheinberg, M.A.; Clarke, A.; Aranow, C.; Wellborne, F.R.; Abud-Mendoza, C.; Hough, D.R.; et al. Belimumab reduces autoantibodies, normalizes low complement levels, and reduces select B cell populations in patients with systemic lupus erythematosus. *Arthritis Rheum.* **2012**, *64*, 2328–2337. [CrossRef]
24. Ramskold, D.; Parodis, I.; Lakshmikanth, T.; Sippl, N.; Khademi, M.; Chen, Y.; Zickert, A.; Mikes, J.; Achour, A.; Amara, K.; et al. B cell alterations during BAFF inhibition with belimumab in SLE. *EBioMedicine* **2019**, *40*, 517–527. [CrossRef] [PubMed]
25. Arends, E.J.; Zlei, M.; Tipton, C.M.; Osmani, Z.; Kamerling, S.; Rabelink, T.; Sanz, I.; Van Dongen, J.J.M.; Van Kooten, C.; Teng, Y.K.O. POS0680 Belimumab Add-On Therapy Mobilises Memory B Cells into the Circulation of Patients with SLE. *Ann. Rheum. Dis.* **2021**, *80*, 585. [CrossRef]
26. Parodis, I.; Tamirou, F.; Houssiau, F.A. Prediction of prognosis and renal outcome in lupus nephritis. *Lupus Sci. Med.* **2020**, *7*, e000389. [CrossRef]
27. Dall'Era, M.; Cisternas, M.G.; Smilek, D.E.; Straub, L.; Houssiau, F.A.; Cervera, R.; Rovin, B.H.; Mackay, M. Predictors of long-term renal outcome in lupus nephritis trials: Lessons learned from the Euro-Lupus Nephritis cohort. *Arthritis Rheumatol.* **2015**, *67*, 1305–1313. [CrossRef] [PubMed]
28. Moroni, G.; Quaglini, S.; Maccario, M.; Banfi, G.; Ponticelli, C. "Nephritic flares" are predictors of bad long-term renal outcome in lupus nephritis. *Kidney Int.* **1996**, *50*, 2047–2053. [CrossRef]
29. Tamirou, F.; Lauwerys, B.R.; Dall'Era, M.; Mackay, M.; Rovin, B.; Cervera, R.; Houssiau, F.A.; Investigators, M.N.T. A proteinuria cut-off level of 0.7 g/day after 12 months of treatment best predicts long-term renal outcome in lupus nephritis: Data from the MAINTAIN Nephritis Trial. *Lupus Sci. Med.* **2015**, *2*, e000123. [CrossRef]
30. Ugolini-Lopes, M.R.; Seguro, L.P.C.; Castro, M.X.F.; Daffre, D.; Lopes, A.C.; Borba, E.F.; Bonfa, E. Early proteinuria response: A valid real-life situation predictor of long-term lupus renal outcome in an ethnically diverse group with severe biopsy-proven nephritis? *Lupus Sci. Med.* **2017**, *4*, e000213. [CrossRef]
31. Parodis, I.; Adamichou, C.; Aydin, S.; Gomez, A.; Demoulin, N.; Weinmann-Menke, J.; Houssiau, F.A.; Tamirou, F. Per-protocol repeat kidney biopsy portends relapse and long-term outcome in incident cases of proliferative lupus nephritis. *Rheumatology (Oxford)* **2020**, *59*, 3424–3434. [CrossRef] [PubMed]
32. Espeli, M.; Bokers, S.; Giannico, G.; Dickinson, H.A.; Bardsley, V.; Fogo, A.B.; Smith, K.G. Local renal autoantibody production in lupus nephritis. *J. Am. Soc. Nephrol.* **2011**, *22*, 296–305. [CrossRef]

33. Gatto, M.; Radu, C.M.; Luisetto, R.; Ghirardello, A.; Bonsembiante, F.; Trez, D.; Valentino, S.; Bottazzi, B.; Simioni, P.; Cavicchioli, L.; et al. Immunization with Pentraxin3 prevents transition from subclinical to clinical lupus nephritis in lupus-prone mice: Insights from renal ultrastructural findings. *J. Autoimmun.* **2020**, *111*, 102443. [CrossRef] [PubMed]
34. Sekine, H.; Watanabe, H.; Gilkeson, G.S. Enrichment of anti-glomerular antigen antibody-producing cells in the kidneys of MRL/MpJ-Fas(lpr) mice. *J. Immunol.* **2004**, *172*, 3913–3921. [CrossRef] [PubMed]
35. Chang, A.; Henderson, S.G.; Brandt, D.; Liu, N.; Guttikonda, R.; Hsieh, C.; Kaverina, N.; Utset, T.O.; Meehan, S.M.; Quigg, R.J.; et al. In situ B cell-mediated immune responses and tubulointerstitial inflammation in human lupus nephritis. *J. Immunol.* **2011**, *186*, 1849–1860. [CrossRef]
36. Hutloff, A.; Buchner, K.; Reiter, K.; Baelde, H.J.; Odendahl, M.; Jacobi, A.; Dorner, T.; Kroczek, R.A. Involvement of inducible costimulator in the exaggerated memory B cell and plasma cell generation in systemic lupus erythematosus. *Arthritis Rheum.* **2004**, *50*, 3211–3220. [CrossRef]
37. Ramanujam, M.; Bethunaickan, R.; Huang, W.; Tao, H.; Madaio, M.P.; Davidson, A. Selective blockade of BAFF for the prevention and treatment of systemic lupus erythematosus nephritis in NZM2410 mice. *Arthritis Rheum.* **2010**, *62*, 1457–1468. [CrossRef]
38. Bekar, K.W.; Owen, T.; Dunn, R.; Ichikawa, T.; Wang, W.; Wang, R.; Barnard, J.; Brady, S.; Nevarez, S.; Goldman, B.I.; et al. Prolonged effects of short-term anti-CD20 B cell depletion therapy in murine systemic lupus erythematosus. *Arthritis Rheum.* **2010**, *62*, 2443–2457. [CrossRef]
39. Jonsdottir, T.; Zickert, A.; Sundelin, B.; Henriksson, E.W.; van Vollenhoven, R.F.; Gunnarsson, I. Long-term follow-up in lupus nephritis patients treated with rituximab–clinical and histopathological response. *Rheumatology (Oxford)* **2013**, *52*, 847–855. [CrossRef]
40. Sfikakis, P.P.; Boletis, J.N.; Lionaki, S.; Vigklis, V.; Fragiadaki, K.G.; Iniotaki, A.; Moutsopoulos, H.M. Remission of proliferative lupus nephritis following B cell depletion therapy is preceded by down-regulation of the T cell costimulatory molecule CD40 ligand: An open-label trial. *Arthritis Rheum.* **2005**, *52*, 501–513. [CrossRef]
41. Furie, R.A.; Aroca, G.; Cascino, M.D.; Garg, J.P.; Rovin, B.H.; Alvarez, A.; Fragoso-Loyo, H.; Zuta-Santillan, E.; Schindler, T.; Brunetta, P.; et al. B-cell depletion with obinutuzumab for the treatment of proliferative lupus nephritis: A randomised, double-blind, placebo-controlled trial. *Ann. Rheum. Dis.* **2022**, *81*, 100–107. [CrossRef] [PubMed]
42. Chan, O.T.; Hannum, L.G.; Haberman, A.M.; Madaio, M.P.; Shlomchik, M.J. A novel mouse with B cells but lacking serum antibody reveals an antibody-independent role for B cells in murine lupus. *J. Exp. Med.* **1999**, *189*, 1639–1648. [CrossRef] [PubMed]
43. Regola, F.; Piantoni, S.; Lowin, T.; Archetti, S.; Reggia, R.; Kumar, R.; Franceschini, F.; Airò, P.; Tincani, A.; Andreoli, L.; et al. Association Between Changes in BLyS Levels and the Composition of B and T Cell Compartments in Patients With Refractory Systemic Lupus Erythematosus Treated With Belimumab. *Front. Pharmacol.* **2019**, *10*, 433. [CrossRef]
44. Huang, W.; Quach, T.D.; Dascalu, C.; Liu, Z.; Leung, T.; Byrne-Steele, M.; Pan, W.; Yang, Q.; Han, J.; Lesser, M.; et al. Belimumab promotes negative selection of activated autoreactive B cells in systemic lupus erythematosus patients. *JCI Insight* **2018**, *3*, e122525. [CrossRef]
45. Staveri, C.; Karokis, D.; Liossis, S.C. New onset of lupus nephritis in two patients with SLE shortly after initiation of treatment with belimumab. *Semin. Arthritis Rheum.* **2017**, *46*, 788–790. [CrossRef]
46. Parodis, I.; Akerstrom, E.; Sjowall, C.; Soltrablan, A.; Jonsen, A.; Gomez, A.; Frodlund, M.; Zickert, A.; Bengtsson, A.A.; Ronnelid, J.; et al. Autoantibody and Cytokine Profiles during Treatment with Belimumab in Patients with Systemic Lupus Erythematosus. *Int. J. Mol. Sci.* **2020**, *21*, 3463. [CrossRef]
47. Furie, R.; Petri, M.; Zamani, O.; Cervera, R.; Wallace, D.J.; Tegzova, D.; Sanchez-Guerrero, J.; Schwarting, A.; Merrill, J.T.; Chatham, W.W.; et al. A phase III, randomized, placebo-controlled study of belimumab, a monoclonal antibody that inhibits B lymphocyte stimulator, in patients with systemic lupus erythematosus. *Arthritis Rheum.* **2011**, *63*, 3918–3930. [CrossRef]
48. Stohl, W.; Schwarting, A.; Okada, M.; Scheinberg, M.; Doria, A.; Hammer, A.E.; Kleoudis, C.; Groark, J.; Bass, D.; Fox, N.L.; et al. Efficacy and Safety of Subcutaneous Belimumab in Systemic Lupus Erythematosus: A Fifty-Two-Week Randomized, Double-Blind, Placebo-Controlled Study. *Arthritis Rheumatol.* **2017**, *69*, 1016–1027. [CrossRef]
49. Zhang, F.; Bae, S.C.; Bass, D.; Chu, M.; Egginton, S.; Gordon, D.; Roth, D.A.; Zheng, J.; Tanaka, Y. A pivotal phase III, randomised, placebo-controlled study of belimumab in patients with systemic lupus erythematosus located in China, Japan and South Korea. *Ann. Rheum. Dis.* **2018**, *77*, 355–363. [CrossRef]
50. Petri, M.; Kim, M.Y.; Kalunian, K.C.; Grossman, J.; Hahn, B.H.; Sammaritano, L.R.; Lockshin, M.; Merrill, J.T.; Belmont, H.M.; Askanase, A.D.; et al. Combined oral contraceptives in women with systemic lupus erythematosus. *N. Engl. J. Med.* **2005**, *353*, 2550–2558. [CrossRef]
51. Furie, R.A.; Petri, M.A.; Wallace, D.J.; Ginzler, E.M.; Merrill, J.T.; Stohl, W.; Chatham, W.W.; Strand, V.; Weinstein, A.; Chevrier, M.R.; et al. Novel evidence-based systemic lupus erythematosus responder index. *Arthritis Rheum.* **2009**, *61*, 1143–1151. [CrossRef] [PubMed]
52. Hay, E.M.; Bacon, P.A.; Gordon, C.; Isenberg, D.A.; Maddison, P.; Snaith, M.L.; Symmons, D.P.; Viner, N.; Zoma, A. The BILAG index: A reliable and valid instrument for measuring clinical disease activity in systemic lupus erythematosus. *QJM Int. J. Med.* **1993**, *86*, 447–458.

53. Gladman, D.; Ginzler, E.; Goldsmith, C.; Fortin, P.; Liang, M.; Urowitz, M.; Bacon, P.; Bombardieri, S.; Hanly, J.; Hay, E.; et al. The development and initial validation of the Systemic Lupus International Collaborating Clinics/American College of Rheumatology damage index for systemic lupus erythematosus. *Arthritis Rheum.* **1996**, *39*, 363–369. [CrossRef]
54. Jacobi, A.M.; Odendahl, M.; Reiter, K.; Bruns, A.; Burmester, G.R.; Radbruch, A.; Valet, G.; Lipsky, P.E.; Dorner, T. Correlation between circulating CD27high plasma cells and disease activity in patients with systemic lupus erythematosus. *Arthritis Rheum.* **2003**, *48*, 1332–1342. [CrossRef] [PubMed]
55. Ellyard, J.I.; Avery, D.T.; Phan, T.G.; Hare, N.J.; Hodgkin, P.D.; Tangye, S.G. Antigen-selected, immunoglobulin-secreting cells persist in human spleen and bone marrow. *Blood* **2004**, *103*, 3805–3812. [CrossRef] [PubMed]
56. Klasener, K.; Jellusova, J.; Andrieux, G.; Salzer, U.; Bohler, C.; Steiner, S.N.; Albinus, J.B.; Cavallari, M.; Suss, B.; Voll, R.E.; et al. CD20 as a gatekeeper of the resting state of human B cells. *Proc. Natl. Acad. Sci. USA* **2021**, *118*, e2021342118. [CrossRef] [PubMed]
57. Sanz, I.; Wei, C.; Jenks, S.A.; Cashman, K.S.; Tipton, C.; Woodruff, M.C.; Hom, J.; Lee, F.E. Challenges and Opportunities for Consistent Classification of Human B Cell and Plasma Cell Populations. *Front. Immunol.* **2019**, *10*, 2458. [CrossRef]

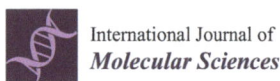

Article

Metabolic Markers and Association of Biological Sex in Lupus Nephritis

Bethany Wolf [1,†], Calvin R. K. Blaschke [2,†], Sandy Mungaray [3], Bryan T. Weselman [2], Mariia Stefanenko [4], Mykhailo Fedoriuk [4], Hongxia Bai [2], Jessalyn Rodgers [3], Oleg Palygin [4], Richard R. Drake [2] and Tamara K. Nowling [3,*]

[1] Department of Public Health Sciences, Medical University of South Carolina, 135 Cannon Street, Suite 303 MSC 835, Charleston, SC 29425, USA; wolfb@musc.edu
[2] Department of Cell and Molecular Pharmacology and Experimental Therapeutics, Medical University of South Carolina, 173 Ashley Avenue Basic Science Building 358, Charleston, SC 29425, USA; btw24@georgetown.edu (B.T.W.); baih@musc.edu (H.B.); draker@musc.edu (R.R.D.)
[3] Division of Rheumatology, Department of Medicine, Medical University of South Carolina, 171 Ashley Avenue, Charleston, SC 29425, USA; mungaray@musc.edu (S.M.); ierardi@musc.edu (J.R.)
[4] Division of Nephrology, Department of Medicine, Medical University of South Carolina, Clinical Sciences Building, 96 Jonathan Lucas Street, Charleston, SC 29425, USA; stefanen@musc.edu (M.S.); fedoriuk@musc.edu (M.F.); palygin@musc.edu (O.P.)
* Correspondence: nowling@musc.edu
† These authors contributed equally to this work.

Abstract: Lupus nephritis (LN) is a serious complication for many patients who develop systemic lupus erythematosus, which primarily afflicts women. Our studies to identify biomarkers and the pathogenic mechanisms underlying LN will provide a better understanding of disease progression and sex bias, and lead to identification of additional potential therapeutic targets. The glycosphingolipid lactosylceramide (LacCer) and N-linked glycosylated proteins (N-glycans) were measured in urine and serum collected from LN and healthy control (HC) subjects (10 females and 10 males in each group). The sera from the LN and HC subjects were used to stimulate cytokine secretion and intracellular Ca^{2+} flux in female- and male-derived primary human renal mesangial cells (hRMCs). Significant differences were observed in the urine of LN patients compared to HCs. All major LacCers species were significantly elevated and differences between LN and HC were more pronounced in males. 72 individual N-glycans were altered in LN compared to HC and three N-glycans were significantly different between the sexes. In hRMCs, Ca^{2+} flux, but not cytokine secretion, was higher in response to LN sera compared to HC sera. Ca^{2+} flux, cytokine secretion, and glycosphingolipid levels were significantly higher in female-derived compared to male-derived hRMCs. Relative abundance of some LacCers and hexosylceramides were higher in female-derived compared to male-derived hRMCs. Urine LacCers and N-glycome could serve as definitive LN biomarkers and likely reflect renal disease activity. Despite higher sensitivity of female hRMCs, males may experience greater increases in LacCers, which may underscore worse disease in males. Elevated glycosphingolipid metabolism may poise renal cells to be more sensitive to external stimuli.

Keywords: glycosylation; N-glycan; glycosphingolipid; lupus nephritis; mesangial cell; sex bias; biomarker

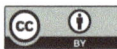

Citation: Wolf, B.; Blaschke, C.R.K.; Mungaray, S.; Weselman, B.T.; Stefanenko, M.; Fedoriuk, M.; Bai, H.; Rodgers, J.; Palygin, O.; Drake, R.R.; et al. Metabolic Markers and Association of Biological Sex in Lupus Nephritis. *Int. J. Mol. Sci.* **2023**, *24*, 16490. https://doi.org/10.3390/ijms242216490

Academic Editors: Ioannis Parodis and Christopher Sjöwall

Received: 6 October 2023
Revised: 8 November 2023
Accepted: 10 November 2023
Published: 18 November 2023

Copyright: © 2023 by the authors. Licensee MDPI, Basel, Switzerland. This article is an open access article distributed under the terms and conditions of the Creative Commons Attribution (CC BY) license (https://creativecommons.org/licenses/by/4.0/).

1. Introduction

Systemic lupus erythematosus (SLE) is an autoimmune disease in which the immune system can attack a variety of organs. Nephritis is a major complication of lupus that occurs in greater than 50% of SLE patients. SLE also exhibits a strong sex bias occurring 9–10 times more frequently in females than males [1]. The underlying mechanisms involved in the development of nephritis in SLE patients are not completely known, nor is the sex bias in disease understood. While many studies have focused on understanding changes in the levels of genes or proteins, few have investigated the changes in lipids or glycosylation with respect to disease or sex bias.

Glycosphingolipids (GSLs) are neutral lipids synthesized from ceramide by the addition of galactose or glucose to generate galactosylceramides (GalCers) or glucosylceramides (GlcCers), which together make up hexosylceramides (HexCers). Lactosylceramides (LacCers) are generated from GlcCers. These GSLs are involved in a wide array of functions in most cell types, including proliferation, apoptosis, and signal transduction [2–6]. We previously demonstrated in a small cohort of subjects that LacCers were significantly elevated in the urine of lupus patients with nephritis compared to lupus patients without nephritis or healthy subjects [7]. Differences in these GSLs were not observed in the serum. While sex differences of the circulating lipidome were recently reported, GSLs (GlcCers and LacCers) were not included [8]. To our knowledge, quantification of circulating or urine GSLs with respect to sex in healthy subjects, or to sex and disease in SLE patients, has not been reported.

Similar to GSLs, N-linked glycosylation of lipids and proteins plays an important role in mediating many different cellular functions including cell interactions and signal transduction. N-linked glycosylation can modulate the activity of proteins including IgG effector function [9]. While changes in the N-glycome are observed in many inflammatory or autoimmune diseases [10,11] including lupus [12–17], global changes in the N-glycome associated with disease or with biologic sex in lupus nephritis are unknown.

In this study, we analyzed differences in the levels of LacCers and N-glycosylated proteins (N-glycans) in urine and serum with respect to disease status and biologic sex. We show that all major LacCers in the urine, but only two major LacCers in the serum, were significantly elevated in LN patients compared to HC subjects in this study cohort. Although no differences were observed in overall levels of urine or serum LacCers with respect to biologic sex, a greater increase in urine LacCers was observed in males when comparing LN to HC. We observed that 75% of the urine N-glycans and 30% of the serum N-glycans were associated with disease status. Three of the urine N-glycans were associated with biologic sex. Activation of primary human renal mesangial cells (hRMCs) to the human sera was observed by measuring intracellular Ca^{2+} flux and cytokine release. Ca^{2+} flux was significantly higher in response to serum from LN patients compared to HC subjects. Intracellular Ca^{2+} flux in hRMCs derived from a female donor was more sensitive and the cells released two-fold to ten-fold higher levels of cytokines in response to sera compared to hRMCs derived from a male donor. Interestingly, the GSLs levels were higher in the female-derived hRMCs compared to the male-derived hRMCs and this may contribute in part to the hyper-response of the female-derived hRMCs.

2. Results

2.1. Comparison of LacCers and N-Linked Glycosylation in Urine of Lupus Nephritis Patients Compared to Healthy Controls and between Sexes

The study population comparing lupus nephritis (LN) patients to healthy controls (HCs) included 20 subjects in each group with equal sex distribution (50% female for each group). LN patients and HCs were similar in age but a larger proportion of LN patients were black relative to HCs. The eGFR and urine creatinine levels were similar in the two groups. Significant differences between LN patients and HCs were observed for UPCr, C3 complement, and C4 complement. Participant demographics by disease status are shown in Table 1. We previously demonstrated that levels of LacCers in the urine of LN patients were significantly higher compared to lupus patients without nephritis and compared to HCs [7]. Similarly, in this study cohort, the levels of the major chain lengths of LacCer (C16, C22, C24:1, and C24), as well as the total of all LacCer chain lengths, were significantly higher in LN patients compared to HCs (Figure 1A). To determine if LacCers levels differed based on biologic sex, we compared LacCers levels in the two groups. Although the differences did not reach statistical significance in this small cohort, the urine LacCers levels tended to be higher in females compared to males in the HC group (Figure 1B). This trend was not observed in the LN group. Thus, the relative increases in LN urine LacCers (C16, C24:1, C24, and total) compared to HC urine was approximately twofold higher in LN males than in LN females (Figure 1C). This suggests that while both sexes with LN experience increases in urine LacCers, males may have a larger increase than females.

Table 1. Demographics and clinical measures of healthy controls (HC) and lupus nephritis (LN) patients.

	HC (N = 20)	LN (N = 20)	p
Sex, male, n (%)	10 (50)	10 (50)	1.000
Age, mean (SD)	34.0 (10.3)	33.2 (11.2)	0.824
Race, n (%)			0.041
Black	10 (50)	16 (80)	
White	10 (50)	3 (15)	
Other	0 (0)	1 (5)	
Estimated Glomerular Filtration Rate, mean (SD)	103.9 (23.9)	93.0 (51.9)	0.455
Urine Creatinine, mg/mL (SD)	1.46 (1.14)	1.24 (0.82)	0.484
Urine Protein: Creatinine, median (IQR)	0.055 (0.033)	1.69 (3.48)	<0.001
Nephritis Class, n (%)			N/A
I	N/A	2 (10)	
II	N/A	2 (10)	
III, IV	N/A	8 (40)	
III + V, IV + V	N/A	3 (15)	
V	N/A	3 (15)	
No biopsy/missing	N/A	2 (10)	
SLEDAI, mean (SD)	N/A	11.85 (5.6)	N/A
Anti-dsDNA, n positive (%)	N/A	15 (75)	N/A
Anti-Sm, n positive (%)	N/A	10 (56)	N/A
Anti-RNP, n positive (%)	N/A	11 (61)	N/A
C3 Complement, mean (SD)	151.0 (16.1)	85.8 (21.5)	<0.001
C4 Complement, mean (SD)	33.9 (11.5)	23.0 (8.18)	0.034

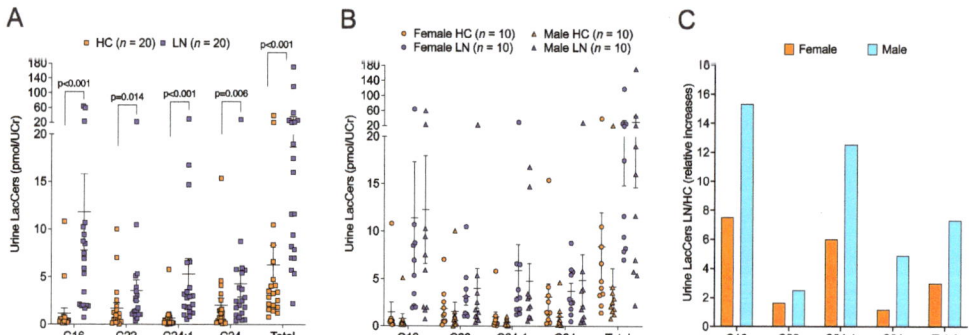

Figure 1. Urine LacCers levels were significantly higher in LN compared to HC. LacCer chain lengths of C14 to C26 were quantified in urine samples of healthy controls (HC) and lupus nephritis patients (LN) and included 10 females and 10 males in each group. (**A**) Levels of the major LacCer chain lengths detected in the urine and the total of all LacCers chain lengths (Total) are shown in the graphs for all HC (*n* = 20) compared to all LN (*n* = 20) subjects. (**B**) Levels of the major LacCer chain lengths by sex in the HC and LN groups. (**C**) Ratio of LacCers levels in LN to HC by sex.

Ninety-six individual N-glycans (peaks) in urine were detectable in most of the samples, summarized in Supplemental Table S2. Nine classes of glycans, which used the sum of the relative frequencies for those peaks in that class, were also considered: mannose, hybrid, biantennary, triantennary, tetrantennary, bisecting, fucosylated, sialylated, and sulfonated. Seven of the N-glycan classes differed significantly between LN patients and HCs after FDR correction (Figure 2A). Of the 96 individual N-glycans detected, the relative abundance of 72 of the N-glycans differed significantly between LN patients and HCs after FDR correction. The top 10 significantly different individual N-glycans are presented in Figure 2C. We also examined sex differences in the relative frequencies of the glycans in these data. The interaction between biologic sex and disease status was not significant in any of the statistical models. Thus, results for disease status are reported across males and females and results for biologic sex are reported across disease status. None of the N-glycan classes differed significantly by sex (Figure 2B) and only three of the individual N-glycans (peaks 2361, 2339, and 2289, Figure 2D) differed significantly by sex after FDR correction. There was a significant increase in the degalactosylated (and desialylated, peak 1485) glycan shown to be associated with IgG that exhibits a more pro-inflammatory function, and significant decreases in the biantennary galactosylated (peaks 1663 and 1809) and sialylated (peaks 2122 and 2435) glycans that are associated with a more anti-inflammatory IgG (Figure 2E). Supplemental Figure S1A shows a heatmap of the 72 glycans found to be associated with disease status and Supplementary Table S2 shows the mean difference and 95% confidence interval in the relative frequencies of all the N-glycan classes and individual peaks between LN patients and HCs as well as between males and females.

We then examined if inclusion of the individual N-glycans in a model that included total urine LacCers level and biologic sex improved discrimination between LN patients and HCs for those N-glycans identified as differing between LN and HC. Models with one N-glycan added were compared to the baseline model for improvements in fit based on the likelihood ratio test. Of the 72 N-glycans identified to be associated with disease, 27 were significant in a model including total urine LacCers and biologic sex (although none retained significance after FDR correction). The primary metric for evaluating discrimination of cases was the AUC statistic. The baseline model including only urine total LacCers and biologic sex had an AUC (95% CI) of 0.87 (0.75, 0.99). Models including one additional N-glycan from among those associated with SLE status improved the AUC relative to the baseline model by between 0 and 0.118 units (i.e., increasing the AUC from 0.870 to between 0.870–0.992). The AUCs, likelihood ratio test p-values (for comparison of a model including the N-glycan versus excluding the N-glycan), and difference in AUCs are shown in Table 2.

Table 2. AUCs, likelihood ratio test (LRT) p-values, and differences in AUC of adding urine N-glycans to a "null" model. The null model included only total urine LacCers and biologic sex. Urine LacCers was natural log transformed prior to fitting the models to meet statistical assumptions. * Inclusion of this glycan yielded perfect separation of the cases and controls.

	AIC	LRT p-Value	AUC (95% CI)	Δ AUC (95% CI)
Null Model	43.12	0.0020	0.870 (0.748, 0.992)	
2669 *	8	0.9970	1 (1, 1)	0.13 (0.008, 0.252)
1419 *	8	0.9976	1 (1, 1)	0.13 (0.008, 0.252)
1581 *	8	0.9987	1 (1, 1)	0.13 (0.008, 0.252)
Mannose *	8	0.9987	1 (1, 1)	0.13 (0.008, 0.252)
1485	33.92	0.0081	0.932 (0.859, 1.00)	0.062 (−0.031, 0.156)
1853	30.1	0.0081	0.945 (0.866, 1.00)	0.075 (−0.025, 0.175)
2174	32.47	0.0085	0.943 (0.876, 1.00)	0.073 (−0.036, 0.181)
1866	31.85	0.0095	0.948 (0.88, 1.00)	0.078 (−0.023, 0.178)
2122	33.54	0.0107	0.943 (0.872, 1.00)	0.073 (−0.047, 0.192)
2158	28.28	0.0108	0.958 (0.903, 1.00)	0.088 (−0.023, 0.198)
1996	31.62	0.0111	0.948 (0.887, 1.00)	0.078 (−0.026, 0.181)
2377	25.13	0.0119	0.970 (0.923, 1.00)	0.100 (−0.019, 0.219)
2361	34	0.0124	0.938 (0.860, 1.00)	0.068 (−0.018, 0.153)
Tetraantennary	33.13	0.0130	0.938 (0.860, 1.00)	0.068 (−0.054, 0.189)
2012	34.74	0.0131	0.917 (0.830, 1.00)	0.047 (−0.062, 0.157)

Table 2. *Cont.*

	AIC	LRT *p*-Value	AUC (95% CI)	Δ AUC (95% CI)
2967	31.54	0.0159	0.943 (0.861, 1.00)	0.073 (−0.042, 0.187)
2289	36.13	0.0170	0.915 (0.828, 1.00)	0.045 (−0.059, 0.149)
Sialylation	35.54	0.0182	0.948 (0.874, 1.00)	0.078 (−0.018, 0.173)
1831	34.34	0.0212	0.932 (0.846, 1.00)	0.062 (−0.014, 0.139)
2056	37.2	0.0225	0.915 (0.829, 1.00)	0.045 (−0.025, 0.115)
1704	33.24	0.0242	0.955 (0.886, 1.00)	0.085 (−0.011, 0.181)
1809	37.7	0.0250	0.917 (0.833, 1.00)	0.047 (−0.036, 0.131)
3770	37.38	0.0264	0.902 (0.805, 1.00)	0.032 (−0.062, 0.127)
2632	38.17	0.0289	0.907 (0.813, 1.00)	0.037 (−0.035, 0.110)
2487	38.8	0.0311	0.897 (0.806, 0.989)	0.027 (−0.065, 0.120)
2267	37.86	0.0314	0.915 (0.830, 1.00)	0.045 (−0.038, 0.128)
1257	20.36	0.0346	0.985 (0.959, 1.00)	0.115 (−0.005, 0.235)
2245	38.88	0.0363	0.902 (0.807, 0.998)	0.032 (−0.034, 0.099)
2852	38.39	0.0367	0.912 (0.823, 1.00)	0.042 (−0.068, 0.153)
1079	39.5	0.0372	0.900 (0.793, 1.00)	0.030 (−0.067, 0.127)
2221	39.48	0.0389	0.902 (0.807, 0.998)	0.032 (−0.047, 0.112)
2638	38.44	0.0406	0.910 (0.809, 1.00)	0.040 (−0.040, 0.120)
3333	38.94	0.0412	0.897 (0.800, 0.995)	0.027 (−0.070, 0.125)
2287	38.33	0.0445	0.902 (0.808, 0.997)	0.032 (−0.040, 0.105)
1663	39.57	0.0477	0.885 (0.774, 0.996)	0.015 (−0.032, 0.062)
1891	19.61	0.0557	0.988 (0.965, 1.00)	0.118 (−0.001, 0.236)
1743	19.12	0.0567	0.985 (0.957, 1.00)	0.115 (0.005, 0.225)
2945	40.2	0.0586	0.897 (0.801, 0.994)	0.027 (−0.032, 0.087)
1905	21.5	0.0604	0.983 (0.954, 1.00)	0.113 (0.001, 0.224)
1444	37.27	0.0657	0.920 (0.831, 1.00)	0.05 (−0.038, 0.138)
2465	41.09	0.0714	0.890 (0.792, 0.988)	0.02 (−0.053, 0.093)
1960	41.41	0.0741	0.887 (0.774, 1.00)	0.017 (−0.038, 0.073)
2523	37.65	0.0813	0.907 (0.809, 1.00)	0.037 (−0.024, 0.099)
3144	40.32	0.0826	0.897 (0.800, 0.995)	0.027 (−0.05, 0.105)
1647	41.44	0.0864	0.895 (0.798, 0.992)	0.025 (−0.04, 0.09)
3646	41.69	0.0948	0.887 (0.787, 0.988)	0.017 (−0.043, 0.078)
2654	41.54	0.1038	0.887 (0.779, 0.996)	0.017 (−0.059, 0.094)
1954	42.03	0.1056	0.892 (0.790, 0.995)	0.022 (−0.036, 0.081)
2610	41.41	0.1125	0.885 (0.777, 0.993)	0.015 (−0.038, 0.068)
2028	42.3	0.1158	0.893 (0.778, 1.00)	0.023 (−0.024, 0.069)
sulfation	42.4	0.1233	0.900 (0.793, 1.00)	0.03 (−0.016, 0.076)
2163	42.2	0.1234	0.882 (0.774, 0.991)	0.012 (−0.062, 0.087)
2923	42.01	0.1353	0.880 (0.774, 0.986)	0.01 (−0.052, 0.072)
1814	42.61	0.1363	0.885 (0.786, 0.984)	0.015 (−0.061, 0.091)
2304	42.78	0.1480	0.887 (0.784, 0.991)	0.017 (−0.057, 0.092)
3092	42.8	0.1579	0.873 (0.754, 0.991)	0.003 (−0.034, 0.039)
1850	42.93	0.1609	0.88 (0.771, 0.989)	0.01 (−0.059, 0.079)
3193	42.38	0.1649	0.885 (0.778, 0.992)	0.015 (−0.042, 0.072)
3113	42.56	0.1651	0.882 (0.769, 0.996)	0.012 (−0.017, 0.042)
3004	42.8	0.1815	0.878 (0.760, 0.995)	0.008 (−0.03, 0.045)
2435	43.22	0.1838	0.875 (0.769, 0.981)	0.005 (−0.06, 0.07)
3093	43.2	0.1933	0.865 (0.740, 0.990)	−0.005 (−0.039, 0.029)
2393	43.16	0.2030	0.880 (0.769, 0.991)	0.010 (−0.042, 0.062)
fucosylation	43.35	0.2073	0.885 (0.780, 0.990)	0.015 (−0.044, 0.074)
2100	43.33	0.2168	0.870 (0.754, 0.986)	0.00 (−0.048, 0.048)
3384	43.18	0.2193	0.873 (0.755, 0.99)	0.003 (−0.044, 0.049)
triantennary	43.7	0.2642	0.870 (0.747, 0.993)	0.00 (−0.052, 0.052)
bisect	43.82	0.2776	0.882 (0.774, 0.991)	0.012 (−0.045, 0.07)
2319	43.58	0.2828	0.882 (0.772, 0.993)	0.012 (−0.036, 0.061)
1875	44.09	0.3257	0.882 (0.769, 0.996)	0.012 (−0.017, 0.042)
2383	44.55	0.4570	0.882 (0.767, 0.998)	0.012 (−0.019, 0.044)
2413	44.69	0.5224	0.863 (0.739, 0.986)	−0.007 (−0.041, 0.026)
1773	44.75	0.5600	0.875 (0.756, 0.994)	0.005 (−0.016, 0.026)

Table 2. Cont.

	AIC	LRT p-Value	AUC (95% CI)	Δ AUC (95% CI)
1611	44.83	0.5933	0.877 (0.762, 0.993)	0.007 (−0.02, 0.035)
2594	44.87	0.6229	0.877 (0.759, 0.996)	0.007 (−0.019, 0.034)
2339	44.89	0.6393	0.875 (0.752, 0.998)	0.005 (−0.019, 0.029)
2341	44.97	0.7073	0.875 (0.758, 0.992)	0.005 (−0.019, 0.029)
2391	45.1	0.9027	0.873 (0.750, 0.995)	0.003 (−0.004, 0.009)

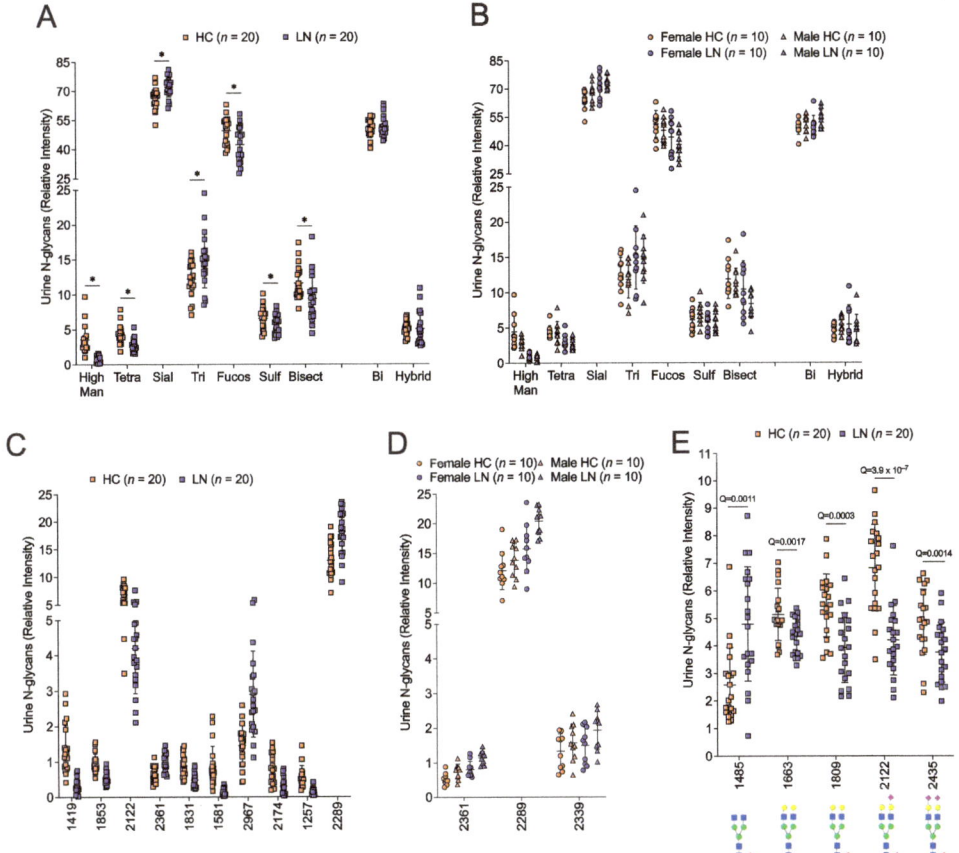

Figure 2. The urine N-glycome was significantly different in LN compared to HC; some differed by sex. N-glycans were quantified in the same urine samples as in Figure 1 of 20 healthy controls (HC) and 20 lupus nephritis patients (LN) and included 10 females and 10 males in each group. N-glycan classes: high mannose (High Man), tetra-antennary (Tetra), sialylated (Sial), tri-antennary (Tri), fucosylated (Fucos), sulfated (Sulf), bisected (Bisect), bi-antennary (Bi), or Hybrid were compared in all HC vs. all LN (**A**) or by sex in each group (**B**). * Significant difference between HC and LN. Specific Q-values are provided in Table S1. Individual N-glycans were compared in all HC vs. all LN (**C**) or by sex in each group (**D**). Of the 72 individual N-glycans that differed significantly between HC and LN, the top 10 are presented in (**C**). Only three N-glycans differed significantly between females and males (**D**). (**E**) N-glycans associated with IgG are significantly different between HC and LN. N-glycan structures shown below the m/z peak values. See Table S2 for a list of all urine N-glycans detected and the adjusted Q values and Table S1 for N-glycans structure information.

2.2. Comparison of LacCers and N-Linked Glycosylation in Serum of Lupus Nephritis Patients Compared to Healthy Controls and between Sexes

Serum samples were analyzed from the same LN patients and HCs from whom urine samples were analyzed above. As we reported previously in a different cohort of subjects [7], we did not observe a significant difference in C16 LacCer levels between LN patients and HCs in this cohort, nor did we observe a difference in the levels of total LacCers (Figure 3A). However, we did observe significant differences in C22 and C24 LacCers between LN patients and HCs. As in the urine LacCers analyses, we did not observe any differences in serum LacCers based on biological sex regardless of disease status (Figure 3B).

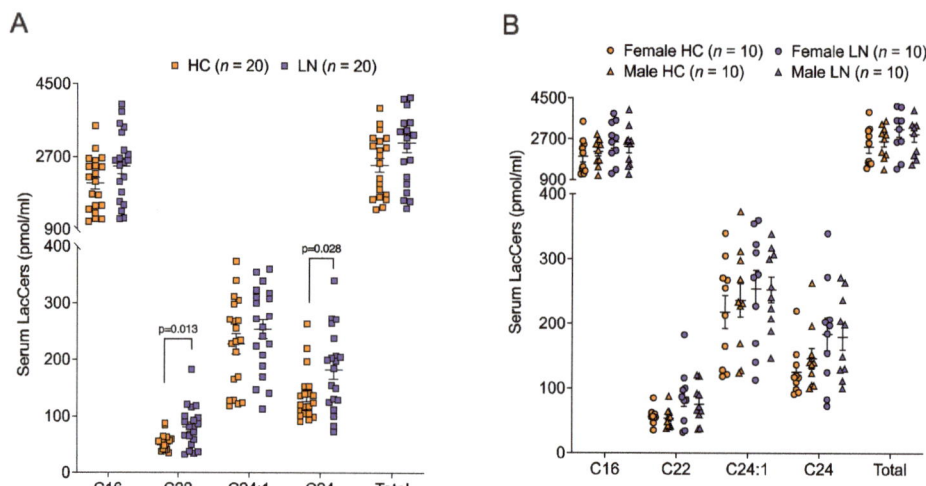

Figure 3. Two serum LacCer species were significantly higher in serum from LN compared to HC. LacCer chain lengths of C14 to C26 were quantified in serum samples of the same HC and LN subjects as in Figure 1 (10 females and 10 males in each group). (**A**) Levels of the major LacCer chain lengths detected in the serum and the total of all LacCers chain lengths (Total) are shown in the graphs for all HC ($n = 20$) compared to all LN ($n = 20$) subjects. (**B**) Levels of the major LacCer chain lengths by sex in the HC and LN groups.

Seventy individual N-glycans (peaks) were detectable in serum in most of the samples. Five N-glycan classes differed significantly between LN patients and HCs after FDR correction (Figure 4A). Of the 70 detected individual N-glycans, the relative abundance of 21 of the N-glycans groups differed significantly between LN patients and HCs after FDR correction. The top 10 significantly different individual N-glycans are shown in Figure 4B. We also examined sex differences in the relative frequencies of the N-glycans in these data; however, none of the N-glycan classes (Figure 4C) or individual N-glycans differed significantly by sex after FDR correction. Only one of the IgG-associated N-glycan peaks, 1809 (desialylated containing a core fucose), in the serum was highly significantly different between the two groups with it being decreased in the LN group (Figure 4D). The mono-sialylated form was also decreased with the difference only just significant at $Q = 0.0449$. Supplementary Figure S1B shows a heatmap of the 26 serum N-glycans (21 individual and 5 classes) associated with disease status. Supplementary Table S3 shows the mean difference and 95% confidence interval in the relative frequencies of the different N-glycan classes or individual N-glycans between LN patients and HCs, and between males and females.

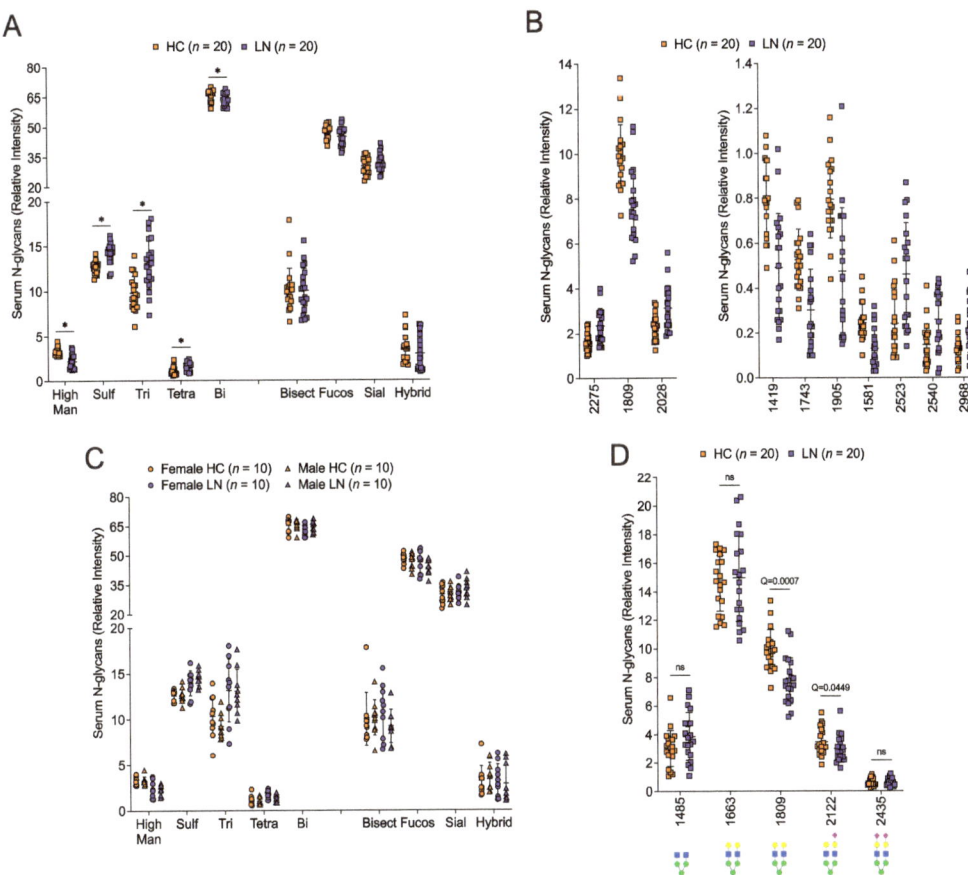

Figure 4. The serum N-glycome was significantly different in LN compared to HC. N-glycans were quantified in the same serum samples as in Figure 3 of 20 healthy controls (HC) and 20 lupus nephritis patients (LN) and included 10 females and 10 males in each group. N-glycan classes: high mannose (High Man), tetra-antennary (Tetra), sialylated (Sial), tri-antennary (Tri), fucosylated (Fucos), sulfated (Sulf), bisected (Bisect), bi-antennary (Bi), or Hybrid were compared in all HC vs. all LN (**A**) or by sex in each group (**C**) * Q < 0.05 (see Table S3 for calculated adjusted Q-values). (**B**) Individual N-glycans were compared in all HC vs. all LN and the top 10 of the 21 individual N-glycans that differed significantly between HC and LN are presented. (**D**) N-glycans associated with IgG (ns, not significant).. N-glycan structures shown below the m/z peak values. See Table S3 for a list of all serum N-glycans detected and the calculated adjusted Q-values and Table S1 for N-glycans structures.

We then examined if inclusion of the individual serum N-glycans in a model including total urine LacCers level and biologic sex improved discrimination between LN and HC for those N-glycans identified as differing between LN patients and HCs. Models with one N-glycan added were compared to the baseline model for improvements in fit base on the likelihood ratio test. Of the 21 individual or 5 classes of N-glycans associated with SLE status, 20 were significant in a model including total urine LacCers and biologic sex (although none retained significance after FDR correction). The baseline model including only urine total LacCers and biologic sex had an AUC (95% CI) of 0.87 (0.75, 0.99). Models including one additional N-glycan from among those identified to be associated with LN status improved the AUC relative to the baseline model by between 0.005 and 0.085 units. The AUCs, likelihood ratio test *p*-values (for comparison of a model including the serum N-glycan versus excluding the N-glycan), and difference in AUCs are shown in Table 3.

Table 3. AUCs, likelihood ratio test (LRT) *p*-values, and differences in AUC of adding serum N-glycans to a "null" model (same null model as in Table 2).

	AIC	LRT *p*-Value	AUC (95% CI)	D AUC
Null Model	43.12	0.002	0.870 (0.748, 0.992)	
mannose	29.08	0.012	0.955 (0.900, 1.00)	0.085 (−0.016, 0.186)
1743	29.71	0.013	0.953 (0.897, 1.00)	0.083 (−0.013, 0.178)
1581	30.74	0.008	0.950 (0.887, 1.00)	0.080 (−0.024, 0.184)
sulfation	32.53	0.006	0.945 (0.875, 1.00)	0.075 (−0.031, 0.181)
1419	32.62	0.006	0.943 (0.876, 1.00)	0.073 (−0.030, 0.175)
triantennary	32.94	0.013	0.935 (0.867, 1.00)	0.065 (−0.041, 0.171)
1809	33.3	0.009	0.938 (0.868, 1.00)	0.068 (−0.039, 0.174)
2275	33.33	0.016	0.927 (0.852, 1.00)	0.057 (−0.041, 0.156)
2540.1	33.69	0.007	0.935 (0.864, 1.00)	0.065 (−0.023, 0.153)
2028	34.96	0.02	0.917 (0.834, 1.00)	0.047 (−0.052, 0.147)
1444	35.96	0.028	0.917 (0.834, 1.00)	0.047 (−0.044, 0.139)
1905	36.12	0.015	0.935 (0.855, 1.00)	0.065 (−0.009, 0.139)
1136	36.24	0.019	0.910 (0.823, 0.997)	0.040 (−0.054, 0.134)
tetraantennary	36.79	0.015	0.915 (0.830, 1.00)	0.045 (−0.049, 0.139)
1257	36.87	0.014	0.920 (0.831, 1.00)	0.050 (−0.044, 0.144)
2319	37.69	0.026	0.900 (0.809, 0.991)	0.030 (−0.072, 0.132)
2122	38.32	0.024	0.910 (0.826, 0.994)	0.040 (−0.053, 0.133)
2633.1	39.17	0.043	0.900 (0.809, 0.991)	0.030 (−0.060, 0.120)
2523.1	39.2	0.036	0.895 (0.799, 0.991)	0.025 (−0.059, 0.109)
2231	40.01	0.053	0.897 (0.803, 0.992)	0.027 (−0.050, 0.105)
2393	40.16	0.04	0.905 (0.813, 0.997)	0.035 (−0.045, 0.115)
2341	40.65	0.066	0.895 (0.799, 0.991)	0.025 (−0.050, 0.100)
biantennary	40.83	0.053	0.897 (0.788, 1.00)	0.027 (−0.036, 0.091)
1647	41.87	0.091	0.890 (0.780, 1.00)	0.020 (−0.037, 0.077)
2968.1	42.67	0.15	0.880 (0.774, 0.986)	0.010 (−0.059, 0.079)
2655.1	42.75	0.158	0.875 (0.767, 0.983)	0.005 (−0.071, 0.081)

2.3. Influence of Disease and Biologic Sex in the Response of Mesangial Cells to Human Sera

The above results showed significant differences in the levels of 21 different N-glycans between LN and HC serum. To determine if renal cells would exhibit differential responses to these sera, primary human renal mesangial cells (hRMCs) were used for the following studies. A preliminary experiment was performed to identify cytokines that may be differentially secreted in response to LN compared to HC sera (see Supplemental methods). We first measured the release of IL-6 and MCP-1 in response to 10% sera collected from 12 HCs, 12 LN patients with active disease, and 12 LN patients with inactive disease (not the same subjects included the LacCers and N-glycan analyses) based on our prior studies in mice. [18,19]. No differences across the three groups were observed in IL-6 or MCP-1 release (Figure S2A). The media from this experiment was then pooled to generate two samples per group and a cytokine array screened to identify cytokines that may be differentially released in response to HC vs. LN Active vs. LN Inactive sera. Results from this array (Figure S2B) suggested that higher levels of CCL5 and CXCL5 were released in response to LN Active sera compared to LN Inactive or HC sera.

To evaluate hRMC response to the sera from the HC subjects and LN patients analyzed in Figures 3 and 4, release of CCL5 and CXCL5 was measured after incubation with 5% serum from each subject. For these studies, we also examined if responses were impacted by the biologic sex from which the hRMCs were derived. No significant differences were observed between HC and LN sera treatments in the levels of CXCL5 (Figure 5A) or CCL5 (Figure 5B) released from the female-derived hRMCs. No significant differences in the release of CXCL5 (Figure 5C) were present in response to sera with respect to biologic sex. However, a trend towards higher levels of CCL5 released in response to female HC compared to male HC sera was observed but not in response to female LN vs. male LN sera (Figure 5D). Similar results were obtained in the male-derived hRMCs (Figure 5E–H), including a trend towards release of higher levels of CCL5 in response to female HC vs. male HC sera (Figure 5G). Interestingly, we observed that the levels of CXCL5 and CCL5 released were ~twenty-fold and ~two-fold higher, respectively, from the female-derived hRMCs (Figure 5A–C) compared to the male-derived hRMCs (Figure 5E–H). These differences were significant ($p < 0.001$ for both CXCL5 and CCL5). These results suggest that the female-derived cells are pre-disposed to be hyper responsive to stimuli compared to the male-derived cells.

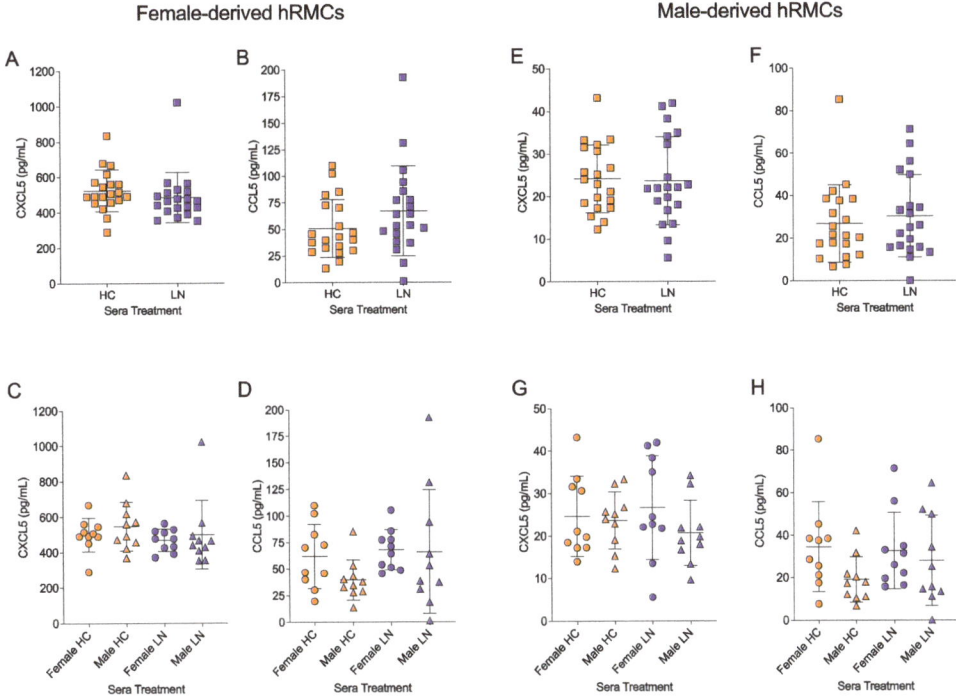

Figure 5. Cytokine release was higher in female-derived compared to male-derived hRMCs in response to sera. hRMCs were treated with 5% serum from 10 female or 10 male HC or from 10 female or 10 male LN subjects. (**A–D**): female-derived hRMCs; and (**E–H**): male-derived hRMCs. (**A,C,E,G**): CXCL5; and (**B,D,F,H**): CCL5 levels in media of sera-treated hRMCs. (**A,B,E,F**): compares HC sera-treated to LN sera-treated (both female- and male-derived sera). (**C,D,G,H**): compares female- and male-derived sera for each group (HC vs. LN). Statistical analyses were performed using unpaired t-tests for comparing HC vs. LN or one-way Anova for comparing female vs. male across the two groups. No significant differences were observed after correcting for multiple comparisons.

To further assess the response of hRMCs to LN versus HC sera and the effect of biological sex of the cells, we measured intracellular calcium $[Ca^{2+}]_i$ flux in response to acute sera applications. Calcium transients in female- or male-derived hRMCs were observed in response to pooled same-sex HC or LN serum. The transient Ca^{2+} response was detected in the range of serum concentrations of 0.001%, 0.01%, 0.1%, 1%, or 5% in 2 mM Ca^{2+} extracellular solution. The lowest concentration of sera 0.001% promotes Ca^{2+} transients with the amplitude around 20% from the saturated values reached at the concentration of

0.01% sera for all groups. Figure 6A illustrates representative confocal fluorescent (Fluo 8 AM) images of intracellular Ca^{2+} levels before and after acute application of 0.001%, 0.01%, or 1% sera. Examples of intracellular Ca^{2+} flux in response to acute application of 5% LN or HC sera in male hRMCs are shown in Figure 6B. Female-derived hRMCs exhibited significantly higher intracellular Ca^{2+} flux in response to LN compared to HC sera in all range of concentrations (Figure 6C), and male-derived cells showed a similar pattern only at the highest tested sera concentrations (5%). This data together with the results presented in Figure 5 suggest that the female-derived hRMCs are more sensitive and respond more robustly to serum stimulation than the male-derived hRMCs.

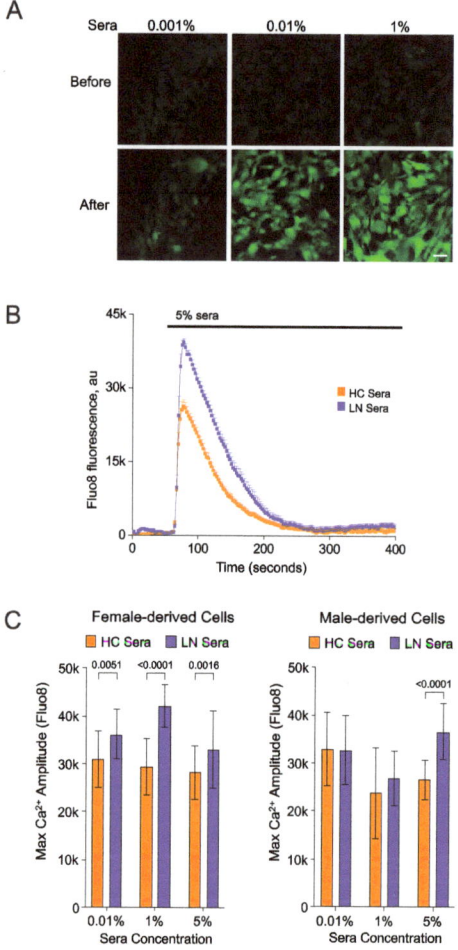

Figure 6. LN sera elicited a higher intracellular Ca^{2+} flux compared to HC sera in hRMCs. Sera was pooled from 10 female or 10 male HC (Control) or from 10 female or 10 male LN subjects and used to stimulate human primary hRMCs. Female-derived hRMCs were treated with HC or LN sera from females. Male-derived hRMCs were treated with HC or LN sera from males. (**A**) Confocal fluorescent images of intracellular Ca^{2+} (Fluo-8 AM) in female hRMCs before and after addition of 0.01%, 0.01%, or 1% female HC sera. Scale bar 50 μm. (**B**) Example of intracellular Ca^{2+} flux in response to acute application of 5% LN or HC sera in male hRMCs. (**C**) Statistical analyses of maximal amplitude of intracellular Ca^{2+} flux in response to acute sera application.

2.4. Differences in LacCers and HexCers Levels and the N-Glycome in Female-Derived and Male-Derived hRMCs

We reported previously that increasing LacCers along with another glycosphingolipid, glucosylceramides (GlcCers), resulted in increased message levels of several cytokines in an immortalized mouse mesangial cell line [19]. We also showed that LacCers and GlcCers (or hexosylceramides, a combination of GlcCers and galactosylceramides) are increased in the renal cortex of lupus prone mice with nephritis [7], and that lupus patients with nephritis that did not respond to therapy had significantly higher levels of LacCers and HexCers prior to beginning treatment [20]. Thus, we measured LacCers and hexosylceramides (HexCers) in our female- and male-derived hRMCs. The levels of both LacCers (Figure 7A) and HexCers (Figure 7B) are higher in the female-derived compared to the male-derived hRMCs prior to any stimulation. The GSLs levels in the cells in Figure 7 were measured in the serum-starved vehicle-treated wells from the experiments in Figure 5. The observed differences in GlcCers and LacCers between the female- and male-derived hRMCs were verified in unmanipulated cells maintained in serum-containing medium at passages 5 and 6 (Figure S3).

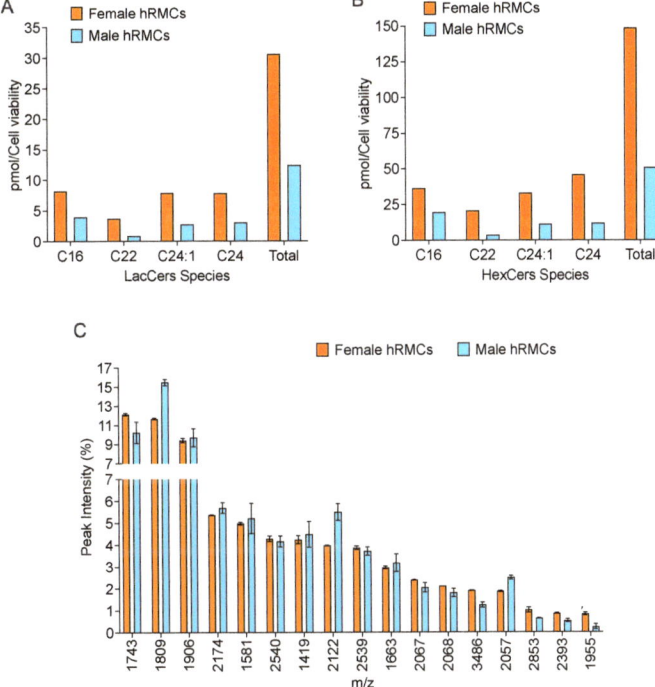

Figure 7. GSL levels were higher in female-derived compared to male-derived hRMCs. LacCers (**A**) and HexCers (**B**) were measured in female-derived and male-derived hRMCs and normalized to cell viability. The major chain lengths expressed in the hRMCs and the total of all chain lengths are shown in the graphs. The vehicle-treated female- or male-derived cells from the respective experiments presented in Figure 5 were scraped and combined to measure GLSs. GlcCers and LacCers levels were normalized to the cell viability determined prior to scraping. (**C**) N-glycans were measured by MALDI-FTICR in female- or male-derived hRMCs plated in duplicate. Individual glycans are presented as the relative peak intensity of the total glycans measured in the individual wells. Means + SD shown on graphs. Statistical analyses were not performed for the GSL or glycan analyses since the measures were performed in hRMCs from only one female donor and one male donor.

We also investigated differences in the N-glycome between the female-derived and male-derived hRMCs. The 17 most abundant N-glycans detected in both the female- and male-derived hRMCs are shown in Figure 7C. The ten most abundant N-glycans comprised >60% of all N-glycans detected in these cells. In comparing the female- and male-derived cells, the type of N-glycans present and relative overall abundance of each of the N-glycans were similar. While several glycans showed trends of being more highly abundant (1743, 3486, 2853, 2393, and 1995) or less abundant (1809, 2122, and 2057) in the female-derived cells relative to the male-derived hRMCs, these differences were not as large as those observed for the GSLs in Figure 7A,B. Thus, the analyses of GSLs and N-glycans in the hRMCs suggest that higher levels of LacCers and HexCers may contribute to a more robust response (higher cytokine release and increased intracellular Ca^{2+} flux) by the female-derived hRMCs following stimulation with sera.

3. Discussion

Given the ~9:1 female:male sex bias in lupus, most studies have focused largely on biologically female subjects (human and mouse studies). While men develop lupus less often than females, men were shown to have more severe disease and a higher risk of progressing to end stage renal disease [21,22]. However, the pathophysiologic mechanisms underlying sex differences are not fully understood. In this study, we determined that the significantly elevated LacCers and altered N-glycome in the urine can discriminate LN patients from HC subjects and could serve as noninvasive definitive markers of LN. Alterations in the serum N-glycome may also be useful in discriminating LN from HC, but ultimately is less informative than the urine N-glycome in this respect. While we observed a few differences in the urine N-glycome in females compared to males, the levels of urine LacCers may be more informative with respect to sex differences. A recent study reported that men with SLE develop disease at a later age [23]. Our results suggest that LN males may experience a greater increase in LacCers than females when comparing the change in LacCers levels from HC to LN. LacCers levels measured in the urine likely are derived from the kidney [24]. Therefore, we hypothesize that lower levels of LacCers may be protective in males and contribute to the later disease onset, but once tolerance is broken and males begin to develop LN, the large increase in LacCers (or possibly glycosphingolipid metabolism in general) may contribute to worse disease.

This hypothesis is supported by our results in primary human mesangial cells (hRMCs) in which the response to stimuli seems to be more dependent on cellular differences rather than on the source of circulating stimuli. hRMCs released significant levels of CXCL5 and CCL5 and exhibited significant increases in intracellular Ca^{2+} in response to human sera. The female-derived hRMCs, which we demonstrated expressed higher levels of the glycosphingolipids (GSLs) LacCers and HexCers, also released significantly more CCL5 and CXCL5 compared to the male-derived hRMCs in response to human serum (regardless of the source). At the lower concentrations of LN or HC sera, the female-derived cells had a higher intracellular Ca^{2+} flux indicating that the female-derived hRMCs have an increased sensitivity to serum stimulation. GSLs modulate cellular functions such as proliferation, apoptosis, migration, and signaling, including Ca^{2+} signaling [6], and defects in GSL metabolism are associated with a variety of human diseases. GSLs expressed on the cell surface form clusters and are widely believed to play roles in the formation and stabilization of lipid domains ("lipid rafts") required to propagate extracellular signals. LacCers were shown to play a role in Lyn-mediated signaling in neutrophils [25–27] and MAPK signaling in cardiomyocytes [28], which leads to superoxide production, phagocytosis, migration, or hypertrophy. In mesangial cells, elevated LacCers and HexCers due to hyperglycemia resulted in hypertrophy, extracellular matrix production, and fibrosis [29]. Our previous studies demonstrated that LN patients that failed to respond to treatment had significantly higher levels of HexCers and LacCers prior to beginning treatment [20]. Together, these observations suggest that renal GSL metabolism plays an important role in the scope (i.e., sensitivity or magnitude) of the initial renal response to stimuli and possibly resistance to therapeutic intervention. Thus, the elevated levels of LacCers and HexCers may poise the female-derived hRMCs to respond more robustly to external stimuli than the male-derived hRMCs. We speculate that altered GSL levels or ratios in the membranes of the hRMCs may contribute in part to the increased response by the female-derived cells since these lipids play important roles in cell signaling. The increased levels in the female-derived cells may be due to differences in expression of the enzymes that modulate GSL metabolism that are regulated in part by ERα as shown in MCF cell lines [30]. Future studies designed to interrogate the expression of GSL metabolic enzymes are needed to address this question.

Post-translational N-linked glycosylation plays an important role in the function of proteins, impacting a variety of cellular functions including discriminating self from non-self. Similar to GSLs, they can play key roles in mediating cell function. Modifications of N-glycosylation, or an altered N-glycome, is associated with several human diseases including lupus [15,31–33]. A recent study showed an abnormal N-glycome in renal biopsy sections of LN patients compared to renal biopsies from healthy tissue or from patients with other types of kidney conditions [16]. Here, we observed a significantly altered N-glycome in the urine of LN patients compared to HC subjects. This included seven of the nine classes and 75% of the individual N-glycans (72 of the 96) detected in urine. Overall, the urine glycan profiles were more informative in regard to disease status as compared with the N-glycans determined in the patient matched serum samples. In the previous study of kidney biopsies, the largest difference was observed in the abundance of mannose-enriched N-glycans, which was higher in the kidneys of LN patients [16]. Conversely, we demonstrated a significant decrease in high mannose-containing N-glycans in the urine of LN patients in this study. The increase in mannose-containing N-glycans reported in the kidney [16] and the decrease we observed in high mannose-containing N-glycans in the urine may be due to differences in how the mannose-containing N-glycans were defined or grouped in the two analyses. Alternatively, differences in levels may be due to tissue versus secreted (into the urine). Future studies with matched urine and renal biopsies to compare levels within the same individuals using the same method of defining N-glycan classes are needed to address this question.

Age, sex, and body mass index (BMI) were associated with changes in the N-glycome [34–39]. Sex differences in the N-glycome reported in the literature are largely associated with IgG glycosylation. Pregnant women were reported to have higher levels of galactosylated and sialylated (anti-inflammatory) forms of IgG, which correlated with estrogen levels [34]. In a lupus study, estrogen was shown to alter IgG sialylation and induce an enzyme that adds sialic acid to N-glycans [40]. In our study, we observed that individual N-glycans in the urine at peaks 2361, 2289, and 2339 differed by sex, with higher levels of all three observed in males compared to females regardless of disease status. However, none of these peaks are associated with IgG. Although we also demonstrated differences in the serum N-glycome between LN and HC, no sex differences were observed. Identifying the proteins from which the three urine N-glycans were derived that differed between sexes is a future goal. Identifying the proteins from which these three N-glycans were derived may lead to a better understanding of sex bias mechanisms in LN. Importantly, inclusion of four of the urine N-glycans associated with LN in a model including total urine LacCers and biologic sex improved the AUC to 1.0, providing perfect separation of LN from HC. Thus, measuring GSLs and N-glycans in the urine could serve as biomarkers of disease. Similarly, inclusion of the serum N-glycans improved the AUC in this model in distinguishing LN patients from HC subjects. Future studies using longitudinal serum samples to survey N-glycans in lupus patients who have not or have developed nephritis to determine if specific serum N-glycans can predict which lupus patients are likely to develop nephritis are of interest.

As mentioned above, many of the differences in glycosylation previously reported relate to IgG. Fc N-linked glycosylation influences the pathogenicity of IgG. Loss of sialic acid and galactose residues from the IgG N-glycome is associated with pro-inflammatory effector functions and autoimmune diseases [9]. Changes in glycosylation of serum IgG autoantibodies in lupus including decreased sialylation and galactosylation were reported previously and an altered IgG glycome was associated with disease status [14]. Here, we observed significant differences in five N-glycans associated with IgG in the urine, and only two of those in the serum, of LN patients. In the urine, there was a significant increase in the degalactosylated (desialylated) glycans associated with pro-inflammatory IgG functions. This was coupled with a corresponding significant decrease in the glycan associated with anti-inflammatory IgG functions, resulting in extensive skewing towards more pro-inflammatory IgG effector functions. Interestingly, we did not observe a skewing to this extent in the serum. Since the serum and urine samples were collected from the same patient at the same visit, it is possible that in LN the more pro-inflammatory forms of IgG are deposited in the kidney (or other target organs), reducing their levels in the circulation. We hypothesize that LN patients with a more skewed pro-inflammatory IgG repertoire may have worse disease or may be more likely to develop nephritis and measuring these glycans could help inform treatment decisions. Longitudinal studies in SLE patients without nephritis that eventually develop nephritis may address whether IgG N-glycans could be used to monitor SLE patients to identify those who will eventually develop kidney disease. Moreover, identification of the individual N-glycans present in the urine may lead to a better understanding of disease mechanisms in LN since most of the proteins present in the urine are likely derived from the kidney.

There were some limitations to this study. The in vitro hRMC studies were performed using cells derived from one female donor and one male donor. Thus, it is possible that the differences observed are due to individual differences that are unrelated to the biologic sex of the donors. Additional analyses will need to be performed in a larger number of female and male donor-derived hRMCs to determine if there is a correlation between biologic sex and GSL metabolism (or N-glycome) and with pathological response. In addition, the female-derived hRMCs showed a significantly higher sensitivity in intracellular Ca^{2+} flux in response to LN sera, specifically at the low concentrations, which was similar to the higher release of CXCL5 and CCL5 in response to sera by the female-derived cells. Thus, future studies are needed to assess differences more globally (i.e., proliferation, apoptosis, or release of other cytokines, growth factors, or extracellular matrix proteins) in the effect of LN vs. HC serum. Another limitation is the small cohort size. GSLs and the N-glycome can vary based on age or can be influenced by ethnicity or environmental factors. The HC and LN groups in this study were matched closely in average age, but the groups were too small to adjust for age, ethnicity, race, or external/environmental factors. In particular, the LN group is 80% Black while the HC group is only 50% Black which may have impacted results since Blacks tend to have worse disease. Thus, the generalizability of our observations is limited. Future studies with a larger cohort will be needed to confirm our observations.

4. Materials and Methods

4.1. Human Samples and Ethics Statement

All results, except those in Supplemental Figure S2, analyzed stored urine and serum samples collected from the same subject at the same visit and included 20 healthy subjects (10 female and 10 male) and 20 lupus nephritis patients (10 female and 10 male). Lupus nephritis (LN) patients met the American College of Rheumatology classification for systemic lupus erythematosus (SLE) with nephritis and samples were collected during active disease. All except two LN patients had biopsy-confirmed nephritis. Healthy subjects (healthy controls, HC) did not have documented autoimmunity, renal disease, an active infection, or an ongoing pregnancy at the time of sample collection. Patient demographics and relevant clinic measures are provided in Table 1. Urine Protein:Creatinine ratio (UPCr), eGFR, C3, and C4 measures were missing for twelve of the HC subjects. The reported values in Table 1 are representative of the eight for whom measures were available. For the autoantibodies, LN patients are reported in Table 1 as having ever been positive for anti-Sm and anti-RNP and positive for anti-dsDNA at the time of sample collection for the samples used in this study. Anti-Sm and anti-RNP measures were not available for two

LN patients. For analyses in Supplemental Figure S2, stored serum samples from 12 HC, 12 LN patients at the time of inactive disease, and 12 LN patients at the time of active disease were used to stimulate mesangial cells as described below. Inclusion and exclusion criteria for HC and LN subjects were the same as described above.

4.2. Cell Culture

Two lots of primary human renal mesangial cells (hRMCs) were commercially obtained from ScienCell (Carlsbad, CA, USA). Each lot was derived from one individual, a 21-week gestation female (referred to as "female-derived") and a 22-week gestation male (referred to as "male-derived") who presumably did not have disease. Cells were negative for HIV-1, HBV, HCV, mycoplasma, bacteria, yeast, and fungi. hRMCs were maintained on poly-l-lysine coated flasks in complete growth mesangial cell media (MCM) (1% penicillin/streptomycin and 1% mesangial cell growth supplement) that was supplemented with 2% FBS in a humidified 5% CO_2 atmosphere at 37 °C according to manufacturer's recommendations (ScienCell). Cells at passages 5 or 6 were used for experiments.

4.3. Lipid Analyses

Glycosphingolipids hexosylceramides (HexCers) and lactosylceramides (LacCers) of individual chain lengths C16, C18, C18:1, C20, C20:1, C22, C22:1, C24, C24:1, C26, and C26:1 were quantified by the Lipidomics Core Facility at MUSC as we described previously [7,20,41]. The most highly expressed ("major") chain lengths in urine, serum, and hRMCs were C16, C22, C24, and C24:1 and quantified levels of these four chain lengths are provided on the graphs. The reported "total" HexCers or LacCers are the sum measures of all 11 chain lengths listed above. For urine, equivalent volumes of urine from each subject were provided and lipid measures were normalized to urine creatinine. Creatinine levels in all urine samples were measured in our laboratory in the same assay by the Jaffe picric acid method [42]. For serum, equivalent volumes of serum from each subject were provided to the core facility and lipids are presented as pmol of lipid per ml of serum. For the hRMCs, lipids were measured in cell pellets and are presented as pmol of lipids normalized to relative cell viability as measured by alamar blue just prior to collecting the cells.

4.4. N-Glycan Analyses

The N-glycan analysis of urine and serum was performed as previously described [43,44]. Serum was diluted 1:2 in 100 mM sodium bicarbonate pH 8.0 and 1 µL spotted on a Nexterion Slide H amine-reactive hydrogel-coated glass slide from Applied Microarrays (Tempe, AZ, USA). Urine samples were buffer exchanged in phosphate buffered saline and concentrated using a 0.5 mL Amicon 10,000 MW centrifugation tube prior to spotting [43]. After a 1-h incubation, salts and lipids were removed using a Carnoy's solution (10% glacial acetic acid, 30% chloroform, 60% ethanol) wash. The samples were then sprayed with the enzyme peptide N-glycosidase F (PNGase F PRIME, N-Zymes Scientific, Doylestown, PA, USA) and incubated for 2 h to cleave N-glycans from the captured glycoproteins. Finally, an α-cyano-4-hydroxycinnamic acid (CHCA) matrix was sprayed onto the slides before performing MALDI-IMS using a Bruker 7T SolariX MALDI-FTICR mass spectrometer for serum and a Bruker MALDI-QTOF timsTOF fleX mass spectrometer for urine.

For cells, N-glycans were quantified as we previously described [18,45]. Briefly, female- or male-derived hRMCs cells were seeded at 6000 cells per well in duplicate wells on 8-well LabTekII chamber slides (Electron Microscopy Sciences, Hatfield, PA, USA). Wells with no cells (media only) were used to determine background levels from media. Cells were washed with PBS, fixed for 30 min in 10% buffered formalin, washed, and stored in PBS until analysis. N-glycans released by PNGase F digestion were detected by MALDI-FTICR as previously reported [18,45].

N-glycan peaks were analyzed using SCiLS Lab (v. 2021b) software (Bruker, Billerica, MA, USA) as previously reported [43]. Mass spectra were normalized to total ion current.

Peaks were selected for N-glycans based on theoretical and established mass values, and maximum mean values for each peak were included in subsequent analyses. Background signal in the blank well was subtracted from each N-glycan measurement to obtain an absolute intensity. Relative intensities of N-glycans were calculated (absolute intensity divided by the intensity of all N-glycans detected in each sample). This accounted for protein concentration differences that could lead to higher signal intensities from sample to sample and allow for detection of low-abundance N-glycans. The sum of relative intensities of the individual N-glycans in a specific class was used to calculate each N-glycan classes (Bi-, Tri-, or Tetra-antennary, bisecting, and hybrid). In addition, each N-glycan was placed into a group based on the absence or presence of mannose, sulfate, sialic acid, or fucose. The sum of relative intensities in these classes/groups were then compared. Sialylated or sulfated N-glycans with multiple sodiated species were included together when comparing the intensities of individual N-glycans across samples. A cumulative peak and structure list of N-glycans used in the statistical analyses is provided in Supplemental Table S1.

4.5. Cytokine Release Experiments

Female-derived or male-derived hRMCs described above were serum-starved for three hours in serum-free complete MCM (without FBS supplementation) when ~80% confluent. Human sera were then added to a final concentration of 5%, incubated for three hours, and refed with fresh serum-free complete MCM. Serum from a single individual was used for all experiments. All treatments were performed in duplicate or triplicate. Media was collected from hRMCs following incubation with human sera. Cell viability was then measured using the Alamar Blue assay (Invitrogen/ThermoFisher, Waltham, MA, USA) following the manufacturer's instructions. ELISA kits from Biolegend (San Diego, CA, USA) were used to measure CCL5 (RANTES) or CXCL5 according to the manufacturer protocol. Relative cell viability (per well) with respect to untreated cells was used to normalize measured cytokine levels per well. For the individual serum analyses, replicates for each serum donor were averaged. The averages for each serum donor are shown on the graphs as individual points.

4.6. Intracellular Ca^{2+} Analyses

The male- and female-derived hRMCs described above were used in confocal fluorescent experiments. The experiments were performed similarly to the previously described protocol [46]. Briefly, cells were grown on glass-bottom dishes (#0 glass, Mattek, Ashland, MA, USA) and loaded with fluorescent Ca^{2+} indicator Fluo-8 AM (AAT Bioquest, Pleasanton, CA, USA). After loading, cells were rinsed and media was replaced with an extracellular solution containing in mM: 2 $CaCl_2$, 145 NaCl, 2 $MgCl_2$, 4.5 KCl, 10 HEPES, pH 7.4 adjusted by NaOH. Confocal imaging was performed using the Leica TCS SP5 laser scanning microscope equipped with an HCX Plan Apochromat $40\times$ 1.25 NA oil objective (Leica Microsystems Inc., Deerfield, IL, USA). Maximum amplitude of intracellular Ca^{2+} transient in individual hRMCs was obtained in response to the application of human sera from LN or HC patients in concentrations from 0.01 to 5% (at least three separate experiments per group). The data were analyzed using ImageJ (NIH) and summarized in OriginPro 2021b software (OriginLab, Northampton, MA, USA).

4.7. Statistical Analyses

Descriptive statistics were determined for participant characteristics by LN status. Differences in patient characteristics for categorical variables were examined using Fisher's exact tests and for continuous or ordinal variables were examined using 2-sample t-tests or Wilcoxon rank sum tests as appropriate.

Comparisons of LacCers or N-glycans in urine and serum by disease status and by biologic sex were examined for associations using a series of linear mixed models. Fixed effects in the models included disease status and biologic sex. We also considered the disease status by biologic sex interaction but only retained if it was statistically significant.

For the N-glycans, all models also included a random batch effect to control for correlation between samples run in the same batch. p-values for the associations between LacCers or N-glycans with disease status or with sex were adjusted using FDR to control for multiple testing. All FDR q-values < 0.05 are considered meaningful. We also evaluated if including individual N-glycans improved prediction of disease status in a model including total urine LacCers and biologic sex using the likelihood ratio test to determine if inclusion of glycans improved prediction and area under the receiver operating characteristics curve (AUC) to examine improvement in ability to discriminate between LN patients and HC subjects.

Differences in CXCL5 and CCL5 production between hRMCs treated with sera from healthy controls versus lupus nephritis were also examined. Additional factors considered included serum source (male or female donors) and cell line biologic sex. Differences between groups in CXCL5 or CCL5 expression were evaluated using a linear model approach. Models included main effects for disease status of the serum donor (HC vs. LN), sex of the serum donor, and sex of the hRMC donor. Two-way interactions between cell type, derived sex, and serum sex were considered but were not significant and thus only main effects were considered. Differences by disease status, serum sex, and derived cell sex were estimated using linear contrasts. p-values were Bonferroni adjusted for the three pairwise comparisons. Model assumptions were checked graphically and transformations were considered as needed.

5. Conclusions

This study demonstrates that altered GSLs and N-glycosylation could serve as effective biomarkers of LN, particularly in urine, and that elevated cellular GSLs levels in the female-derived hRMCs were associated with a greater response (higher levels of cytokine secretion and intracellular Ca^{2+} flux) to human sera. GSLs and N-glycans also warrant further investigation as potential predictive biomarkers of LN and future studies are needed to determine if the elevated levels of GSLs in the female-derived cells are due to sex differences or other individual donor differences. Elucidating the mechanisms by which GSLs and an altered N-glycome contribute to disease, and specifically the response of renal cells to external stimuli, could provide a better understanding of disease pathology.

Supplementary Materials: The supporting information can be downloaded at https://www.mdpi.com/article/10.3390/ijms242216490/s1.

Author Contributions: B.W. performed the statistical analyses and assisted in the interpretation of results; C.R.K.B. and B.T.W. performed the urine and serum N-glycan analyses; S.M. performed the mesangial cell experiments and ELISAs; M.S., M.F. and O.P. designed and performed the Ca^{2+} imaging experiments; H.B. performed the N-glycan analyses of the mesangial cells; J.R. assisted with the processing of urine and serum samples and measured creatinine in the urine samples; R.R.D. assisted with the design and performance of all N-glycan analyses and the interpretation of results; T.K.N. conceived and designed the study, and assisted with the design and performance of experiments, and interpretation of results. All coauthors contributed to the drafting and editing of the manuscript. B.T.W., C.R.K.B. and S.M. contributed equally to this study. All authors have read and agreed to the published version of the manuscript.

Funding: This work was supported in part by funding from the following sources: Department of Defense (DoD) Congressionally Directed Medical Research Programs (W81XWH-16-1-0640 and W81XWH-22-1-0330 awarded to T.K.N.). Opinions, interpretations, and recommendations are those of the authors and are not necessarily endorsed by the DoD. National Institutes of Health grants R01 DK126720 and DK129227 (to O.P.) and U01 CA242096 (to R.R.D.), and MUSC COMETS-PPG (to O.P.).

Institutional Review Board Statement: This study was approved by the MUSC Institutional Review Board and/or by the Department of Defense Human Research Protection Office (Approval Code: Pro00069547). All volunteers provided informed consent for the use of their samples in research.

Informed Consent Statement: All subjects were seen at the Medical University of South Carolina (MUSC) clinics and provided informed consent for their samples to be used for research. These studies were approved by the Institutional Review Board at MUSC. All samples were obtained from the Core Center for Clinical Research (CCCR) biorepository at MUSC and were provided in a coded manner.

Data Availability Statement: All data supporting the conclusions of this study are available upon request to the corresponding author.

Acknowledgments: The authors acknowledge the Lipidomics Shared Resource, Hollings Cancer Center, MUSC (P30 CA138313 and P30 GM103339); the Core Center for Clinical Research (CCCR) at the MUSC (P30 AR072582) and its director Jim Oates, M.D. for assistance in identifying subjects and providing samples for this study; and Sophia LeClerc for assisting laboratory personnel in culturing and collecting hRMCs and in the performance of ELISAs.

Conflicts of Interest: The authors declare no conflict of interest.

References

1. Izmirly, P.M.; Parton, H.; Wang, L.; McCune, W.J.; Lim, S.S.; Drenkard, C.; Ferucci, E.D.; Dall'Era, M.; Gordon, C.; Helmick, C.G.; et al. Prevalence of Systemic Lupus Erythematosus in the United States: Estimates from a Meta-Analysis of the Centers for Disease Control and Prevention National Lupus Registries. *Arthritis Rheumatol.* **2021**, *73*, 991–996. [CrossRef]
2. Lingwood, C.A. Glycosphingolipid functions. *Cold Spring Harb. Perspect. Biol.* **2011**, *3*, a004788. [CrossRef]
3. Jennemann, R.; Grone, H.J. Cell-specific in vivo functions of glycosphingolipids: Lessons from genetic deletions of enzymes involved in glycosphingolipid synthesis. *Prog. Lipid Res.* **2013**, *52*, 231–248. [CrossRef]
4. Head, B.P.; Patel, H.H.; Insel, P.A. Interaction of membrane/lipid rafts with the cytoskeleton: Impact on signaling and function: Membrane/lipid rafts, mediators of cytoskeletal arrangement and cell signaling. *Biochim. Biophys. Acta* **2014**, *1838*, 532–545. [CrossRef]
5. Zhang, T.; de Waard, A.A.; Wuhrer, M.; Spaapen, R.M. The Role of Glycosphingolipids in Immune Cell Functions. *Front. Immunol.* **2019**, *10*, 90. [CrossRef]
6. Weesner, J.A.; Annunziata, I.; van de Vlekkert, D.; d'Azzo, A. Glycosphingolipids within membrane contact sites influence their function as signaling hubs in neurodegenerative diseases. *FEBS Open Bio* **2023**, *13*, 1587–1600. [CrossRef] [PubMed]
7. Nowling, T.K.; Mather, A.R.; Thiyagarajan, T.; Hernandez-Corbacho, M.J.; Powers, T.W.; Jones, E.E.; Snider, A.J.; Oates, J.C.; Drake, R.R.; Siskind, L.J. Renal glycosphingolipid metabolism is dysfunctional in lupus nephritis. *J. Am. Soc. Nephrol. JASN* **2015**, *26*, 1402–1413. [CrossRef] [PubMed]
8. Tabassum, R.; Ruotsalainen, S.; Ottensmann, L.; Gerl, M.J.; Klose, C.; Tukiainen, T.; Pirinen, M.; Simons, K.; Widen, E.; Ripatti, S. Lipidome- and Genome-Wide Study to Understand Sex Differences in Circulatory Lipids. *J. Am. Heart Assoc.* **2022**, *11*, e027103. [CrossRef]
9. Buhre, J.S.; Becker, M.; Ehlers, M. IgG subclass and Fc glycosylation shifts are linked to the transition from pre- to inflammatory autoimmune conditions. *Front. Immunol.* **2022**, *13*, 1006939. [CrossRef]
10. Radovani, B.; Gudelj, I. N-Glycosylation and Inflammation; the Not-So-Sweet Relation. *Front. Immunol.* **2022**, *13*, 893365. [CrossRef] [PubMed]
11. Lu, H.; Wei, Z.; Wang, C.; Guo, J.; Zhou, Y.; Wang, Z.; Liu, H. Redesigning Vina@QNLM for Ultra-Large-Scale Molecular Docking and Screening on a Sunway Supercomputer. *Front. Chem.* **2021**, *9*, 750325. [CrossRef]
12. Tomana, M.; Schrohenloher, R.E.; Reveille, J.D.; Arnett, F.C.; Koopman, W.J. Abnormal galactosylation of serum IgG in patients with systemic lupus erythematosus and members of families with high frequency of autoimmune diseases. *Rheumatol. Int.* **1992**, *12*, 191–194. [CrossRef] [PubMed]
13. Pilkington, C.; Yeung, E.; Isenberg, D.; Lefvert, A.K.; Rook, G.A. Agalactosyl IgG and antibody specificity in rheumatoid arthritis, tuberculosis, systemic lupus erythematosus and myasthenia gravis. *Autoimmunity* **1995**, *22*, 107–111. [CrossRef] [PubMed]
14. Vuckovic, F.; Kristic, J.; Gudelj, I.; Teruel, M.; Keser, T.; Pezer, M.; Pucic-Bakovic, M.; Stambuk, J.; Trbojevic-Akmacic, I.; Barrios, C.; et al. Association of systemic lupus erythematosus with decreased immunosuppressive potential of the IgG glycome. *Arthritis Rheumatol.* **2015**, *67*, 2978–2989. [CrossRef]
15. Sjowall, C.; Zapf, J.; von Lohneysen, S.; Magorivska, I.; Biermann, M.; Janko, C.; Winkler, S.; Bilyy, R.; Schett, G.; Herrmann, M.; et al. Altered glycosylation of complexed native IgG molecules is associated with disease activity of systemic lupus erythematosus. *Lupus* **2015**, *24*, 569–581. [CrossRef] [PubMed]
16. Alves, I.; Santos-Pereira, B.; Dalebout, H.; Santos, S.; Vicente, M.M.; Campar, A.; Thepaut, M.; Fieschi, F.; Strahl, S.; Boyaval, F.; et al. Protein Mannosylation as a Diagnostic and Prognostic Biomarker of Lupus Nephritis: An Unusual Glycan Neoepitope in Systemic Lupus Erythematosus. *Arthritis Rheumatol.* **2021**, *73*, 2069–2077. [CrossRef]
17. Wang, Y.; Lin, S.; Wu, J.; Jiang, M.; Lin, J.; Zhang, Y.; Ding, H.; Zhou, H.; Shen, N.; Di, W. Control of lupus activity during pregnancy via the engagement of IgG sialylation: Novel crosstalk between IgG sialylation and pDC functions. *Front. Med.* **2023**, *17*, 549–561. [CrossRef] [PubMed]
18. Sundararaj, K.; Rodgers, J.; Angel, P.; Wolf, B.; Nowling, T.K. The role of neuraminidase in TLR4-MAPK signalling and the release of cytokines by lupus serum-stimulated mesangial cells. *Immunology* **2021**, *162*, 418–433. [CrossRef]

19. Sundararaj, K.; Rodgers, J.I.; Marimuthu, S.; Siskind, L.J.; Bruner, E.; Nowling, T.K. Neuraminidase activity mediates IL-6 production by activated lupus-prone mesangial cells. *Am. J. Physiol. Ren. Physiol.* **2018**, *314*, F630–F642. [CrossRef]
20. Troyer, B.; Rodgers, J.; Wolf, B.J.; Oates, J.C.; Drake, R.R.; Nowling, T.K. Glycosphingolipid Levels in Urine Extracellular Vesicles Enhance Prediction of Therapeutic Response in Lupus Nephritis. *Metabolites* **2022**, *12*, 134. [CrossRef] [PubMed]
21. Tan, T.C.; Fang, H.; Magder, L.S.; Petri, M.A. Differences between male and female systemic lupus erythematosus in a multiethnic population. *J. Rheumatol.* **2012**, *39*, 759–769. [CrossRef]
22. Ramirez Sepulveda, J.I.; Bolin, K.; Mofors, J.; Leonard, D.; Svenungsson, E.; Jonsen, A.; Bengtsson, C.; Consortium, D.; Nordmark, G.; Rantapaa Dahlqvist, S.; et al. Sex differences in clinical presentation of systemic lupus erythematosus. *Biol. Sex. Differ.* **2019**, *10*, 60. [CrossRef]
23. Trentin, F.; Signorini, V.; Manca, M.L.; Cascarano, G.; Gualtieri, L.; Schiliro, D.; Valevich, A.; Cardelli, C.; Carli, L.; Elefante, E.; et al. Gender differences in SLE: Report from a cohort of 417 Caucasian patients. *Lupus Sci. Med.* **2023**, *10*, e000880. [CrossRef] [PubMed]
24. McCluer, R.H.; Williams, M.A.; Gross, S.K.; Meisler, M.H. Testosterone effects on the induction and urinary excretion of mouse kidney glycosphingolipids associated with lysosomes. *J. Biol. Chem.* **1981**, *256*, 13112–13120. [CrossRef]
25. Chiricozzi, E.; Ciampa, M.G.; Brasile, G.; Compostella, F.; Prinetti, A.; Nakayama, H.; Ekyalongo, R.C.; Iwabuchi, K.; Sonnino, S.; Mauri, L. Direct interaction, instrumental for signaling processes, between LacCer and Lyn in the lipid rafts of neutrophil-like cells. *J. Lipid Res.* **2015**, *56*, 129–141. [CrossRef] [PubMed]
26. Iwabuchi, K.; Prinetti, A.; Sonnino, S.; Mauri, L.; Kobayashi, T.; Ishii, K.; Kaga, N.; Murayama, K.; Kurihara, H.; Nakayama, H.; et al. Involvement of very long fatty acid-containing lactosylceramide in lactosylceramide-mediated superoxide generation and migration in neutrophils. *Glycoconj. J.* **2008**, *25*, 357–374. [CrossRef]
27. Iwabuchi, K.; Nagaoka, I. Lactosylceramide-enriched glycosphingolipid signaling domain mediates superoxide generation from human neutrophils. *Blood* **2002**, *100*, 1454–1464. [CrossRef]
28. Mishra, S.; Chatterjee, S. Lactosylceramide promotes hypertrophy through ROS generation and activation of ERK1/2 in cardiomyocytes. *Glycobiology* **2014**, *24*, 518–531. [CrossRef] [PubMed]
29. Subathra, M.; Korrapati, M.; Howell, L.A.; Arthur, J.M.; Shayman, J.A.; Schnellmann, R.G.; Siskind, L.J. Kidney glycosphingolipids are elevated early in diabetic nephropathy and mediate hypertrophy of mesangial cells. *Am. J. Physiol. Ren. Physiol.* **2015**, *309*, F204–F215. [CrossRef] [PubMed]
30. Zhang, X.; Wu, X.; Su, P.; Gao, Y.; Meng, B.; Sun, Y.; Li, L.; Zhou, Z.; Zhou, G. Doxorubicin influences the expression of glucosylceramide synthase in invasive ductal breast cancer. *PLoS ONE* **2012**, *7*, e48492. [CrossRef]
31. Chui, D.; Sellakumar, G.; Green, R.; Sutton-Smith, M.; McQuistan, T.; Marek, K.; Morris, H.; Dell, A.; Marth, J. Genetic remodeling of protein glycosylation in vivo induces autoimmune disease. *Proc. Natl. Acad. Sci. USA* **2001**, *98*, 1142–1147. [CrossRef] [PubMed]
32. Green, R.S.; Stone, E.L.; Tenno, M.; Lehtonen, E.; Farquhar, M.G.; Marth, J.D. Mammalian N-glycan branching protects against innate immune self-recognition and inflammation in autoimmune disease pathogenesis. *Immunity* **2007**, *27*, 308–320. [CrossRef] [PubMed]
33. Hashii, N.; Kawasaki, N.; Itoh, S.; Nakajima, Y.; Kawanishi, T.; Yamaguchi, T. Alteration of N-glycosylation in the kidney in a mouse model of systemic lupus erythematosus: Relative quantification of N-glycans using an isotope-tagging method. *Immunology* **2009**, *126*, 336–345. [CrossRef] [PubMed]
34. Ercan, A.; Kohrt, W.M.; Cui, J.; Deane, K.D.; Pezer, M.; Yu, E.W.; Hausmann, J.S.; Campbell, H.; Kaiser, U.B.; Rudd, P.M.; et al. Estrogens regulate glycosylation of IgG in women and men. *JCI Insight* **2017**, *2*, e89703. [CrossRef]
35. Ding, N.; Nie, H.; Sun, X.; Sun, W.; Qu, Y.; Liu, X.; Yao, Y.; Liang, X.; Chen, C.C.; Li, Y. Human serum N-glycan profiles are age and sex dependent. *Age Ageing* **2011**, *40*, 568–575. [CrossRef]
36. Kristic, J.; Lauc, G.; Pezer, M. Immunoglobulin G glycans—Biomarkers and molecular effectors of aging. *Clin. Chim. Acta* **2022**, *535*, 30–45. [CrossRef]
37. Yu, X.; Wang, Y.; Kristic, J.; Dong, J.; Chu, X.; Ge, S.; Wang, H.; Fang, H.; Gao, Q.; Liu, D.; et al. Profiling IgG N-glycans as potential biomarker of chronological and biological ages: A community-based study in a Han Chinese population. *Medicine* **2016**, *95*, e4112. [CrossRef]
38. Nikolac Perkovic, M.; Pucic Bakovic, M.; Kristic, J.; Novokmet, M.; Huffman, J.E.; Vitart, V.; Hayward, C.; Rudan, I.; Wilson, J.F.; Campbell, H.; et al. The association between galactosylation of immunoglobulin G and body mass index. *Prog. Neuropsychopharmacol. Biol. Psychiatry* **2014**, *48*, 20–25. [CrossRef]
39. Mertins, P.; Tang, L.C.; Krug, K.; Clark, D.J.; Gritsenko, M.A.; Chen, L.; Clauser, K.R.; Clauss, T.R.; Shah, P.; Gillette, M.A.; et al. Reproducible workflow for multiplexed deep-scale proteome and phosphoproteome analysis of tumor tissues by liquid chromatography-mass spectrometry. *Nat. Protoc.* **2018**, *13*, 1632–1661. [CrossRef]
40. Engdahl, C.; Bondt, A.; Harre, U.; Raufer, J.; Pfeifle, R.; Camponeschi, A.; Wuhrer, M.; Seeling, M.; Martensson, I.L.; Nimmerjahn, F.; et al. Estrogen induces St6gal1 expression and increases IgG sialylation in mice and patients with rheumatoid arthritis: A potential explanation for the increased risk of rheumatoid arthritis in postmenopausal women. *Arthritis Res. Ther.* **2018**, *20*, 84. [CrossRef]

41. Nowling, T.K.; Rodgers, J.; Thiyagarajan, T.; Wolf, B.; Bruner, E.; Sundararaj, K.; Molano, I.; Gilkeson, G. Targeting glycosphingolipid metabolism as a potential therapeutic approach for treating disease in female MRL/lpr lupus mice. *PLoS ONE* **2020**, *15*, e0230499. [CrossRef]
42. Toora, B.D.; Rajagopal, G. Measurement of creatinine by Jaffe's reaction—Determination of concentration of sodium hydroxide required for maximum color development in standard, urine and protein free filtrate of serum. *Indian J. Exp. Biol.* **2002**, *40*, 352–354. [PubMed]
43. Blaschke, C.R.K.; Hartig, J.P.; Grimsley, G.; Liu, L.; Semmes, O.J.; Wu, J.D.; Ippolito, J.E.; Hughes-Halbert, C.; Nyalwidhe, J.O.; Drake, R.R. Direct N-Glycosylation Profiling of Urine and Prostatic Fluid Glycoproteins and Extracellular Vesicles. *Front. Chem.* **2021**, *9*, 734280. [CrossRef] [PubMed]
44. Blaschke, C.R.K.; Black, A.P.; Mehta, A.S.; Angel, P.M.; Drake, R.R. Rapid N-Glycan Profiling of Serum and Plasma by a Novel Slide-Based Imaging Mass Spectrometry Workflow. *J. Am. Soc. Mass Spectrom.* **2020**, *31*, 2511–2520. [CrossRef] [PubMed]
45. Angel, P.M.; Saunders, J.; Clift, C.L.; White-Gilbertson, S.; Voelkel-Johnson, C.; Yeh, E.; Mehta, A.; Drake, R.R. A Rapid Array-Based Approach to N-Glycan Profiling of Cultured Cells. *J. Proteome Res.* **2019**, *18*, 3630–3639. [CrossRef]
46. Palygin, O.; Klemens, C.A.; Isaeva, E.; Levchenko, V.; Spires, D.R.; Dissanayake, L.V.; Nikolaienko, O.; Ilatovskaya, D.V.; Staruschenko, A. Characterization of purinergic receptor 2 signaling in podocytes from diabetic kidneys. *iScience* **2021**, *24*, 102528. [CrossRef]

Disclaimer/Publisher's Note: The statements, opinions and data contained in all publications are solely those of the individual author(s) and contributor(s) and not of MDPI and/or the editor(s). MDPI and/or the editor(s) disclaim responsibility for any injury to people or property resulting from any ideas, methods, instructions or products referred to in the content.

Article

Limited Association between Antibodies to Oxidized Low-Density Lipoprotein and Vascular Affection in Patients with Established Systemic Lupus Erythematosus

Lina Wirestam [1,†], Frida Jönsson [1,†], Helena Enocsson [1], Christina Svensson [2], Maria Weiner [3], Jonas Wetterö [1], Helene Zachrisson [2], Per Eriksson [1] and Christopher Sjöwall [1,*]

1 Department of Biomedical and Clinical Sciences, Division of Inflammation and Infection, Linkoping University, SE-581 85 Linkoping, Sweden
2 Department of Clinical Physiology, University Hospital and Department of Health, Medicine and Caring Sciences, Linkoping University, SE-581 85 Linkoping, Sweden
3 Department of Nephrology in Linkoping, Department of Health, Medicine and Caring Sciences, Linköping University, SE-581 85 Linkoping, Sweden
* Correspondence: christopher.sjowall@liu.se
† These authors contributed equally to this work.

Abstract: Patients with systemic lupus erythematosus (SLE) are at an increased risk of cardiovascular disease. We aimed to evaluate whether antibodies to oxidized low-density lipoprotein (anti-oxLDL) were associated with subclinical atherosclerosis in patients with different SLE phenotypes (lupus nephritis, antiphospholipid syndrome, and skin and joint involvement). Anti-oxLDL was measured by enzyme-linked immunosorbent assay in 60 patients with SLE, 60 healthy controls (HCs) and 30 subjects with anti-neutrophil cytoplasmic antibody-associated vasculitis (AAV). Intima-media thickness (IMT) assessment of vessel walls and plaque occurrence were recorded using high-frequency ultrasound. In the SLE cohort, anti-oxLDL was again assessed in 57 of the 60 individuals approximately 3 years later. The levels of anti-oxLDL in the SLE group (median 5829 U/mL) were not significantly different from those in the HCs group (median 4568 U/mL), while patients with AAV showed significantly higher levels (median 7817 U/mL). The levels did not differ between the SLE subgroups. A significant correlation was found with IMT in the common femoral artery in the SLE cohort, but no association with plaque occurrence was observed. The levels of anti-oxLDL antibodies in the SLE group were significantly higher at inclusion compared to 3 years later (median 5707 versus 1503 U/mL, $p < 0.0001$). Overall, we found no convincing support for strong associations between vascular affection and anti-oxLDL antibodies in SLE.

Keywords: SLE; anti-oxidized low-density lipoprotein; biomarkers; intima-media thickness; cardiovascular disease

1. Introduction

Despite pronounced advances in treatment, cerebrovascular and cardiovascular disease (CVD), e.g., coronary heart disease and stroke, still constitute leading causes of death worldwide. Atherosclerosis remains as a key role in CVD. The initial process involves the trapping of low-density lipoproteins (LDL) in the sub-endothelial space of medium- and large-sized arteries [1]. Apolipoprotein-B-containing lipoproteins (e.g., LDL) become oxidized and internalized by macrophages which transform the macrophages into foam cells [2]. Induction of foam cells later leads to plaque lipid core development, foam cell apoptosis/necrosis, and inflammation with cytokine production [3]. Ultimately, advanced lesions may cause stenosis with ischaemic symptoms or plaque rupture and infarction of the affected area [1]. The atherosclerotic process is regarded as a slowly progressing inflammatory disease [2].

Increased intima-media thickness (IMT) in arteries signifies the first stages of atherosclerosis. Carotid artery IMT measured by ultrasound is a common method to assess early atherosclerosis [2,4]. Depending on the cause of vascular affection, the vessel wall will have different appearances and high-frequency ultrasound (US) can distinguish vessel wall atherosclerosis from inflammation caused by arteritis [5]. Detection of plaques by US indicates more advanced atherosclerosis [4].

In general, the risk of CVD is increased in patients with rheumatic diseases [6]. The risk is particularly high in systemic lupus erythematosus (SLE), where the overall relative risk of CVD is increased by 2- to 10-fold. Younger patients with SLE have been estimated to have an up to 50-fold higher relative risk of stroke and myocardial infarction [7,8]. Accelerated atherosclerosis is considered one of the primary causes of increased CVD risk in SLE [7].

Recently, antibodies targeting oxidized LDL (oxLDL) have attracted increased interest in relation to CVD [9]. Assessment of anti-oxLDL antibodies has been suggested to aid in the stratification of CVD risk [3] and as a potential pharmaceutical target [10]. However, contradictory data have been reported [1,3,11]. Previous studies have demonstrated increased levels of anti-oxLDL antibodies in patients with SLE [12,13] and associations with biological markers of disease activity as well as with anti-cardiolipin antibodies [13–15].

The aims of the current study were to evaluate whether the plasma levels of IgG anti-oxLDL antibodies associate with (i) the signs of CVD detected with US, (ii) traditional risk factors for atherosclerosis and CVD, and (iii) SLE disease phenotypes, disease activity, or antinuclear antibody (ANA) fine specificities. To pursue this, we included 60 well-characterized patients with SLE, 60 matched healthy controls (HC), and 30 patients with antineutrophil cytoplasmic antibody-associated (ANCA) vasculitis (AAV). Blood samples from patients with SLE and matched controls were collected at the same time-point as the US examinations were performed. Approximately 3 years later, another blood sample was collected and analyzed for anti-oxLDL antibodies.

2. Results

2.1. Anti-oxLDL Antibodies in the SLE, AAV, and HC Groups

The demographics, laboratory data, and ongoing medical therapies of patients with SLE and HC are detailed in Table 1. The levels of anti-oxLDL antibodies did not differ significantly between the SLE group (median 5829 U/mL, interquartile range (IQR) 5025) and the HCs (median 4568 U/mL, IQR 2973). AAV showed significantly higher anti-oxLDL levels (median 7817 U/mL, IQR 15186) compared to the HCs ($p = 0.0013$), but not compared to the SLE group (Figure 1A). In addition, no clear differences were observed between the SLE subgroups: antiphospholipid syndrome (APS) (median 6283 U/mL, IQR 4624), lupus nephritis (LN) (median 5122 U/mL, IQR 5180), and skin and joint involvement only (median 5519 U/mL, IQR 5845) (Figure 1B).

2.2. Anti-oxLDL Antibodies over Time

A total of 57 of the 60 patients with SLE provided a second blood sample approximately 3 years after the first sample was drawn. The levels of anti-oxLDL antibodies were significantly higher on the first occasion (median 5707 U/mL, IQR 4950) compared to the second occasion (median 1503 U/mL, IQR 745), $p < 0.0001$ (Figure 1C). No significant differences were observed between the SLE subgroups on the second occasion: APS (median 1503 U/mL, IQR 741), LN (median 1314 U/mL, IQR 666), and skin and joint involvement only (median 1536 U/mL, IQR 855) (Figure 1D). During the 3-year follow-up visit, the anti-oxLDL levels in patients with SLE were significantly lower than in the HCs assessed on the first occasion ($p < 0.0001$). None of the patients on immunosuppressive therapy, daily glucocorticoid doses, or statins were different between the sampling occasions.

Table 1. Characteristics of the included patients with SLE and the HCs.

	SLE: All (Inclusion) (n = 60)	SLE: APS (n = 20)	SLE: LN (n = 20)	SLE: Skin and Joint (n = 20)	Healthy Controls (n = 60)	SLE: All 3 Years Later (n = 57)
Background variables median (range)						
Age at examination (years)	44 (23–63)	47.5 (24–63)	41 (25–63)	43.5 (23–58)	43 (23–63)	48 (27–67)
Female gender, n (%)	52 (87)	15 (75)	18 (90)	19 (95)	52 (87)	50 (88)
Duration of SLE (years)	8 (1–35)	14 (1–35)	8 (1–27)	7 (1–19)	N/A	12 (5–39)
SLEDAI-2K (score)	2 (0–10)	2 (0–10)	2 (0–4)	1 (0–8)	N/A	2 (0–22)
SDI (score)	0 (0–4)	1 (0–4)	0 (0–3)	0 (0–1)	N/A	1 (0–5)
Traditional risk factors and laboratory data, median (range)						
Body mass index (kg/m^2)	25.0 (19.7–38)	25.1 (19.7–35.5)	26.1 (22.4–33.2)	24.5 (20.1–38)	23.3 (16.8–35.1)	26.6 (19.6–40.5)
Waist circumference (cm)	90 (71–123)	90 (71–116)	90 (79–119)	88.5 (76–123)	83 (64–117)	87 (73–129)
Ever smoker (former or current), n (%)	14 (23)	3 (15)	4 (20)	7 (35)	0	20 (35)
Diabetes, n (%)	1 (2)	1 (5)	0	0	0	0
eGFR (mL/min/1.73 m^2)	86.5 (35–100)	77.5 (35–100)	87 (53–100)	88.5 (61–100)	N/A	88.0 (31–100)
Total cholesterol (mmol/L)	4.6 (3–7)	4.8 (3.6–6.8)	4.4 (3–6.8)	4.8 (3.2–7)	4.7 (2.9–8.3)	4.7 (2.7–7.4)
Triglycerides (mmol/L)	0.93 (0.33–4.7)	1.0 (0.39–4.7)	1.15 (0.52–3.3)	0.80 (0.33–1.8)	1.15 (0.45–2.9)	1.1 (0.6–6.9)
HDL (mmol/L)	1.5 (0.87–2.8)	1.7 (0.87–2.8)	1.35 (1–2.7)	1.5 (1.2–2.8)	1.6 (1–2.8)	1.6 (0.93–2.9)
LDL (mmol/L)	2.4 (1–4.8)	2.3 (1.7–4.8)	2.4 (1–3.9)	2.65 (1.6–4.2)	2.4 (1–6)	2.5 (1.1–4.1)
CRP (mg/L)	1.2 (0.08–15)	1.3 (0.08–14)	1 (0.08–4.1)	1.7 (0.5–15)	0.95 (0.2–24)	1.3 (0.08–26)
Complement protein C3 (g/L)	0.94 (0.63–1.7)	0.92 (0.67–1.4)	0.96 (0.63–1.4)	0.95 (0.69–1.7)	N/A	0.96 (0.59–1.7)
Complement protein C4 (g/L)	0.15 (0.05–0.55)	0.16 (0.06–0.55)	0.14 (0.05–0.29)	0.16 (0.07–0.32)	N/A	0.16 (0.04–0.41)
Anti-dsDNA (positive), n (%)	21 (35)	7 (35)	10 (50)	4 (20)	N/A	22 (39)
Anti-dsDNA (IU/mL)	40 (40–1366)	40 (40–352)	40 (40–494)	40 (40–1366)	N/A	40 (40–2510)
IL-6 (above cut-off), n (%)	33 (55)	9 (45)	13 (65)	11 (55)	16 (27)	28 (49)
IL-6 (ng/L)	1.6 (0.75–34)	0.75 (0.75–6)	1.6 (0.75–34)	1.6 (0.75–7.1)	0.75 (0.75–12)	0.75 (0.75–18)
Medical treatment, ongoing, n (%)						
Antimalarials	54 (90)	16 (80)	20 (100)	18 (90)	0	50 (88)
Antihypertensives	20 (33)	6 (30)	11 (55)	3 (15)	0	21 (37)
Glucocorticoids	31 (52)	9 (45)	12 (60)	10 (50)	0	25 (44)
Daily prednisolone dose (mg)	2.5 (0–10)	0 (0–5)	4.5 (0–10)	1.25 (0–5)	0	0 (0–135)
Warfarin	11 (18)	10 (50)	1 (5)	0	0	15 (26)
Antiplatelet	11 (18)	6 (30)	5 (25)	0	0	11 (19)
Statins	5 (8)	3 (15)	2 (10)	0	0	8 (14)
Mycophenolate mofetil	16 (27)	4 (20)	11 (55)	1 (5)	0	11 (19)
Methotrexate	5 (8)	1 (5)	0	4 (20)	0	5 (9)
Leflunomide	0	0	0	0	0	1 (2)
Azathioprine	3 (5)	2 (10)	0	1 (5)	0	4 (7)
Sirolimus	2 (3)	1 (5)	0	1 (5)	0	2 (4)
Dehydroepiandrosterone	1 (2)	0	1 (5)	0	0	2 (4)
Bortezomib	1 (2)	0	1 (5)	0	0	1 (2)
Rituximab	2 (3)	0	1 (5)	1 (5)	0	0 (0)
Belimumab	2 (3)	1 (5)	1 (5)	0	0	5 (9)

AAV = anti-neutrophil cytoplasmic antibody-associated vasculitis, ANCA = anti-neutrophil cytoplasmic antibody, APS = antiphospholipid syndrome, BVAS = Birmingham Vasculitis Activity Score, CRP = C-reactive protein, dsDNA = double stranded deoxyribonucleic acid, eGFR = estimated glomerular filtration rate, HCs = healthy controls, HDL = high-density lipoproteins, IL = interleukin, LDL = low-density lipoprotein, LN = lupus nephritis, MPO = myeloperoxidase, N/A = not assessed, PR3 = proteinase 3, SDI = Systemic Lupus International Collaborating Clinics/American College of Rheumatology damage index, SLE = systemic lupus erythematosus, and SLEDAI-2K = systemic lupus erythematosus disease activity index 2000.

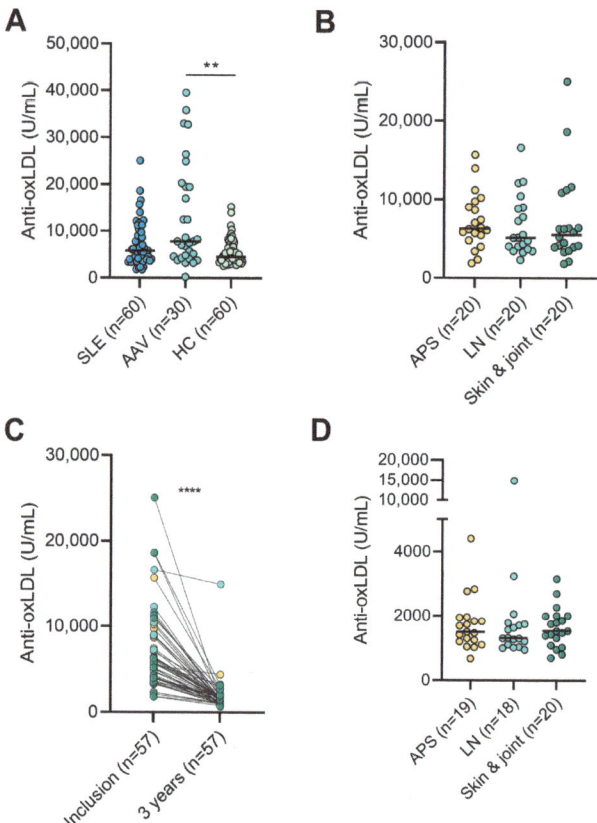

Figure 1. Plasma anti-oxidized LDL antibody levels in (**A**) patients with systemic lupus erythematosus (SLE), anti-neutrophil cytoplasmic antibody (ANCA)-associated vasculitis (AAV), and healthy controls (HC). (**B**) Subgroups of SLE with antiphospholipid syndrome (APS), lupus nephritis (LN), or the skin and joint disease phenotype. (**C**) Patients with SLE at study inclusion and after approximately 3 years. (**D**) Subgroups of SLE after approximately 3 years. ** $p < 0.01$; **** $p < 0.0001$.

2.3. Anti-oxLDL Antibodies versus the IMT and Plaque Occurrence

All patients with SLE and the HCs underwent US examination. Atherosclerotic plaques were verified by US in 15 out of 60 patients with SLE, but no significant difference in the levels of anti-oxLDL was found between those with and without plaques. The correlations between anti-oxLDL and IMT are demonstrated in Table 2. A weak inverse correlation between anti-oxLDL levels was observed for IMT of the common femoral artery (CFA) (rho -0.29, $p = 0.026$) among the HCs. A univariate general linear model was used to evaluate the association between anti-oxLDL levels and the IMT in the different vessel, but no significant associations were found. All p-values were >0.1 and thus, it was not possible to proceed with a multiple regression analysis.

Table 2. Spearman's correlations between the levels of anti-oxLDL antibodies (Units/mL) and background variables, traditional CVD risk factors, laboratory data, IMT measurements, and ongoing medication in patients with SLE and the HCs.

Variables	All SLE: Inclusion (n = 60)		Healthy Controls (n = 60)		All SLE: 3 Years Later (n = 57)	
	rho	p-Value	rho	p-Value	rho	p-Value
Background variables						
Age at evaluation (years)	−0.091	0.45	−0.24	0.064	0.15	0.26
SLE duration (years)	0.024	0.86	N/A	N/A	0.17	0.21
SLEDAI-2K	0.15	0.24	N/A	N/A	**0.38**	**0.004**
SDI	−0.066	0.62	N/A	N/A	0.19	0.15
Traditional risk factors for CVD and laboratory data						
BMI (kg/m^2)	−0.056	0.67	−0.071	0.59	−0.085	0.53
Waist circumference (cm)	−0.10	0.44	−0.071	0.59	−0.010	0.94
eGFR (mL/min/1.73 m^2)	0.081	0.54	N/A	N/A	−0.043	0.75
Total cholesterol (mmol/L)	0.075	0.57	−0.16	0.23	−0.14	0.30
Triglycerides (mmol/L)	−0.11	0.40	−0.17	0.20	−0.13	0.34
HDL (mmol/L)	−0.078	0.56	−0.061	0.64	−0.067	0.62
LDL (mmol/L)	0.12	0.35	−0.097	0.46	−0.049	0.72
CRP (mg/L)	0.12	0.36	0.16	0.24	0.018	0.90
IL-6 (ng/L)	0.092	0.49	0.093	0.48	0.035	0.80
C3 (g/L)	−0.19	0.14	N/A	N/A	−0.22	0.10
C4 (g/L)	−0.25	0.054	N/A	N/A	**−0.33**	**0.01**
Anti-dsDNA (IU/mL)	0.16	0.21	N/A	N/A	**0.34**	**0.01**
High frequency ultrasound						
IMT CCA, mean	0.14	0.28	−0.22	0.091	N/A	N/A
IMT ICA, mean	−0.05	0.71	−0.15	0.26	N/A	N/A
IMT SCA, mean	0.034	0.80	−0.13	0.33	N/A	N/A
IMT AxA, mean	0.092	0.48	−0.029	0.83	N/A	N/A
IMT CFA, mean	−0.10	0.46	**−0.29**	**0.026**	N/A	N/A
IMT SFA, mean	−0.029	0.83	−0.064	0.63	N/A	N/A
IMT aortic arc	0.023	0.86	−0.19	0.14	N/A	N/A
Medical treatment						
Daily glucocorticoid dose (prednisolone; mg)	−0.083	0.53	N/A	N/A	−0.053	0.69

AxA = axillary artery, BMI = body mass index, C = complement protein, CCA = common carotid artery, CFA = common femoral artery, CRP = C-reactive protein, CVD = cardiovascular disease, dsDNA = double stranded deoxyribonucleic acid, eGFR = estimated glomerular filtration rate, HDL = high-density lipoproteins, ICA = internal carotid artery, IL = interleukin, IMT = intima-media thickness, LDL = low-density lipoprotein, SCA = subclavian artery, SDI = Systemic Lupus International Collaborating Clinics/American College of Rheumatology damage index, SFA = superficial femoral artery, SLE = systemic lupus erythematosus, and SLEDAI-2K = systemic lupus erythematosus disease activity index 2000. Rho and p in bold format are statistically significant.

2.4. Anti-oxLDL versus Background Variables and Pharmacotherapy

No significant correlations were obtained between age and anti-oxLDL levels in either the SLE group or the HCs (Table 2). Women showed a non-significant tendency towards higher levels of anti-oxLDL, both in the SLE group (women 5961 U/mL, IQR 4946; men median 4532 U/mL, IQR 7214), the AAV group (women median 8458 U/mL, IQR 15276; men median 7442 U/mL, IQR 16166), and the HCs (women median 4638 U/mL, IQR 3967; men median 4428 U/mL, IQR 3749). The duration of SLE (years) showed no significant correlation with the levels of anti-oxLDL (Table 2).

No significant correlation was found between anti-oxLDL levels and SLE disease activity index 2000 (SLEDAI-2K) nor for global organ damage (Systemic Lupus International Collaborating Clinics/American College of Rheumatology Damage Index: SDI). We further separately examined the presence of organ damage in the cardiovascular, neuropsychiatric, and peripheral vascular domains of SDI, without detecting any significant differences in the levels of anti-oxLDL (Figure 2). For the AAV group, neither myeloperoxidase (MPO) or proteinase-3 (PR3) ANCA levels (rho = 0.09, p = 0.63 and rho = -0.035, p = 0.85, respectively) nor the Birmingham Vasculitis Activity Score (BVAS) (rho = 0.017, p = 0.93) significantly correlated with anti-oxLDL antibody levels.

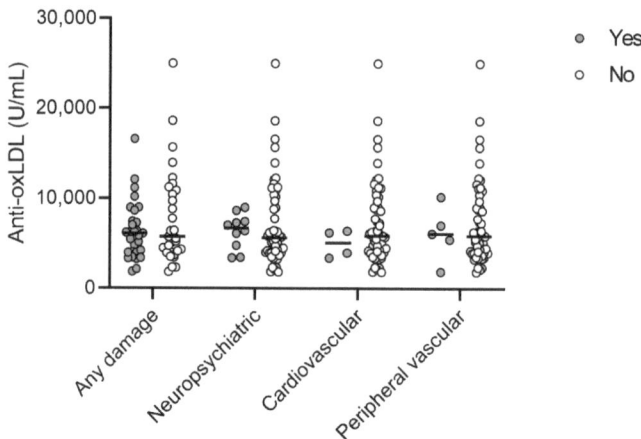

Figure 2. Plasma anti-oxidized LDL levels in patients with SLE at inclusion with or without global organ damage according to the SLICC/ACR Damage Index (SDI), as well as specifically in the neuropsychiatric, cardiovascular, and peripheral vascular domains.

Ongoing medical treatments are detailed in Table 1. By comparing anti-oxLDL antibody levels in the different treatment groups, no significant differences were found for the SLE group. Patients with SLE who had received B-cell targeted therapies (e.g., rituximab, belimumab and cyclophosphamide [16]) did not have lower levels of anti-oxLDL (median 3443 U/mL, IQR 14086) than the others (5832 U/mL, IQR 4978), p = 0.47. In contrast, patients with AAV without ongoing immunosuppressive therapy showed higher anti-oxLDL levels (median 10,551 U/mL, IQR 17769) compared to patients with ongoing immunosuppression (median 4453 U/mL, IQR 6752), p = 0.028. The mean glucocorticoid dose did not correlate to the anti-oxLDL levels, neither in the SLE group, nor in the AAV group.

The cut-off level for positive tests based on the 95th percentile results from the HCs was determined to be 11,178 U/mL. Approximately 10 patients with SLE (16.7%) and 12 patients with AAV (40%) were then judged to be anti-oxLDL antibody positive. By applying the cut-off level, no additional associations were observed for the positive patients.

2.5. Anti-oxLDL Antibodies versus Traditional Risk Factors and Laboratory Data

Anti-oxLDL did not correlate with body mass index (BMI) (Table 1), and no significant difference in anti-oxLDL levels was found when comparing the two patient groups with a BMI above or below 25. The estimated glomerular filtration rate (eGFR) showed no correlation with anti-oxLDL levels in either the SLE group or the AAV group. Among the patients with SLE, 'ever smokers' showed a higher median anti-oxLDL (6550 U/mL, IQR 9718) compared to 'never smokers' (5767 U/mL, IQR 4739), but this was not statistically significant (p = 0.15).

2.6. Anti-oxLDL Antibodies during the 3-Year Follow-Up

During the visit 3 years after inclusion, anti-oxLDL levels correlated significantly with SLEDAI-2K (rho = 0.38, p = 0.004). SLEDAI-2K was slightly increased on the second sample occasion (mean 2.3, median 2, range 0–22) compared to the first sample occasion (mean 2, median 2, range 0–10). An inverse correlation was found for complement protein C4 (rho = −0.33, p = 0.012), but not for C3. Anti-oxLDL antibody levels correlated positively with anti-dsDNA (rho = 0.34, p = 0.01). During this visit, we also had access to ANA fine specificities. However, anti-oxLDL levels did not coincide with any specific ANA specificity (Figure 3).

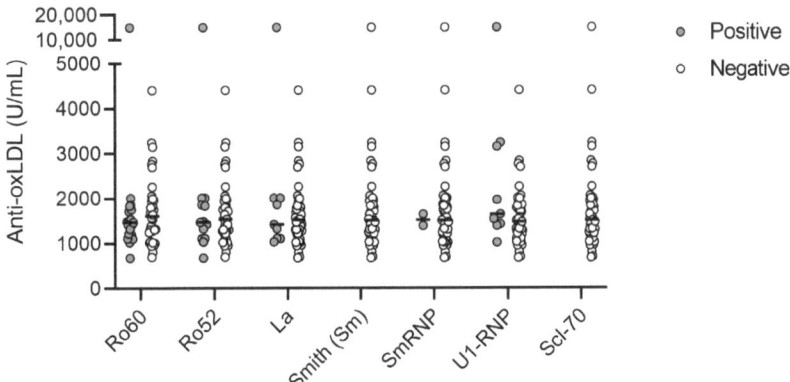

Figure 3. Plasma anti-oxidized LDL levels in patients with SLE stratified by antinuclear antibody (ANA) fine specificities during the second visit (approximately 3 years after inclusion).

3. Discussion

CVD continues to be a leading cause of morbidity and mortality in the general population and especially among patients with SLE. Therefore, it is of upmost importance to find and treat possible risk factors for the development of atherosclerosis, and new biomarkers are wanted. In the present study, it was evaluated whether IgG anti-oxLDL levels are associated with subclinical atherosclerosis in SLE with different disease phenotypes. Anti-oxLDL antibody levels were essentially similar between the SLE and HC groups, as well as between groups with different SLE manifestations. Only one weak association was found with IMT, but none with the occurrence of plaque.

Ultrasonography-determined IMT is used for atherosclerosis detection. Svensson et al. showed that thicker IMT was found in several vessels in patients with SLE compared to HC, but the pathogenetic mechanisms beyond increased IMT in SLE remains unclear [4]. In the current study, we found a weak negative correlation between anti-oxLDL levels and mean IMT values for the common femoral artery in the HCs group, but no other associations. A total of 15 out of the 60 patients with SLE (25%) had US-verified atherosclerotic plaques, but no significant difference was shown in anti-oxLDL levels with or without plaques. In the current study, we could not find any significant correlation between anti-oxLDL and traditional risk factors such as BMI, hypertension, age, and glucocorticoid therapy. Statin therapy did not influence the anti-oxLDL levels, in line with a recent meta-analysis [17].

The median levels of anti-oxLDL were similar between individuals with SLE during the first visit and the controls, even though the range was larger among patients with SLE and AAV compared to the HCs. Elevated anti-oxLDL titres have previously been shown in SLE [18,19]. Unexpectedly, we observed no differences in anti-oxLDL between the SLE disease phenotypes at any timepoint. However, we cannot exclude that this could be related to low statistical power. Both primary APS and secondary APS in SLE have previously shown elevated anti-oxLDL [20,21]. Hayem et al. reported high anti-oxLDL in patients with deep venous thrombosis but not with arterial thrombosis [21]. We could not find any association with organ damage (all domains) or when we analyzed the presence of damage in the cardiovascular and neuropsychiatric domains separately. Previous studies have shown contradictory results regarding the value of anti-oxLDL in CVD risk determination [1,3,11]. Associations between anti-oxLDL antibodies and the extent of CVD has been shown, while experimental data on the other hand indicate a possible protective role of the antibodies [19,22]. In our study, IgG anti-oxLDL antibodies were measured. The isotype appears important since IgM antibodies indicate protection from CVD whilst IgG shows divergent results [3]. Moreover, different subclasses of IgG have different effector functions which could also contribute to heterogeneous results [19,23].

The presence of antibodies against Ro/SSA and La/SSB has previously been shown to be associated with the development of anti-oxLDL by others [24]. However, in our study, anti-oxLDL levels did not discriminate between ANA fine specificities.

Unexpectedly, anti-oxLDL levels were considerably lower among patients with SLE during the second visit compared to the first visit. The reason for this finding is not entirely clear, but the overall disease activity was in fact slightly higher during the second visit and we cannot exclude that this might have affected the anti-oxLDL results. As a reflection of this, we observed associations of anti-oxLDL with low complement and higher disease activity (only for the second visit) which is in line with previous studies [13,14]. Increased SLE disease activity is often a consequence of increased immune complex formation. Hence, circulating autoantibodies may seemingly decrease but still exist in immune complexes [25,26]. Furthermore, the antibody-mediated removal of oxLDL may limit inflammation in atherosclerotic lesions and decreased antibody levels could thus contribute to accumulation of antigen, loss of tolerance, and increased inflammation in vascular tissues [23,27].

Interestingly, recombinant human oxLDL antibodies mediate the uptake of oxLDL in monocytes via Fc receptors in both healthy individuals [28] as well as in patients with SLE [10], suggesting atheroprotective properties. From that perspective, high levels of anti-oxLDL could be atheroprotective. Similarly, patients with SLE have lower levels of apolipoprotein B antibodies compared to controls, and patients with manifest CVD have lower levels of apolipoprotein B antibodies than patients without CVD [23]. Whether the decreased levels of anti-oxLDL among the patients with SLE examined herein will lead to an increased risk of future myocardial infarction and stroke will be assessed during the future clinical follow-up. Further prospective studies measuring anti-oxLDL in relation to CVD risk in SLE are warranted.

The main strength of our study is the inclusion of healthy controls age- and sex-matched to the SLE group and well characterized populations. We also included a disease control group, AAV, to compare with another rheumatic disease. Many of the included patients were newly diagnosed with AAV, as compared to the SLE cohort where the median disease duration was 8 years during the first visit. In addition, samples from patients with AAV were not similar in terms of the sample matrix and were not examined after overnight fasting which was a limitation. Although the SLE study population was well characterized, the number of included subjects overall was relatively low. This limits the statistical power and decreases the possibilities to draw firm conclusions.

To conclude, the levels of anti-oxLDL antibodies were similar in the SLE group in comparison to the healthy and diseased controls, and no differences were found between the SLE disease phenotypes. Compared to 3 years later, the levels of anti-oxLDL antibodies in the SLE group were significantly higher at inclusion. Nevertheless, we could not find any strong correlations with increased IMT, the occurrence of plaque, or to traditional CVD risk factors. Further studies are needed to determine the use of anti-oxLDL as a possible biomarker in CVD risk stratification, especially in SLE populations.

4. Material and Methods

4.1. Study Population and Sampling

The study population, consisting of subjects with SLE and HCs based at the University Hospital of Linköping, Sweden, has previously been described in detail [29]. In short, 60 patients (52 women and 8 men) with SLE as well as 60 healthy age- and sex-matched controls were included. The diagnosis of SLE was based on fulfilment of the 1982 American College of Rheumatology (ACR) and/or the 2012 Systemic Lupus International Collaborating Clinics (SLICC) classification criteria [30]. Patients above 63 years of age were excluded due to the higher risk of age-related atherosclerosis and those below 23 years of age were excluded due to short SLE duration. The 60 patients with SLE were divided into 3 subgroups based on disease phenotypes. These subgroups were matched with each other according to age and sex and included: 20 patients with LN, meeting the ACR criterion for renal disorder in the absence of APS; 20 patients had SLE with APS without LN; and 20 patients with primarily skin and joint involvement without LN or APS.

Blood samples were collected after 12 h overnight fasting immediately after the US examination, peripheral venous blood was drawn from everyone, and plasma was prepared and stored at $-70\,°C$ until analyzed. A total of 57 of the 60 patients with SLE (95%) provided a second blood sample 45 months (range 43–47) after the first sample was drawn.

In addition, 30 patients with AAV serving as disease controls were included from the regional vasculitis register based at the University Hospital of Linköping, Sweden [31]. The patients were recruited between 2013 and 2020, had a clinical diagnosis of either microscopic polyangiitis (MPA) or granulomatosis with polyangiitis (GPA) and were classified according to the European Medicined Agency algorithm [32]. Disease activity was assessed using the BVAS [33].

4.2. High Frequency Ultrasound (US)

A GE Logic E9 US system (LOGIQ E9 XD clear 2.0 General Electric Medical Systems US, Wauwatosa, Wisconsin, USA) was used for the US measurements. IMT was measured in the common carotid artery (CCA), the internal carotid artery (ICA), the subclavian artery (SCA), the axillary artery (AxA), the common femoral artery (CFA), the superficial femoral artery (SFA), and the aortic arc. Both the right and left side were measured, and each side was measured twice to gain a mean IMT. All individuals went through a standardized examination procedure and the same vascular sonographer performed all of the examinations and measurements [4]. The mean IMT values of the right and left were used. US measurements were determined during the first visit.

4.3. Variables

For the subjects with SLE and the HCs, we had access to data regarding length, weight, waist circumference, age, sex, smoking habits, ongoing pharmacotherapy, blood pressure, and laboratory measurements (total cholesterol, triglycerides, high density lipoproteins (HDL), low LDL, high sensitivity C-reactive protein (hsCRP), and interleukin (IL)-6). For patients with SLE, we also had access to plasma creatinine, serological data (complement protein C3 and C4 as well as anti-dsDNA antibodies), SLE duration, SLEDAI-2K, and SDI divided into separate organ domains [4]. During the second sampling occasion, ANA fine specificities using addressable laser bead immunoassay (ALBIA) and FIDIS™ Connective profile Solonium software ver. 1.7.1.0 (Theradiag, Croissy-Beaubourg, France) were analyzed at the Clinical Immunology Laboratory, Linköping [34]. For anti-dsDNA antibody levels (cut-off level for a positive test = 80 IU/mL) and IL-6 (cut-off = 1.5 ng/L); all results below the cut-offs were given half the cut-off value.

For patients with AAV, we had access to sex, age at inclusion in the cohort, creatinine levels at inclusion, ongoing pharmacotherapy, levels of MPO- and PR3-ANCA, AAV duration, and disease activity assessed by the Birmingham Vasculitis Activity Score (BVAS). Levels of IgG ANCA (MPO and PR3) were analyzed at the Clinical Immunology Laboratory, Linköping, using flouroenzyme immunoassays [35].

4.4. Anti-oxLDL Antibodies

An enzyme-linked immunosorbent assay (ELISA) kit (Immundiagnostik AG, Bensheim, Germany) [36,37] was used for the quantitative determination of IgG ox LDL antibodies in plasma (K7809; lot number K7809-200928). The samples were analyzed in duplicate according to the manufacturer's specifications. Briefly, samples diluted at a ratio of 1:10,000 were added to ELISA plates pre-coated with oxLDL and incubated 2 h in room temperature (RT) at 500 rpm shaking. After washing, the peroxidase-labelled conjugate was added and incubated for 1 h in RT at 500 rpm shaking. After additional washing, tetramethylbenzidine was added and incubated in the dark at RT for 20 min. The reaction was terminated with acidic stop solution, and the optical density was read at 450 nm. To avoid interassay variation between the two sample occasions, all samples were adjusted according to the recovery of an assay control sample with a known anti-oxLDL concentration (supplied by the manufacturer).

4.5. Statistical Methods

The statistical analyses were performed using SPSS statistics V.27 (IBM, Armonk, New York, NY, USA), and GraphPad Prism, V.9 (GraphPad Software, La Jolla, CA, USA) was used for the graphical illustrations. Correlations were calculated using Spearman's test. Possible differences between two groups were analyzed using the Mann–Whitney U test. The Kruskal–Wallis test with Dunn's multiple comparison test was applied when analyzing three or more groups. The chi-squared test was used for analyzing two dichotomous variables. The Wilcoxon matched pairs signed rank test was used to test differences in anti-oxLDL levels between the two time points. The univariate general linear model was used to evaluate the impact of anti-oxLDL levels on the IMT in the different vessels. All variables with a p-value of 0.1 or less were combined in a multiple regression analysis. A two-sided p-value < 0.05 was considered significant.

Author Contributions: Conceptualization, C.S. (Christopher Sjöwall) and P.E.; methodology, L.W., F.J. and C.S. (Christina Svensson); software, L.W., F.J., H.E. and C.S. (Christina Svensson); formal analysis, L.W., F.J., H.E. and C.S. (Christina Svensson); investigation, L.W., F.J., H.E., C.S. (Christina Svensson), M.W., J.W., H.Z., P.E. and C.S. (Christopher Sjöwall); resources, C.S. (Christopher Sjöwall); data curation, C.S. (Christina Svensson), M.W. and C.S. (Christopher Sjöwall); writing—original draft preparation, L.W. and F.J.; writing—review and editing, L.W., F.J., H.E., C.S. (Christina Svensson), M.W., J.W., H.Z., P.E. and C.S. (Christopher Sjöwall); visualization, L.W.; supervision, C.S. (Christopher Sjöwall), H.Z. and P.E.; project administration, C.S. (Christopher Sjöwall); funding acquisition, C.S. (Christopher Sjöwall). All authors have read and agreed to the published version of the manuscript.

Funding: This work has been supported by grants from the Swedish Rheumatism Association (Grant nr R-939149), the Region Östergötland (ALF Grants; Grant nr RÖ-960604), the Gustafsson Foundation (Grant nr 2023-36), the King Gustaf V's 80-year Anniversary Foundation (Grant nr FAI-2020-0663), and the King Gustaf V and Queen Victoria's Freemasons Foundation (Grant nr 2021). The funders had no role in the design of the study, the collection, analysis, or interpretation of the data, or in writing of the manuscript.

Institutional Review Board Statement: The study was conducted in accordance with the Declaration of Helsinki and approved by the Regional Ethics Board in Linköping (ref. M75-08, 2010/205-31 and 2017/572-32).

Informed Consent Statement: Oral and written informed consent was obtained from all patients and control subjects involved in the study.

Data Availability Statement: All datasets generated for this study are included in the article.

Acknowledgments: The authors wish to thank Marianne Petersson and Anna-Lena Åblad for the bio-bank administration.

Conflicts of Interest: The authors declare no conflict of interest.

References

1. Hartley, A.; Haskard, D.; Khamis, R. Oxidized LDL and anti-oxidized LDL antibodies in atherosclerosis-Novel insights and future directions in diagnosis and therapy. *Trends Cardiovasc. Med.* **2019**, *29*, 22–26. [CrossRef]
2. Nowak, B.; Madej, M.; Luczak, A.; Malecki, R.; Wiland, P. Disease Activity, Oxidized-LDL Fraction and Anti-Oxidized LDL Antibodies Influence Cardiovascular Risk in Rheumatoid Arthritis. *Adv. Clin. Exp. Med.* **2016**, *25*, 43–50. [CrossRef]
3. Van den Berg, V.J.; Vroegindewey, M.M.; Kardys, I.; Boersma, E.; Haskard, D.; Hartley, A.; Khamis, R. Anti-Oxidized LDL Antibodies and Coronary Artery Disease: A Systematic Review. *Antioxidants* **2019**, *8*, 484. [CrossRef]
4. Svensson, C.; Eriksson, P.; Zachrisson, H.; Sjowall, C. High-Frequency Ultrasound of Multiple Arterial Areas Reveals Increased Intima Media Thickness, Vessel Wall Appearance, and Atherosclerotic Plaques in Systemic Lupus Erythematosus. *Front. Med.* **2020**, *7*, 581336. [CrossRef] [PubMed]
5. Zachrisson, H.; Svensson, C.; Dremetsika, A.; Eriksson, P. An extended high-frequency ultrasound protocol for detection of vessel wall inflammation. *Clin. Physiol. Funct. Imaging* **2018**, *38*, 586–594. [CrossRef] [PubMed]
6. Alhusain, A.; Bruce, I.N. Cardiovascular risk and inflammatory rheumatic diseases. *Clin. Med.* **2013**, *13*, 395–397. [CrossRef] [PubMed]
7. Yazdany, J.; Pooley, N.; Langham, J.; Nicholson, L.; Langham, S.; Embleton, N.; Wang, X.; Desta, B.; Barut, V.; Hammond, E. Systemic lupus erythematosus; stroke and myocardial infarction risk: A systematic review and meta-analysis. *RMD Open* **2020**, *6*, e001247. [CrossRef] [PubMed]
8. Enocsson, H.; Karlsson, J.; Li, H.Y.; Wu, Y.; Kushner, I.; Wettero, J.; Sjowall, C. The Complex Role of C-Reactive Protein in Systemic Lupus Erythematosus. *J. Clin. Med.* **2021**, *10*, 5837. [CrossRef]
9. Tektonidou, M.G. Cardiovascular disease risk in antiphospholipid syndrome: Thrombo-inflammation and atherothrombosis. *J. Autoimmun.* **2022**, *128*, 102813. [CrossRef]
10. Yao Mattisson, I.; Rattik, S.; Bjorkbacka, H.; Ljungcrantz, I.; Terrinoni, M.; Lebens, M.; Holmgren, J.; Fredrikson, G.N.; Gullstrand, B.; Bengtsson, A.A.; et al. Immune responses against oxidized LDL as possible targets for prevention of atherosclerosis in systemic lupus erythematosus. *Vasc. Pharmacol.* **2021**, *140*, 106863. [CrossRef] [PubMed]
11. Iseme, R.A.; McEvoy, M.; Kelly, B.; Agnew, L.; Walker, F.R.; Handley, T.; Oldmeadow, C.; Attia, J.; Boyle, M. A role for autoantibodies in atherogenesis. *Cardiovasc. Res.* **2017**, *113*, 1102–1112. [CrossRef]
12. Nowak, B.; Szmyrka-Kaczmarek, M.; Durazinska, A.; Plaksej, R.; Borysewicz, K.; Korman, L.; Wiland, P. Anti-ox-LDL antibodies and anti-ox-LDL-B2GPI antibodies in patients with systemic lupus erythematosus. *Adv. Clin. Exp. Med.* **2012**, *21*, 331–335.
13. Ye, Y.; Wu, T.; Zhang, T.; Han, J.; Habazi, D.; Saxena, R.; Mohan, C. Elevated oxidized lipids, anti-lipid autoantibodies and oxidized lipid immune complexes in active SLE. *Clin. Immunol.* **2019**, *205*, 43–48. [CrossRef] [PubMed]
14. Gomez-Zumaquero, J.M.; Tinahones, F.J.; De Ramon, E.; Camps, M.; Garrido, L.; Soriguer, F.J. Association of biological markers of activity of systemic lupus erythematosus with levels of anti-oxidized low-density lipoprotein antibodies. *Rheumatology* **2004**, *43*, 510–513. [CrossRef]
15. Vaarala, O.; Alfthan, G.; Jauhiainen, M.; Leirisalo-Repo, M.; Aho, K.; Palosuo, T. Crossreaction between antibodies to oxidised low-density lipoprotein and to cardiolipin in systemic lupus erythematosus. *Lancet* **1993**, *341*, 923–925. [CrossRef] [PubMed]
16. Parodis, I.; Stockfelt, M.; Sjowall, C. B Cell Therapy in Systemic Lupus Erythematosus: From Rationale to Clinical Practice. *Front. Med.* **2020**, *7*, 316. [CrossRef] [PubMed]
17. Jamialahmadi, T.; Baratzadeh, F.; Reiner, Z.; Mannarino, M.R.; Cardenia, V.; Simental-Mendia, L.E.; Pirro, M.; Watts, G.F.; Sahebkar, A. The Effects of Statin Therapy on Oxidized LDL and Its Antibodies: A Systematic Review and Meta-Analysis. *Oxid. Med. Cell Longev.* **2022**, *2022*, 7850659. [CrossRef]
18. Wu, R.; Svenungsson, E.; Gunnarsson, I.; Haegerstrand-Gillis, C.; Andersson, B.; Lundberg, I.; Elinder, L.S.; Frostegard, J. Antibodies to adult human endothelial cells cross-react with oxidized low-density lipoprotein and beta 2-glycoprotein I (beta 2-GPI) in systemic lupus erythematosus. *Clin. Exp. Immunol.* **1999**, *115*, 561–566. [CrossRef] [PubMed]
19. Shoenfeld, Y.; Wu, R.; Dearing, L.D.; Matsuura, E. Are anti-oxidized low-density lipoprotein antibodies pathogenic or protective? *Circulation* **2004**, *110*, 2552–2558. [CrossRef]
20. Zhao, D.; Ogawa, H.; Wang, X.; Cameron, G.S.; Baty, D.E.; Dlott, J.S.; Triplett, D.A. Oxidized low-density lipoprotein and autoimmune antibodies in patients with antiphospholipid syndrome with a history of thrombosis. *Am. J. Clin. Pathol.* **2001**, *116*, 760–767. [CrossRef] [PubMed]
21. Hayem, G.; Nicaise-Roland, P.; Palazzo, E.; de Bandt, M.; Tubach, F.; Weber, M.; Meyer, O. Anti-oxidized low-density-lipoprotein (OxLDL) antibodies in systemic lupus erythematosus with and without antiphospholipid syndrome. *Lupus* **2001**, *10*, 346–351. [CrossRef] [PubMed]
22. Salonen, J.T.; Yla-Herttuala, S.; Yamamoto, R.; Butler, S.; Korpela, H.; Salonen, R.; Nyyssonen, K.; Palinski, W.; Witztum, J.L. Autoantibody against oxidised LDL and progression of carotid atherosclerosis. *Lancet* **1992**, *339*, 883–887. [CrossRef] [PubMed]
23. Svenungsson, E.; Engelbertsen, D.; Wigren, M.; Gustafsson, J.T.; Gunnarsson, I.; Elvin, K.; Jensen-Urstad, K.; Fredrikson, G.N.; Nilsson, J. Decreased levels of autoantibodies against apolipoprotein B-100 antigens are associated with cardiovascular disease in systemic lupus erythematosus. *Clin. Exp. Immunol.* **2015**, *181*, 417–426. [CrossRef]
24. Kurien, B.T.; Fesmire, J.; Anderson, C.J.; Scofield, R.H. Anti-Ro and Concomitant Anti-La Autoantibodies Strongly Associated With Anti-oxLDL or Anti-Phospholipid Antibody in Systemic Lupus Erythematosus. *J. Clin. Rheumatol.* **2016**, *22*, 418–425. [CrossRef] [PubMed]

25. Bengtsson, A.; Nezlin, R.; Shoenfeld, Y.; Sturfelt, G. DNA levels in circulating immune complexes decrease at severe SLE flares-correlation with complement component C1q. *J. Autoimmun.* **1999**, *13*, 111–119. [CrossRef] [PubMed]
26. Sohrabian, A.; Parodis, I.; Carlstromer-Berthen, N.; Frodlund, M.; Jönsen, A.; Zickert, A.; Sjöwall, C.; Bengtsson, A.A.; Gunnarsson, I.; Ronnelid, J. Increased levels of anti-dsDNA antibodies in immune complexes before treatment with belimumab associate with clinical response in patients with systemic lupus erythematosus. *Arthritis Res. Ther.* **2019**, *21*, 259. [CrossRef]
27. Sturfelt, G.; Bengtsson, A.; Klint, C.; Nived, O.; Sjöholm, A.; Truedsson, L. Novel roles of complement in systemic lupus erythematosus–hypothesis for a pathogenetic vicious circle. *J. Rheumatol.* **2000**, *27*, 661–663.
28. Schiopu, A.; Bengtsson, J.; Soderberg, I.; Janciauskiene, S.; Lindgren, S.; Ares, M.P.; Shah, P.K.; Carlsson, R.; Nilsson, J.; Fredrikson, G.N. Recombinant human antibodies against aldehyde-modified apolipoprotein B-100 peptide sequences inhibit atherosclerosis. *Circulation* **2004**, *110*, 2047–2052. [CrossRef]
29. Wirestam, L.; Saleh, M.; Svensson, C.; Compagno, M.; Zachrisson, H.; Wettero, J.; Sjowall, C. Plasma osteopontin versus intima media thickness of the common carotid arteries in well-characterised patients with systemic lupus erythematosus. *Lupus* **2021**, *30*, 1244–1253. [CrossRef]
30. Tan, E.M.; Cohen, A.S.; Fries, J.F.; Masi, A.T.; McShane, D.J.; Rothfield, N.F.; Schaller, J.G.; Talal, N.; Winchester, R.J. The 1982 revised criteria for the classification of systemic lupus erythematosus. *Arthritis Rheum.* **1982**, *25*, 1271–1277. [CrossRef]
31. Eriksson, P.; Jacobsson, L.; Lindell, A.; Nilsson, J.A.; Skogh, T. Improved outcome in Wegener's granulomatosis and microscopic polyangiitis? A retrospective analysis of 95 cases in two cohorts. *J. Intern. Med.* **2009**, *265*, 496–506. [CrossRef] [PubMed]
32. Watts, R.; Lane, S.; Hanslik, T.; Hauser, T.; Hellmich, B.; Koldingsnes, W.; Mahr, A.; Segelmark, M.; Cohen-Tervaert, J.W.; Scott, D. Development and validation of a consensus methodology for the classification of the ANCA-associated vasculitides and polyarteritis nodosa for epidemiological studies. *Ann. Rheum. Dis.* **2007**, *66*, 222–227. [CrossRef] [PubMed]
33. Mukhtyar, C.; Lee, R.; Brown, D.; Carruthers, D.; Dasgupta, B.; Dubey, S.; Flossmann, O.; Hall, C.; Hollywood, J.; Jayne, D.; et al. Modification and validation of the Birmingham Vasculitis Activity Score (version 3). *Ann. Rheum. Dis.* **2009**, *68*, 1827–1832. [CrossRef]
34. Enocsson, H.; Wirestam, L.; Dahle, C.; Padyukov, L.; Jönsen, A.; Urowitz, M.B.; Gladman, D.D.; Romero-Diaz, J.; Bae, S.C.; Fortin, P.R.; et al. Soluble urokinase plasminogen activator receptor (suPAR) levels predict damage accrual in patients with recent-onset systemic lupus erythematosus. *J. Autoimmun.* **2020**, *106*, 102340. [CrossRef] [PubMed]
35. Karlsson, J.; Wettero, J.; Weiner, M.; Ronnelid, J.; Fernandez-Botran, R.; Sjowall, C. Associations of C-reactive protein isoforms with systemic lupus erythematosus phenotypes and disease activity. *Arthritis Res. Ther.* **2022**, *24*, 139. [CrossRef]
36. Kopprasch, S.; Bornstein, S.R.; Bergmann, S.; Graessler, J.; Hohenstein, B.; Julius, U. Long-term follow-up of circulating oxidative stress markers in patients undergoing lipoprotein apheresis by Direct Adsorption of Lipids (DALI). *Atheroscler. Suppl.* **2017**, *30*, 115–121. [CrossRef]
37. Zdanowska, N.; Owczarczyk-Saczonek, A.; Czerwińska, J.; Nowakowski, J.; Kozera-Żywczyk, A.; Owczarek, W.; Zdanowski, W.; Swacha, Z.; Placek, W. Methotrexate decreases oxidized low-density lipoprotein serum levels in patients with plaque psoriasis—Results of a preliminary study. *Acta Pol. Pharm.-Drug Res.* **2021**, *78*, 121–127. [CrossRef]

Disclaimer/Publisher's Note: The statements, opinions and data contained in all publications are solely those of the individual author(s) and contributor(s) and not of MDPI and/or the editor(s). MDPI and/or the editor(s) disclaim responsibility for any injury to people or property resulting from any ideas, methods, instructions or products referred to in the content.

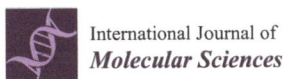

Article

Role of Advanced Glycation End Products as New Biomarkers in Systemic Lupus Erythematosus

Irene Carrión-Barberà [1,2,3,4,†], Laura Triginer [3,†], Laura Tío [3,*], Carolina Pérez-García [1,3,4], Anna Ribes [3], Victoria Abad [1,4], Ana Pros [1,4], Marcelino Bermúdez-López [5,6], Eva Castro-Boqué [5], Albert Lecube [7,8,9], José Manuel Valdivielso [5], ILERVAS Project Group [‡], Jordi Monfort [1,3,4,§] and Tarek Carlos Salman-Monte [1,3,4,§]

1. Rheumatology Department, Hospital del Mar, 08003 Barcelona, Spain
2. Medicine Department, Medicine Faculty, Universitat Autònoma de Barcelona, 08193 Bellaterra, Spain
3. Inflammation and Cartilage Cellular Research Group, Hospital del Mar Research Institute (IMIM), C/Dr. Aigüader 88, 08003 Barcelona, Spain
4. Clinical Expertise Unit (UEC) in Systemic Autoimmune Diseases and Vasculitis, Hospital del Mar, 08003 Barcelona, Spain
5. Grupo de Investigación Translacional Vascular y Renal, IRBLleida, 25198 Lleida, Spain
6. Departament de Medicina Experimental, Universitat de Lleida, 25198 Lleida, Spain
7. Departament d'Endocrinologia i Nutrició, Hospital Universitari Arnau de Vilanova, 25198 Lleida, Spain
8. Grup de Recerca Obesitat i Metabolisme (ODIM), IRBLleida, Universitat de Lleida, 25198 Lleida, Spain
9. Centro de Investigación Biomédica en Red de Diabetes y Enfermedades Metabólicas Asociadas (CIBERDEM), Instituto de Salud Carlos III (ISCIII), 28029 Madrid, Spain
* Correspondence: ltio@researchmar.net; Tel.: +34-933-160-445
† These authors contributed equally to this work.
‡ A full list of the ILERVAS Project collaborators is provided in Appendix A.
§ Both authors supervised equally to this work.

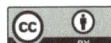

Citation: Carrión-Barberà, I.; Triginer, L.; Tío, L.; Pérez-García, C.; Ribes, A.; Abad, V.; Pros, A.; Bermúdez-López, M.; Castro-Boqué, E.; Lecube, A.; et al. Role of Advanced Glycation End Products as New Biomarkers in Systemic Lupus Erythematosus. *Int. J. Mol. Sci.* **2024**, *25*, 3022. https://doi.org/10.3390/ijms25053022

Academic Editors: Christopher Sjöwall and Ioannis Parodis

Received: 26 January 2024
Revised: 27 February 2024
Accepted: 28 February 2024
Published: 5 March 2024

Copyright: © 2024 by the authors. Licensee MDPI, Basel, Switzerland. This article is an open access article distributed under the terms and conditions of the Creative Commons Attribution (CC BY) license (https://creativecommons.org/licenses/by/4.0/).

Abstract: Advanced glycation end-products (AGEs) may play a relevant role as inducers in the chronic inflammatory pathway present in immune-mediated diseases, such as systemic lupus erythematosus (SLE). AGEs concentrations have been associated, with discrepant results to date, with some parameters such as disease activity or accrual damage, suggesting their potential usefulness as biomarkers of the disease. Our objectives are to confirm differences in AGEs levels measured by cutaneous autofluorescence between SLE patients and healthy controls (HC) and to study their correlation with various disease parameters. Cross-sectional study, where AGEs levels were measured by skin autofluorescence, and SLE patients' data were compared with those of sex- and age-matched HC in a 1:3 proportion through a multiple linear regression model. Associations of AGEs levels with demographic and clinical data were analyzed through ANOVA tests. Both analyses were adjusted for confounders. AGEs levels in SLE patients were significantly higher than in HC ($p < 0.001$). We found statistically significant positive associations with SLE disease activity index (SLEDAI) and damage index (SDI), physician and patient global assessment, C-reactive protein, leukocyturia, complement C4, IL-6 and oral ulcers. We also found a negative statistically significant association with current positivity of anti-nuclear and anti-Ro60 antibodies. AGEs seem to have a contribution in LES pathophysiology, being associated with activity and damage and having a role as a new management and prognosis biomarker in this disease. The association with specific antibodies and disease manifestations may indicate a specific clinical phenotype related to higher or lower AGEs levels.

Keywords: systemic lupus erythematosus; advanced glycation end products; cardiovascular disease; biomarkers

1. Background

Advanced glycation end-products (AGEs) are a set of compounds whose formation is a complicated molecular process resulting from the non-enzymatic interaction of reducing sugars and associated metabolites with peptides, proteins, and amino acids [1]. AGEs can accumulate under hyperglycaemic and pro-oxidative conditions, and it has been postulated that they have a role in inflammation.

The mechanisms of toxicity of AGEs are mainly related to two facts. On the one hand, glycation favors cross-links between the modified proteins, causing structural alterations and resulting in gradual deterioration in cell and tissue function and the generation of new immunological epitopes [2]. On the other hand, AGEs are recognized by their own receptor (RAGE), which is expressed in multiple cells from the immune system [3]. RAGE is divided into extracellular, transmembrane, and intracellular segments [4]. The interaction of AGEs with RAGE can activate the downstream nuclear factor kappa-B (NF-κB) signaling pathway and promote the secretion of several cytokines.

Soluble RAGE (sRAGE is variant of RAGE, a positively charged 48-kDa cleavage product from RAGE that keeps the ligand binding site but loses the other two domains [5]. sRAGE binding to ligands terminates intracellular signal transduction due to the loss of the transmembrane and intracellular fragments and inhibits the proinflammatory processes mediated by RAGE and its ligands by acting as a decoy which competitively binds to RAGE ligands [6]. sRAGE and not RAGE levels have been studied and linked to inflammation [7] as sRAGE is soluble and easy measurable, while RAGE is a cell–bound receptor and hence tissues are required for its measurement.

So far, more than 20 AGEs have been described in tissues [8]. Due to their stability, the most measured AGEs are serum or plasmatic Nε-(carboxymethyl)lysine (CML) and pentosidine. However, a part of the AGEs has the characteristic of being fluorescent, so it is possible to quantify them in a single measurement using an autofluorescence reader. This technique that measures accumulated AGEs in the skin, makes this assessment more appropriate to quantify the concentration of AGEs in an individual throughout their life than that of a single specific moment in relation to an acute process. So that, skin AGEs may better correlate with disease control, duration, and complications than serum AGEs [9]. As a validation method, it has been described that this autofluorescent measurement correlates with the concentration of AGEs, both fluorescent and not fluorescent, measured in skin biopsies [10]. Some of the advantages of measuring skin AGEs vs serum or plasmatic ones consist of having non-invasive, real-time data, easily available and affordable.

In systemic autoimmune diseases, such as systemic lupus erythematosus (SLE), increased AGEs formation can be expected, as inflammation is one of the hallmarks of the disease. Chronic inflammation in SLE appears to be associated with an intensified glycation process and the formation of AGEs, having higher values compared to healthy controls (HC) been demonstrated in some studies [11–15]. At the same time, AGEs are also involved in the generation of more inflammation and reactive oxygen species, creating positive feedback that enhances inflammation and AGEs levels.

Regarding atherosclerosis, AGEs have been linked to increased vascular rigidity and atherosclerosis [16–18]. In SLE, the presence of accelerated atherosclerosis that cannot be fully explained by traditional risk factors for cardiovascular disease is a well-recorded phenomenon [19]. Some studies have suggested that increased levels of AGEs might contribute to the development of this accelerated atherosclerosis in SLE and, therefore, could be used as early markers for cardiovascular disease in this pathology [14,15].

Lately, there has been increased attention on the potential of RAGE and AGEs to target chronic inflammatory diseases such as SLE. Some studies have expounded on their usefulness as biomarkers of SLE diagnosis and prognosis, their relationship with accelerated atherosclerosis, as well as their potential place as targets for new treatments. However, we find some controversial results in the literature, showing that more and better studies are needed to fully elucidate their role in SLE.

Taking into account that the relation between skin AGEs and SLE has only been reported in one previous paper, the purpose of this work is to try to elucidate the role of AGEs in SLE as potential biomarkers of the disease, as well as their application in routine clinical practice as a tool for improving the diagnosis, monitoring, and/or prognosis of the disease, or as surrogate markers for the assessment of cardiovascular risk in this population. Our study involved describing AGEs concentrations in SLE and comparing them to age- and sex-matched HC; searching for correlations between AGEs concentrations and SLE characteristics such as specific manifestations, indexes of activity or accrual damage, or patient reported outcomes (PROs); and finally, exploring AGEs relationship with cardiovascular disease and cardiovascular risk factors (CVRF).

2. Results

2.1. Characteristics of Patients and Controls

The differences between the 189 HC and 62 cases are shown in Table 1: HC had a higher BMI and a higher incidence of dyslipidemia (both in total cholesterol and low-density lipoprotein values), obesity, hypertension, and active smoking. Patients with SLE had higher AGEs values and creatinine concentrations.

Table 1. Descriptive characteristics of cases and healthy controls and bivariate analysis between both groups. As we are exploring confounding variables p-value was widened and considered statistically significant if <0.1 (highlighted in bold in the text). AGEs: advanced glycation end products; HDL: High-density lipoprotein; LDL: Low-density lipoprotein.

	Controls	Cases	p-Value
	N = 189	N = 62	
Ethnicity			<0.001
Caucasian	189 (100%)	46 (74.2%)	
Other	0 (0.00%)	16 (25.8%)	
Age	56.0 [52.0; 62.0]	55.0 [51.0; 61.8]	0.193
Sex: Female	180 (95.2%)	58 (93.5%)	0.748
Hypertension	73 (38.6%)	14 (22.6%)	**0.032**
Obesity	61 (32.3%)	12 (19.4%)	**0.075**
Dyslipidemia	85 (45.0%)	9 (14.5%)	**<0.001**
Smoking			**0.054**
Never	79 (41.8%)	24 (38.7%)	
Former (>1 year)	54 (28.6%)	27 (43.5%)	
Active	56 (29.6%)	11 (17.7%)	
Body mass index	28.9 (5.98)	25.6 (4.65)	**<0.001**
Creatinine	0.70 [0.61; 0.77]	0.74 [0.64; 0.90]	**0.006**
Uric acid	4.90 (1.27)	4.70 (1.62)	0.365
Cholesterol	210 (37.5)	187 (39.5)	**<0.001**
HDL	61.9 (14.0)	65.9 (15.7)	0.125
LDL	138 (29.3)	112 (34.6)	**<0.001**
Triglycerides	123 [95.8; 160]	92.0 [70.0; 159]	**0.003**
Antidyslipidemics	27 (14.3%)	11 (17.7%)	0.649
Antihypertensives	61 (32.3%)	16 (25.8%)	0.424
AGEs	1.98 (0.45)	2.71 (0.56)	**<0.001**
AGEs in tertiles			**<0.001**
[1.0, 1.9)	83 (43.9%)	3 (4.84%)	
[1.9, 2.4)	74 (39.2%)	13 (21.0%)	
[2.4, 4.2]	32 (16.9%)	46 (74.2%)	

2.2. Comparison of AGEs in SLE Patients vs. Healthy Controls

According to all of the data explored, the multivariate model was adjusted with age, smoking, dyslipidemia, creatinine. The model reported a statistically significant difference between SLE and HC in AGEs values, showing that AGEs values in SLE patients were 0.721

(95% confidence interval (CI) [0.566; 0.876]) units higher ($p < 0.001$) than HC. See Table 2 for the analysis of covariance of fixed effects and Supplementary Figure S3 for the effects graphic.

Table 2. Fixed-effects analysis of covariance (ANCOVA) model to study differences in AGEs levels between cases and healthy controls. y: years.

	Est.	2.5%	97.5%	t Val.	p-Value
Intercept	1.9418	1.8450	2.0385	39.5252	<0.0001
Group: Cases	0.7210	0.5660	0.8759	9.1645	<0.0001
Age (57.5 years)	0.0168	0.0081	0.0254	3.8359	0.0002
Smoking (Yes)	0.3265	0.1945	0.4585	4.8724	<0.0001
Creatinine (0.72 mg/dL)	0.2110	−0.1763	0.5983	1.0732	0.2843
Dyslipidemia (Yes)	−0.1240	−0.2544	0.0065	−1.8720	0.0624
(Group: Cases) + (Dyslipidemia (Yes))	0.1286	−0.2227	0.4799	0.7211	0.4715

2.3. Characteristics of SLE Patients According to AGEs Levels: Bivariate Analysis

A total of 122 SLE patients were included. All of the variables that showed statistically significant differences according to AGEs tertiles in the bivariate analysis are depicted in Table 3, adjusted by age (p-value M1) and by both age and smoking (p-value M2). The demographic characteristics and other SLE variables of interest are detailed in Supplementary Table S3.

Table 3. Variables that showed statistically significant differences according to AGEs tertiles in the bivariate analysis. M1: adjusted by age, M2: adjusted by age and smoking. "c" indicates variables which have been categorized as stated in Section 4. Bold indicates p-value < 0.1 and * indicates values according to the blood test performed in the study. p-val: p-value; SLEDAI: SLE disease activity index; SDI: systemic Lupus International Collaborating Clinics/American College of Rheumatology (SLICC/ACR) Damage Index; PGA: Physician global assessment; FACIT: Functional Assessment of Chronic Illness Therapy—Fatigue Scale; PtGA: Patient global assessment; GPT: Glutamic-pyruvic transaminase; CRP: C-reactive protein; IL-6: interleukin-6; ANA: antinuclear antibodies; C4: complement C4; GC: glucocorticoids; IS: Immunosuppressants (includes treatment with methotrexate, leflunomide, tacrolimus, mycophenolic acid or mycophenolate mofetil, azathioprine, cyclophosphamide, cyclosporine, rituximab or belimumab).

Variables	All	1st Tertile [1.2, 2.3)	2nd Tertile [2.3, 2.8)	3rd Tertile [2.8, 4.6]	p-Val M1	p-Val M2
	N = 122	N = 44	N = 41	N = 37		
Age	50.4 (14.9)	41.8 (13.8)	49.9 (12.2)	61.2 (11.9)		<0.001
Smoker	32 (26.2%)	10 (22.7%)	11 (26.8%)	11 (29.7%)	<0.001	
cDisease duration (years)					0.082	0.090
0–5	50 (41.0%)	19 (43.2%)	18 (43.9%)	13 (35.1%)		
6–10	16 (13.1%)	7 (15.9%)	6 (14.6%)	3 (8.11%)		
11–20	33 (27.0%)	13 (29.5%)	11 (26.8%)	9 (24.3%)		
>20	23 (18.9%)	5 (11.4%)	6 (14.6%)	12 (32.4%)		
Classificatory Criteria and Other Clinical and Serological Data						
Oral ulcers ever	50 (41.0%)	13 (29.5%)	18 (43.9%)	19 (51.4%)	0.022	0.033
Arthritis ever	92 (75.4%)	31 (70.5%)	32 (78.0%)	29 (78.4%)	0.070	0.092
Renal disease ever	8 (6.56%)	2 (4.55%)	1 (2.44%)	5 (13.5%)	0.067	0.054
cNumber of manifestations					0.032	0.069
[3, 7)	58 (47.5%)	19 (43.2%)	21 (51.2%)	18 (48.6%)		
7	24 (19.7%)	10 (22.7%)	8 (19.5%)	6 (16.2%)		
[8, 12]	40 (32.8%)	15 (34.1%)	12 (29.3%)	13 (35.1%)		
Disease Activity Indexes						
SLEDAI	4.00 [2.00; 6.00]	4.00 [0.00; 6.00]	4.00 [2.00; 6.00]	6.00 [2.00; 8.00]	0.016	0.041

Table 3. Cont.

Variables	All	1st Tertile [1.2, 2.3)	2nd Tertile [2.3, 2.8)	3rd Tertile [2.8, 4.6]	p-Val M1	p-Val M2
	N = 122	N = 44	N = 41	N = 37		
cSLEDAI					0.003	0.008
Remission/Mild	71 (58.7%)	29 (67.4%)	25 (61.0%)	17 (45.9%)		
Moderate	39 (32.2%)	11 (25.6%)	14 (34.1%)	14 (37.8%)		
Severe	11 (9.09%)	3 (6.98%)	2 (4.88%)	6 (16.2%)		
SDI	0.00 [0.00; 1.00]	0.00 [0.00; 1.00]	0.00 [0.00; 1.00]	1.00 [0.00; 2.00]	0.026	0.007
cSDI_3					0.052	0.017
0–2	110 (90.9%)	41 (95.3%)	38 (92.7%)	31 (83.8%)		
3–4	8 (6.61%)	2 (4.65%)	2 (4.88%)	4 (10.8%)		
5–6	3 (2.48%)	0 (0.00%)	1 (2.44%)	2 (5.41%)		
PGA	2.00 [1.00; 3.00]	1.50 [1.00; 2.00]	2.00 [1.00; 3.00]	2.00 [1.00; 2.00]	0.083	0.051
cPGA					0.051	0.029
<1	18 (14.9%)	7 (16.3%)	6 (14.6%)	5 (13.5%)		
1–2	69 (57.0%)	27 (62.8%)	19 (46.3%)	23 (62.2%)		
>2	34 (28.1%)	9 (20.9%)	16 (39.0%)	9 (24.3%)		
Patient Reported Outcomes						
FACIT	17.5 [10.0; 27.0]	14.0 [9.00; 23.0]	22.0 [13.0; 30.0]	18.0 [10.0; 28.0]	0.099	0.138
PtGA	2.75 [1.00; 5.00]	2.00 [1.00; 3.00]	3.00 [2.00; 5.00]	3.00 [1.00; 5.00]	0.028	0.042
cPtGA					0.112	0.121
[0.0, 2.5)	57 (46.7%)	26 (59.1%)	14 (34.1%)	17 (45.9%)		
[2.5, 4.5)	28 (23.0%)	9 (20.5%)	12 (29.3%)	7 (18.9%)		
[4.5, 8.0]	37 (30.3%)	9 (20.5%)	15 (36.6%)	13 (35.1%)		
Serological variables						
GPT *	17.0 [13.0; 22.0]	16.0 [12.0; 22.5]	16.0 [13.0; 20.0]	18.0 [15.0; 23.0]	0.095	0.068
Total cholesterol *	181 (37.7)	172 (29.6)	174 (38.0)	201 (39.5)	0.046	0.093
cCRP *					0.058	0.053
[0.03, 0.12)	45 (37.2%)	24 (55.8%)	8 (19.5%)	13 (35.1%)		
[0.12, 0.28)	36 (29.8%)	11 (25.6%)	17 (41.5%)	8 (21.6%)		
[0.28, 3.92]	40 (33.1%)	8 (18.6%)	16 (39.0%)	16 (43.2%)		
cIL-6 *					0.049	0.025
[0.63, 1.88)	36 (33.3%)	18 (48.6%)	12 (31.6%)	6 (18.2%)		
[1.88, 3.33)	36 (33.3%)	11 (29.7%)	14 (36.8%)	11 (33.3%)		
[3.33, 144.10]	36 (33.3%)	8 (21.6%)	12 (31.6%)	16 (48.5%)		
ANA+ *	112 (92.6%)	43 (100%)	38 (92.7%)	31 (83.8%)	0.027	0.036
Anti-Ro60+ *	45 (37.8%)	17 (40.5%)	19 (47.5%)	9 (24.3%)	0.183	0.164
C4 *	19.8 (8.23)	18.5 (7.97)	18.7 (7.09)	22.4 (9.23)	0.025	0.017
Leukocyturia *	0.00 [0.00; 1.00]	0.00 [0.00; 0.00]	0.00 [0.00; 1.00]	1.00 [0.00; 2.00]	0.004	0.001
Hematuria *	0.00 [0.00; 0.00]	0.00 [0.00; 0.00]	0.00 [0.00; 0.00]	0.00 [0.00; 1.00]	0.031	0.067
cLeukocyturia *					0.052	0.024
0	72 (60.0%)	33 (78.6%)	24 (58.5%)	15 (40.5%)		
1	25 (20.8%)	6 (14.3%)	11 (26.8%)	8 (21.6%)		
[2, 5]	23 (19.2%)	3 (7.14%)	6 (14.6%)	14 (37.8%)		
Treatments						
GC	30 (24.6%)	7 (15.9%)	11 (26.8%)	12 (32.4%)	0.004	<0.001
Current dose of GC	5.00 [2.50; 10.0]	7.50 [3.75; 10.0]	5.00 [2.50; 12.5]	5.00 [2.50; 6.25]	0.050	0.029
Tacrolimus	1 (0.82%)	0 (0.00%)	0 (0.00%)	1 (2.70%)	0.147	0.083
cTreatment2					0.077	0.092
No IS	66 (54.1%)	27 (61.4%)	20 (48.8%)	19 (51.4%)		
IS	56 (45.9%)	17 (38.6%)	21 (51.2%)	18 (48.6%)		

2.4. Correlations between AGEs and SLE Characteristics: Multivariate Analysis

After adjustment for confounding variables, several SLE characteristics showed associations with AGEs levels. First of all, two of the most important SLE disease indexes, SLE disease activity index (SLEDAI) and SLE damage index (SDI), were significantly associated with AGEs levels. While for the SLEDAI we found a progressive increase in AGEs values as the SLEDAI activity escalated (AGEs values in patients with moderate and severe activity were 0.2 (95% CI [0.0006; 0.4], $p = 0.0493$) and 0.52 (95% CI [0.177; 0.86], $p = 0.003$) units higher than patients in remission/mild, respectively, we only found differences in SDI between those with low (0–2) and high scores (5, 6) (AGEs values 0.717 (95% CI [0.139; 1.295], $p = 0.0156$) units higher). This association with disease activity is also reflected in both the physician global assessment (PGA) and the patient global assessment (PtGA). In those cases, values higher than 1 (PGA) or 3 (PtGA) were associated with an AGEs increase. PGA score of 1–2 and a PGA score higher than 2 had AGEs levels 0.033 (95% CI [0.058; 0.61], $p = 0.018$) and 0.39 (95% CI [0.094; 0.694], $p = 0.01$) units higher than patients with a PGA of 0, respectively; and patients with a PtGA score >3 had AGEs levels 0.26 (95% CI [0.063; 0.46], $p = 0.01$) units higher than patients with PtGA score ≤ 3.

Regarding serum biomarkers, we observed an increment in AGEs levels as C-reactive protein (CRP) and IL-6 increased, but significant differences were only detected between the 3rd and 1st tertile: 0.259 (95% CI [0.035; 0.48], $p = 0.02$) units higher for CRP and 0.352 (95% CI [0.1; 0.6], $p = 0.006$) for IL-6. The same tendency was observed in the level of leukocyturia (0.369, 95% CI [0.112; 0.626], $p = 0.005$) and C4 complement, although in this last one, significant differences with the 2nd tertile were also observed (0.25 (95% CI [0.02; 0.48], $p = 0.0335$) units higher for the 2nd tertile; and 0.28 (95% CI [0.056; 0.514], $p = 0.015$) for the 3rd one).

With reference to autoantibodies, a negative association was found between AGEs levels and both the presence of ANA or anti-Ro60 antibodies in the blood test performed for the study, where AGEs values were 0.496 (95% CI [0.937; 0.054], $p = 0.028$) and 0.26 (95% CI [0.5; 0.017], $p = 0.035$) units lower, respectively.

Finally, patients which had ever presented oral ulcers, a prevalent SLE manifestation, had AGEs values 0.216 (95% CI [0.02; 0.41], $p = 0.03$) units higher than patients who had never. All of these data are depicted, according to the prediction of each model, in Figures 1 and 2 which graphically represent the mean and its corresponding 95% CI of AGEs for each category of variables. p-values < 0.05 indicate significant differences between the categories and the reference level of each variable. Also, the fixed-effects ANCOVA model between AGEs and each of the variables are provided Supplementary Table S4.

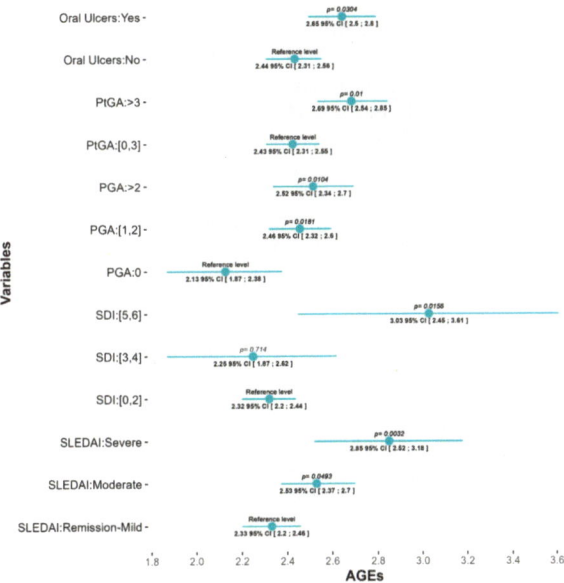

Figure 1. Statistically significant associations between AGEs levels and SLE characteristics and indexes. *p*-values < 0.05 (bold) indicate significant differences between the categories and the reference level of each variable; *p*-values not in bold indicate associations not statistically significant. PtGA: patient global assessment; PGA: physician global assessment; SDI: SLE damage index; SLEDAI: SLE disease activity index.

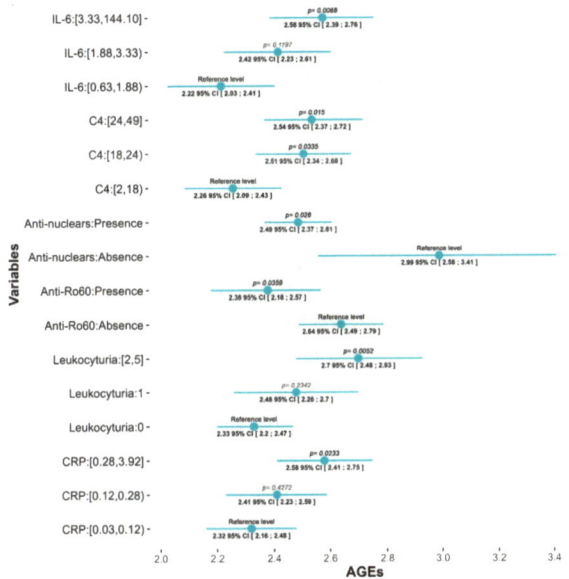

Figure 2. Statistically significant correlations between AGEs levels and SLE serological parameters. The change in AGEs values is depicted according to the reference category of each variable. *p*-value is considered significant if <0.05 (bold). IL-6: interleukin 6 (pg/mL); C4: complement 4 (mg/dL); CRP: C-reactive protein (mg/dL).

3. Discussion

We observed statistically significant differences between AGEs values measured by skin autofluorescence in SLE patients vs. HC. This difference has only been studied in two previous works [14,15] with small sample sizes (55 and 30 cases respectively, matched 1:1 with HC), and our research builds upon these studies in the following ways. First, we have increased the sample size, especially the HC sample, by matching cases with HC in a 1:3 proportion instead of a 1:1 proportion, making the study more robust. Secondly, we selected HC that had at least one CVRF, so they would be more comparable to our patients who at least have one CVRF, being that the disease itself. This is based on the well-reported knowledge that AGEs are related to inflammation and cardiovascular risk on the one hand and, on the other, that patients with autoimmune diseases such as rheumatoid arthritis, have an increased risk of cardiovascular disease that makes necessary to add a fixed multiplier of 1.5 to 2 to the established cardiovascular disease prediction general algorithms in order to adjust for the increased risk due to the disease [20]. Nienhuis et al. [14] selected a second control population with essential hypertension (EH), apart from the one conformed by HC. They found statistically significant differences in AGEs levels between SLE patients and HC but not between the SLE and the EH cohort, suggesting that finding differences when selecting HC with at least one CVRF could traduce a higher statistical power and a reduced probability of committing a type I error. Furthermore, they selected an SLE population with inactive disease, which might not reflect the reality of SLE patients in terms of disease characteristics in the way our patients might, which were included independently of their disease activity.

Additionally, we carefully examined all possible confounding factors to avoid drawing premature conclusions. Two controversial points were raised during the analysis. First, we observed only a positive trend shown by creatinine in the bivariate analysis of AGEs levels in the whole sample [21]. We discussed if that trend could have a fictitious origin since patients with SLE had higher creatinine levels (although in normal range) and were mostly located in the third AGEs tertile, and also since the trend was not observed when we analyzed the two groups separately. However, we finally decided to include creatinine in the model since there is ample evidence of a higher accumulation of AGEs in patients with renal failure [22] and lupus nephritis [12], and a difference could exist between groups since renal disease was an exclusion criterion in the HC group. Secondly, we found a negative association between dyslipidemia and AGEs, which was observed both in the combined analysis of the whole sample and in the HC separately (suggesting that such association comes from the HC group). The only data in the literature that could explain this negative association comes from the reported effect of lipid-lowering drugs in reducing AGEs levels [23]. Among HC, only 27 of the 85 with dyslipidemia (32%) were being treated with lipid-lowering agents, so we hypothesized that the rest could be controlling it with a lower-fat diet, which has also been associated with reduced AGEs levels [24]. Hence, we ended up including dyslipidemia in the model.

As for the interaction term between the main effect and dyslipidemia, although it was not found to be significant in the model, graphically the interaction seemed clear, especially in the group of SLE patients (Supplementary Figure S2). This could be due to a lack of statistical power, since in the group of SLE patients there were only 8 dyslipidemic cases, unlike the 85 dyslipidemic HC. Therefore, the statistical power to detect this difference was much lower in the patient group, generating a less precise CI to reject the alternative hypothesis and leading to a lack of significance.

Regarding the study of AGEs relationship with SLE characteristics, we have found associations between AGEs levels and some disease activity indexes: SLEDAI, PGA, PtGA, CRP, and IL-6. As reflected in Section 2, the rise of AGEs levels with the increase of SLEDAI, which is the activity index most frequently used for SLE in clinical practice nowadays, showed a robust correlation. This association was also observed with other markers of activity commonly used to assess the disease state: PGA, PtGA, and IL-6. PGA is a part of the main indexes used currently to define remission or low disease activity in SLE. PtGA may be a more subjective parameter which can be influenced by external factors but that is clearly related to quality of life in SLE patients. IL-6 is not used routinely in the follow-up of SLE patients but its role in inflammation it is widely known generally and in rheumatic diseases in particular.

In the case of CRP, a significant association was only found between the upper tertile (0.28–3.92 mg/dL) and the first (<0.12), suggesting that the highest levels of AGEs were found among the patients with higher CRP values, both with values considered normal and abnormal (normal reference values in our laboratory <0.5 mg/dL). However, this correlation is only supported up to CRP values < 0.7 ($R2 = 0.42$, $p < 0.0001$), as graphically reflected in Supplementary Figure S4. No correlation was found with higher CRP levels, which could be justified by a small number of patients with abnormal CRP levels. There was also a positive association with higher C4 levels, which draws attention since low C4 levels are the ones traditionally associated with high disease activity. However, although a decrease in complement levels is included in SLE classificatory criteria, there is wide controversy in the literature about the limited usefulness of the current techniques and types of complement measured in SLE and their ability to reflect disease activity [25]. Other uncertainties about complement are whether low levels should be persistent or combined (both C3 and C4) to be significant [26,27]. In our study, C3 levels showed a statistically significant direct correlation with C4 values ($p \leq 0.001$) but not with AGEs levels. There was no association between having normal C4 levels at the moment of the study and not having had hypocomplementemia ever: 43% of the patients with current normal C4 levels had history of hypocomplementemia and 57% did not, while 77% of the patients with history of low C4 had now normal levels. This could traduce either fluctuant titers or normalized levels of C4 in response to treatment/lower disease activity and a need for further studies to elucidate the relation between complement and AGEs.

We also found a relationship between AGEs and indexes of accrual damage, the SDI. There is only a previous work in the literature that analyzed this association [15]. They found a correlation between AGEs and SDI in the univariate analysis that was lost after adjusting for age as well as in the multivariate analysis. In our case, the association persisted after adjusting for age and smoking status and any other possible confounding factor in the multivariate analysis. Considering this association, measuring AGEs levels could have a high impact in the prognosis of the disease helping to identify a subtype of patients with a more serious disease marked by higher accrual damage, which would be susceptible of a stricter follow-up and intensive treatment regimen, and subsequently allowing to improve these patients' outcomes.

Specific manifestations (oral ulcers) or autoantibodies profile (less frequent anti-Ro60+ antibodies), could indicate a different clinical phenotype in SLE patients with less inflammation and thus, with lower AGEs levels. In clinical practice, it is very common to find overlaps of autoimmune diseases in the same patient, being especially frequent in SLE its overlap with Sjögren syndrome (SjS). It is known that both diseases have different inflammatory profiles [28], which could explain why there could be differences in AGEs levels between patients anti-Ro60 positive and negative. AGEs concentrations have been scarcely studied in SjS and efforts have not been directed to skin AGEs but RAGE and sRAGE with conflicting results [29–31], so more studies are needed to investigate AGEs levels in SjS and their differences both with SLE patients and with patients with a SLE-SjS overlap. Unfortunately, we could not validate this hypothesis in our study as the presence of SjS was recorded together with other autoimmune diseases as presence of overlapping syndrome in general, making studying the association only in SjS not possible. Furthermore, some patients had ongoing diagnostic SjS tests at the moment of our work. Similarly, oral ulcers are much more frequent in SLE than other autoimmune disease, potentially traducing a more typical SLE disease than in those without, which might justify differences in AGEs levels.

Regarding the negative relation found between AGEs and ANA antibodies, all patients were ANA+ at SLE diagnosis but 10 of them (8.2%) converted during disease follow-up and were ANA− at the moment of the study. It has been reported that the reduction of ANA responses might reflect the natural history of the disease as well as the effects of therapy [32]. Accordingly, these patients could have increased AGEs levels due to longer disease duration or more intense need for therapy due to more severe disease, and consequent more accrual damage and potentially higher AGEs levels. In our cohort, currently ANA− patients showed higher disease duration (15 vs. 10 years) and higher SDI (same levels of p25 and p50 but differences in p75: 1.56 vs. 0.68) although the differences were not statistically significant, probably due to lack of statistical power on account of the small sample size, also shown by the wide CI of this variable Supplementary Table S4. We didn't observe differences in terms of taking immunosuppressants in the moment of the study between ANA+ and ANA− patients, but we did not retrieve data of the therapy history of patients, so we cannot rule out differences in the number of immunosuppressants or time taking therapy between both groups.

Despite the known relationship between AGEs and atherosclerosis, we did not find any correlation between AGEs levels and either CVRF or cardiovascular events (CVE). However, the p-value in the bivariate analysis was <0.1 and, considering that we have a small number of patients with CVE (N = 9), it is likely that our results are limited by a lack of statistical power which prevents us from drawing conclusions about the role of AGEs in cardiovascular risk. Furthermore, we assessed cardiovascular disease only through traditional CVRF or CVE and did not perform additional tests such as the intima-media thickness of the common carotid artery measured by ultrasound [15] or the small artery elasticity measured by pulse-wave analysis using tonometric recordings of the radial artery [14], both of which have been associated with AGEs levels in previous works. We also reassessed the correlation between AGEs and SDI excluding all variables related to cardiovascular disease (expressed as CVE in our study) as De Leeuw et al. do in their work [15]. They found a correlation in the bivariate analysis between skin AGEs and SDI, also after correction for the damage caused by CV disease. This association was not seen after adjusting for age or in the multivariate analysis. In our cohort, this new analysis did not alter the statistical correlation between SDI and AGEs, indicating that the association is not attributable to AGEs being associated to CV damage.

Only one of the two previous works studying skin AGEs in SLE have analyzed their association with disease characteristics, finding an association with age, creatinine, disease duration, the intima-media thickness of the common carotid artery, and the SDI in the univariate analysis, and only with age and disease duration in the multivariate one [15]. Our work has carried out a much more extensive analysis considering a great amount of demographic and clinical variables and performing a more complex statistical analysis considering all possible confounding factors, which provides a much deeper knowledge into these relationships and opens the door to the feasibility of using AGEs as a clinical tool for SLE management and prognosis.

Our study presents several limitations. Firstly, due to the retrospective nature of the study some data could not be retrieved such as the cumulative glucocorticoid (GC) dose that the patients had taken throughout the disease, and we could only assess the impact of GC through the current dose at the moment of the study. Likewise, the design makes it impossible to assess causality, which warrants future prospective studies. Secondly, and in order to clarify the effect on longstanding disease and therapy in AGEs levels, studies in newly diagnosed patients should be performed. Another limitation is that we did not check for all of the factors that have been described to influence AGEs levels such as diet [24].

To our knowledge, this is the second work to study and the first to find an association between SLE activity parameters and skin AGEs. We have found a correlation with, not one, but several SLE activity biomarkers and, also, with damage indexes. Furthermore, we have described, for the first time, skin AGEs associations with specific serological and clinical parameters that could define more precisely a specific type of patients in whom AGEs could have a particularly meaningful contribution. Therefore, our results are innovative and indicative of the promising role of AGEs and the AGEs skin reader as a tool to be implemented in daily clinical practice as a noninvasive, fast, real-time surrogate biomarker of SLE disease activity, damage, and specific manifestations.

4. Methodology

4.1. Subjects

This was a cross-sectional study conducted at the Hospital del Mar where patients of all ages who were visited at the SLE outpatient clinic, met the 1997 American College of Rheumatology (ACR) [33] or the 2012 Systemic Lupus International Collaborating Clinics (SLICC) classificatory criteria [34] for SLE, accepted to participate and signed the informed consent were randomly included. The exclusion criteria were pregnancy, diabetes mellitus (DM), treatment with corticosteroids at a dose equivalent to prednisone >20 mg/day, active malignancy, and fibromyalgia. Patients and the public were not involved in the design, conduct, reporting, or dissemination of this work.

4.2. Healthy Controls

The control population was selected from the ILERVAS cohorts (Vascular and Renal Translational Research Group, IRBLleida), which includes HC selected from primary care health centers, with at least one traditional CVRF and aged between 50 and 70 years if women or between 45 and 65 years if men. The traditional CVRF included were arterial hypertension (AHT) and/or dyslipidemia (DLP) and/or obesity (defined as a body mass index (BMI) > 30 kg/m^2), and/or history in first-degree relatives of premature cardiovascular disease (men before 65-year-old and women before 60 years-old) and/or smokers and former smokers (<10 years since quitting). Exclusion criteria were as follows: history of cardiovascular disease (angina, myocardial infarction, cerebrovascular accident, peripheral arterial disease, intestinal ischemia or ischemia of some other territory), history of carotid surgery or surgery of arteries from other territories, DM and/or chronic renal disease (CRD), institutionalized population, population on long-term home-care, active neoplastic processes, life expectancy < 18 months [35]. AGEs levels were measured by autofluorescence in all of the HC.

4.3. Assessment of AGES Accumulation

In all patients, accumulated AGEs were measured non-invasively in the skin by an autofluorescence reader (Age Reader Mu Connect®, DiagnOptics Technologies BV, Groningen, The Netherlands) as described previously in the literature [10]. A light source emitting light at a wavelength of 320 to 400 nm excites fluorescent moieties in compounds in the skin to produce fluorescence at a wavelength of 420 to 600 nm (peak 440 nm). The output represents the ratio between autofluorescence in the range 420 to 600 nm and excitation light in the range 320 to 400 nm and is reported in arbitrary units (AU). Three consecutive AGEs measurements were taken from the ventral (anterior) surface of the forearm of each participant 10 cm below the elbow fold, avoiding any tattoos or heavily pigmented areas of skin. Measurements were performed at room temperature, while patients were in a seated position [36] (see Supplementary Figure S1). The mean value of the three measures was calculated and compared with AGEs values from age-matched HC obtained from previous works [10].

4.4. Statistical Methods

4.4.1. Comparison of Accumulated AGEs between Patients and Controls

A random sample of 60 individuals with systemic lupus erythematosus and of 183 healthy controls was calculated to be sufficient to estimate, with 95% confidence, a beta risk of 0.2 in a two-sided test, and an accuracy of ±0.25 units, the population mean of values (with an expected standard deviation of about 0.6 units [15]). HC were sex- and age-matched with a factor of approximately 3:1 to each of the SLE patients and selected according to the common variables between both groups. Due to the limited age range of our control group, some of the SLE patients had to be excluded as it was not possible to age-match them with HC. In addition, SLE patients with cardiovascular disease could not be included in the analysis due to it being an exclusion criterion in the HC sample. Difference of AGEs between SLE cases and HC was assessed through a fixed-effects analysis of covariance (ANCOVA) model adjusted for the confounding factors.

In order to identify potentially confounding variables, in addition to a bibliographic review about previously reported factors related to AGEs, a bivariate analysis was performed separating by cases and HC, and by tertiles of AGEs. Categorical data were described with absolute and relative frequencies, whereas continuous variables were displayed as mean (standard deviation), or as median (interquartile range) if non-normally distributed. In the case of categorical variables, we employed the Fisher's exact test for variables with small frequencies and the χ^2 test for the rest. For normal continuous variables, the Student's t-test was used when analyzing two groups and the analysis of variance (ANOVA) when there were more than two. For non-normal continuous variables, the test used was the Mann-Whitney U test to compare two groups and the Kruskal-Wallis' test to compare more than two. The significance level for these explorative analyses of confounding variables was taken to be <0.1.

Variables with statistically significant differences both between groups and with the AGEs response variable were considered potential confounders and were examined through interaction graphs before including them in the final model.

In the specific case of comparing AGEs levels between cases and controls and, as all of the HC were Caucasian, we performed a sensitivity analysis to assess the influence of ethnicity, testing only Caucasian patients against HC. We did not find any differences, so we kept all of the ethnicities in the final analysis.

Later on, we explored the associations between AGEs levels (stratified in tertiles) and data of all of the participants of the study (both SLE patients and HC), in order to evaluate possible confounding factors. The bivariate analysis showed a significant positive relationship between smoking and AGEs levels, while creatinine showed a trend in that same direction. On the contrary, the presence of dyslipidemia was associated with lower values of AGEs (Supplementary Table S1).

According to these results and the differences found between SLE patients and HC, interaction graphs were created to visually assess smoking, age, dyslipidemia, and creatinine as cofounding variables. We found differences in the slopes of age and dyslipidemia (Supplementary Figure S2) which were then evaluated in the fixed-effects analysis of covariance model (Supplementary Figure S3). Smoking was also added to the model due to extensive literature linking it to AGEs values. Furthermore, in the smoking interaction graph we observed that the slopes of non-smokers and former smokers behaved similarly, with only a slight increase in mean cumulative AGEs in non-smokers with SLE, but apparently insignificant, so we unified non-smokers and former smokers in the same group vs. active smokers to increase statistical power (Supplementary Figure S2a).

According to all of the data explored, the multivariate model was adjusted with age, smoking, dyslipidemia, creatinine, and the interaction terms. None of the interaction terms were statistically significant so they were finally removed from the model except for the interaction between dyslipidemia and group (SLE or HC). This one, was not omitted since it allowed us to observe the effect ($p = 0.062$) of dyslipidemia, granting a better estimation of the AGEs value (Table 2). This was verified by adjusting it without the interaction, where the main effect of dyslipidemia was lost. Dyslipidemia was also adjusted for age and smoking (since HC with dyslipidemia were younger and smoked less), and its effect remained unchanged, ruling out that it was confused by other variables (Supplementary Table S2).

4.4.2. Relation between Characteristics of SLE and Accumulated AGEs

An exploratory analysis was conducted using ANOVA tests adjusted for both age and current smoking status to investigate the association between SLE patient characteristics and the level of accumulated AGEs, including all patients from the cross-sectional study.

For a better analysis, skewed variables of interest were categorized into tertiles or according to non-linear patterns, evaluated with general additive models. Associations with a p value < 0.1 were considered significant and, if consistent, were examined individually. First of all, the identification of potentially confounding variables was performed as described in the previous analysis (D.1.). Then multiple lineal regression models studying association between AGEs levels and each variable of interest were fitted considering the corresponding confounding factors, to avoid spurious associations. In this case, the significance level was taken to be <0.05.

In both analysis, continuous variables included in the final models were mean centered to facilitate interpretation. The assumptions of linearity, homoscedasticity and normality of the residuals were verified and the presence of influential points in each model was evaluated. All statistical work was carried out4 using R version 4.1.2.

5. Conclusions

SLE patients present higher skin AGEs levels than HC, supporting the hypothesis of the association between AGEs and SLE. Furthermore, the correlation observed between skin AGEs levels and SLE activity and damage markers indicate that AGEs seem to have a role as a new biomarker in this disease related to management and prognosis, which would have enormous implications in a field currently uncovered in SLE. The association with specific antibodies and disease manifestations may indicate a particular clinical phenotype related to higher AGEs levels, unveiling another potential clinical use of these products.

Supplementary Materials: The supporting information can be downloaded at: https://www.mdpi.com/article/10.3390/ijms25053022/s1.

Author Contributions: Conceptualization, L.T. (Laura Tío), C.P.-G., J.M. and T.C.S.-M.; Methodology, L.T. (Laura Triginer); Formal analysis, L.T. (Laura Triginer); Investigation, I.C.-B., L.T. (Laura Triginer), C.P.-G. and A.R.; Resources, I.C.-B., C.P.-G., V.A., A.P., M.B.-L., E.C.-B., A.L., J.M.V., ILERVAS Project Group and T.C.S.-M.; Data curation, L.T. (Laura Triginer); Writing—original draft, I.C.-B.; Writing—review & editing, L.T. (Laura Triginer), L.T. (Laura Tío), C.P.-G., J.M. and T.C.S.-M.; Supervision, L.T. (Laura Tío), J.M. and T.C.S.-M.; Project administration, L.T. (Laura Tío); Funding acquisition, L.T. (Laura Tío), J.M. and T.C.S.-M. All authors have read and agreed to the published version of the manuscript.

Funding: This work was supported by the Instituto de Salud Carlos III (ISCIII) and the European Union (Grants number PI18/00059, PI23/00185, RETIC RD16/0009/0011), as well as by the Fundación Española de Reumatología through the Ayuda a la Intensificación de la Actividad Investigadora awarded in 2021, the Diputació de Lleida and Ministerio de Ciencia, Innovación y Universidades (IJC2018-037792-I) and the Societat Catalana de Reumatologia.

Institutional Review Board Statement: The protocol for our study was consistent with the provisions of the Declaration of Helsinki and was approved by the ethics committee of the Hospital del Mar (CEIm-PSMAR 2018/7907/I on 12 July 2018).

Informed Consent Statement: Informed consent was obtained from all subjects involved in the study.

Data Availability Statement: The data presented in this study are available on request from the corresponding author. The data are not publicly available due to ongoing research analysis.

Acknowledgments: We gratefully acknowledge all investigators who form part of the ILERVAS project. We would also like to thank the PhD program of the Universitat Autònoma de Barcelona, Isaac Alarcón Valero, Andrea Toloba and María Grau Magaña for their support throughout the research process. The authors would like to thank to Virtudes María, Marta Elias, Teresa Molí, Cristina Domínguez, Noemí Nova, Alba Prunera, Núria Sans, Meritxell soria, Francesc Pons, Rebeca Senar, Pau Guix, Fundació Renal Jaume Arnó, and the Primary Care teams of the province of Lleida for recruiting participants and their efforts in the accurate development of the ILERVAS project. Samples were obtained with support from IRBLleida Biobank (B.0000682) and Plataforma Biobancos PT17/0015/0027.

Conflicts of Interest: The authors declare that they have no competing interests.

Abbreviations

AGEs	Advanced glycation end-products
ANA	antinuclear antibodies
ANCOVA	analysis of covariance
BMI	body mass index
CVRF	cardiovascular risk factors
HC	healthy controls
LDL	low-density lipoproteins
PGA	physician global assessment
PROs	patient reported outcomes
PtGA	patient global assessment
RAGE	receptor for advanced glycation end-products
SDI	systemic lupus erythematosus damage index
SjS	Sjögren syndrome
SLE	systemic lupus erythematosus
SLEDAI	systemic lupus erythematosus disease activity index
SLICC	Systemic Lupus International Collaborating Clinics

Appendix A

Collaborating author names for the ILERVAS project group are:

Cristina Farràs [1], Ferrán Barbé [2], Reinald Pamplona [3], Dídac Mauricio [4,5,6], Elvira Fernández [7], Eva Miquel [1], Marta Ortega [1], Jessica González [2], Jordi de Batlle [2], Silvia Barril [2], Manuel Sánchez-de-la-Torre [2], Manuel Portero-Otín [6], Mariona Jové [6], Marta Hernández [4,8], Ferran Rius [4,8], Josep Franch-Nadal [4,5], Esmeralda Castelblanco [4,5], Pere Godoy [9], Montse Martinez-Alonso [10].

[1] Centre d'Atenció Primària Cappont. Gerència Territorial de Lleida, Institut Català de la Salut, Barcelona, Spain. Research Support Unit Lleida, Fundació Institut Universitari per a la recerca a l'Atenció Primària de Salut Jordi Gol i Gorina (IDIAPJGol), Barcelona, Spain.

[2] Departament de Medicina Respiratòria, Hospital Universitari Arnau de Vilanova, Grup Recerca Translational Medicina Respiratòria, IRBLleida, Universitat de Lleida, Lleida, CIBER de enfermedades respiratorias (CIBERES), Madrid, Spain.

[3] Departament de Medicina Experimental, IRBLleida, Universitat de Lleida, Lleida, Spain.

[4] Centro de Investigación Biomédica en Red de Diabetes y Enfermedades Metabólicas Asociadas (CIBERDEM), Instituto de Salud Carlos III (ISCIII), Madrid, Spain.

[5] Departament d'Endocrinologia i Nutrició, Hospital de la Santa Creu i Sant Pau, Institut de Recerca Biomèdica Sant Pau (IIB Sant Pau), Barcelona, Spain.

[6] Faculty of Medicine, University of Vic & Central University of Vic, Vic, Spain.

[7] Grupo de investigación Translacional vascular y Renal, IRBLleida, Red de Investigación Renal (RedInRen). ISCIII), Lleida, Spain.

[8] Departament d'Endocrinologia i Nutrició, Hospital Universitari Arnau de Vilanova, Grup de Recerca Obesitat i Metabolisme (ODIM), IRBLleida, Universitat de Lleida, Lleida, Spain.

[9] Agència de Salut Pública de Catalunya, Departament de Salut, IRBLleida, Universitat de Lleida, Lleida, Spain, CIBER de Epidemiología y Salud Pública (CIBERESP), Madrid, Spain.

[10] Unitat de Bioestadística, IRBLleida, Departament de ciències Mèdiques Bàsiques, Universitat de Lleida, Lleida, Spain.

References

1. Rabbani, N.; Thornalley, P.J. Advanced Glycation End Products in the Pathogenesis of Chronic Kidney Disease. *Kidney Int.* **2018**, *93*, 803–813. [CrossRef] [PubMed]
2. Kurien, B.T.; Hensley, K.; Bachmann, M.; Scofield, R.H. Oxidatively Modified Autoantigens in Autoimmune Diseases. *Free Radic. Biol. Med.* **2006**, *41*, 549–556. [CrossRef] [PubMed]

3. Pullerits, R.; Bokarewa, M.; Dahlberg, L.; Tarkowski, A. Decreased Levels of Soluble Receptor for Advanced Glycation End Products in Patients with Rheumatoid Arthritis Indicating Deficient Inflammatory Control. *Arthritis Res. Ther.* **2005**, *7*, R817–R824. [CrossRef] [PubMed]
4. Hudson, B.I.; Lippman, M.E. Targeting RAGE Signaling in Inflammatory Disease. *Annu. Rev. Med.* **2018**, *69*, 349–364. [CrossRef]
5. Sárkány, Z.; Ikonen, T.P.; Ferreira-da-Silva, F.; Saraiva, M.J.; Svergun, D.; Damas, A.M. Solution Structure of the Soluble Receptor for Advanced Glycation End Products (SRAGE). *J. Biol. Chem.* **2011**, *286*, 37525–37534. [CrossRef]
6. Geroldi, D.; Falcone, C.; Emanuele, E. Soluble Receptor for Advanced Glycation End Products: From Disease Marker to Potential Therapeutic Target. *Curr. Med. Chem.* **2006**, *13*, 1971–1978. [CrossRef] [PubMed]
7. Nienhuis, H.L.; De Leeuw, K.; Bijzet, J.; Smit, A.; Schalkwijk, C.G.; Graaff, R.; Kallenberg, C.G.; Bijl, M. Skin Autofluorescence Is Increased in Systemic Lupus Erythematosus but Is Not Reflected by Elevated Plasma Levels of Advanced Glycation Endproducts. *Rheumatology* **2008**, *47*, 1554–1558. [CrossRef]
8. Thorpe, S.R.; Baynes, J.W. Maillard Reaction Products in Tissue Proteins: New Products and New Perspectives. *Amino Acids* **2003**, *25*, 275–281. [CrossRef]
9. Coll, J.-C.; Turcotte, A.-F.; Garceau, É.; Michou, L.; Weisnagel, S.J.; Mac-Way, F.; Morin, S.N.; Rabasa-Lhoret, R.; Gagnon, C. Skin and Serum Advanced Glycation End Products in Adults With Type 1 Diabetes. *Can. J. Diabetes* **2022**, *46*, S25. [CrossRef]
10. Meerwaldt, R.; Graaf, R.; Oomen, P.H.N.; Links, T.P.; Jager, J.J.; Alderson, N.L.; Thorpe, S.R.; Baynes, J.W.; Gans, R.O.B.; Smit, A.J. Simple Non-Invasive Assessment of Advanced Glycation Endproduct Accumulation. *Diabetologia* **2004**, *47*, 1324–1330. [CrossRef]
11. Nowak, A.; Przywara-Chowaniec, B.; Damasiewicz-Bodzek, A.; Blachut, D.; Nowalany-Kozielska, E.; Tyrpień-Golder, K. Advanced Glycation End-Products (Ages) and Their Soluble Receptor (Srage) in Women Suffering from Systemic Lupus Erythematosus (Sle). *Cells* **2021**, *10*, 3523. [CrossRef] [PubMed]
12. Ene, C.D.; Georgescu, S.R.; Tampa, M.; Matei, C.; Mitran, C.I.; Mitran, M.I.; Penescu, M.N.; Nicolae, I. Cellular Response against Oxidative Stress, a Novel Insight into Lupus Nephritis Pathogenesis. *J. Pers. Med.* **2021**, *11*, 693. [CrossRef] [PubMed]
13. Chen, D.Y.; Chen, Y.M.; Lin, C.C.; Hsieh, C.W.; Wu, Y.C.; Hung, W.T.; Chen, H.H.; Lan, J.L. The Potential Role of Advanced Glycation End Products (AGEs) and Soluble Receptors for AGEs (SRAGE) in the Pathogenesis of Adult-Onset Still's Disease. *BMC Musculoskelet. Disord.* **2015**, *16*, 111. [CrossRef]
14. Nienhuis, H.L.A.; de Leeuw, K.; Bijzet, J.; van Doormaal, J.J.; van Roon, A.M.; Smit, A.J.; Graaff, R.; Kallenberg, C.G.M.; Bijl, M. Small Artery Elasticity Is Decreased in Patients with Systemic Lupus Erythematosus without Increased Intima Media Thickness. *Arthritis Res. Ther.* **2010**, *12*, R181. [CrossRef]
15. De Leeuw, K.; Graaff, R.; de Vries, R.; Dullaart, R.P.; Smit, A.J.; Kallenberg, C.G.; Bijl, M. Accumulation of Advanced Glycation Endproducts in Patients with Systemic Lupus Erythematosus. *Rheumatology* **2007**, *46*, 1551–1556. [CrossRef] [PubMed]
16. Quyyumi, A.A. Inflamed Joints and Stiff Arteries. *Circulation* **2006**, *114*, 1137–1139. [CrossRef]
17. Makita, Z.; Yanagisawa, K.; Kuwajima, S.; Bucala, R.; Vlassara, H.; Koike, T. The Role of Advanced Glycosylation End-Products in the Pathogenesis of Atherosclerosis. *Nephrol. Dial. Transplant.* **1996**, *11*, 31–33. [CrossRef]
18. Vekic, J.; Vujcic, S.; Bufan, B.; Bojanin, D.; Al-Hashmi, K.; Al-Rasadi, K.; Stoian, A.P.; Zeljkovic, A.; Rizzo, M. The Role of Advanced Glycation End Products on Dyslipidemia. *Metabolites* **2023**, *13*, 77. [CrossRef]
19. De Leeuw, K.; Freire, B.; Smit, A.J.; Bootsma, H.; Kallenberg, C.G.; Bijl, M. Traditional and Non-Traditional Risk Factors Contribute to the Development of Accelerated Atherosclerosis in Patients with Systemic Lupus Erythematosus. *Lupus* **2006**, *15*, 675–682. [CrossRef]
20. Peters, M.J.L.; Symmons, D.P.M.; McCarey, D.; Dijkmans, B.A.C.; Nicola, P.; Kvien, T.K.; McInnes, I.B.; Haentzschel, H.; Gonzalez-Gay, M.A.; Provan, S.; et al. EULAR Evidence-Based Recommendations for Cardiovascular Risk Management in Patients with Rheumatoid Arthritis and Other Forms of Inflammatory Arthritis. *Ann. Rheum. Dis.* **2010**, *69*, 325–331. [CrossRef]
21. Cotton, T.; Fritzler, M.J.; Choi, M.Y.; Zheng, B.; Niaki, O.Z.; Pineau, C.A.; Lukusa, L.; Bernatsky, S. Serologic Phenotypes Distinguish Systemic Lupus Erythematosus Patients Developing Interstitial Lung Disease and/or Myositis. *Lupus* **2022**, *31*, 1477–1484. [CrossRef]
22. Raj, D.S.; Choudhury, D.; Welbourne, T.C. Advanced Glycation End Products: A Nephrologist's Perspective. *Am. J. Kidney Dis.* **2000**, *35*, 365–380. [CrossRef]
23. Sourris, K.C.; Watson, A.; Jandeleit-Dahm, K. Inhibitors of Advanced Glycation End Product (AGE) Formation and Accumulation. *Handb. Exp. Pharmacol.* **2021**, *264*, 395–423. [CrossRef]
24. Goldberg, T.; Cai, W.; Peppa, M.; Dardaine, V.; Baliga, B.S.; Uribarri, J.; Vlassara, H. Advanced Glycoxidation End Products in Commonly Consumed Foods. *J. Am. Diet. Assoc.* **2004**, *104*, 1287–1291. [CrossRef] [PubMed]
25. Weinstein, A.; Alexander, R.V.; Zack, D.J. A Review of Complement Activation in SLE. *Curr. Rheumatol. Rep.* **2021**, *23*, 16. [CrossRef] [PubMed]
26. Gandino, I.J.; Scolnik, M.; Bertiller, E.; Scaglioni, V.; Catoggio, L.J.; Soriano, E.R. Complement Levels and Risk of Organ Involvement in Patients with Systemic Lupus Erythematosus. *Lupus Sci. Med.* **2017**, *4*, e000209. [CrossRef] [PubMed]
27. Li, H.; Lin, S.; Yang, S.; Chen, L.; Zheng, X. Diagnostic Value of Serum Complement C3 and C4 Levels in Chinese Patients with Systemic Lupus Erythematosus. *Clin. Rheumatol.* **2015**, *34*, 471–477. [CrossRef]
28. Lee, K.E.; Mun, S.; Kim, S.M.; Shin, W.; Jung, W.; Paek, J.; Lee, J.; Erin, H.; Welsey, H.L.; Han, K.; et al. The Inflammatory Signature in Monocytes of Sjögren's Syndrome and Systemic Lupus Erythematosus, Revealed by the Integrated Reactome and Drug Target Analysis. *Genes Genom.* **2022**, *44*, 1215–1229. [CrossRef]

29. Stewart, C.; Cha, S.; Caudle, R.M.; Berg, K.; Katz, J. Decreased Levels of Soluble Receptor for Advanced Glycation End Products in Patients with Primary Sjögren's Syndrome. *Rheumatol. Int.* **2008**, *28*, 771–776. [CrossRef]
30. Katz, J.; Stavropoulos, F.; Bhattacharyya, I.; Stewart, C.; Perez, F.M.; Caudle, R.M. Receptor of Advanced Glycation End Product (RAGE) Expression in the Minor Salivary Glands of Patients with Sjögren's Syndrome: A Preliminary Study. *Scand. J. Rheumatol.* **2004**, *33*, 174–178. [CrossRef]
31. Kanne, A.M.; Jülich, M.; Mahmutovic, A.; Tröster, I.; Sehnert, B.; Urbonaviciute, V.; Voll, R.E.; Kollert, F. Association of High Mobility Group Box Chromosomal Protein 1 and Receptor for Advanced Glycation End Products Serum Concentrations with Extraglandular Involvement and Disease Activity in Sjögren's Syndrome. *Arthritis Care Res.* **2018**, *70*, 944–948. [CrossRef] [PubMed]
32. Pisetsky, D.S.; Lipsky, P.E. New Insights into the Role of Antinuclear Antibodies in Systemic Lupus Erythematosus. *Nat. Rev. Rheumatol.* **2020**, *16*, 565–579. [CrossRef] [PubMed]
33. Hochberg, M.C. Updating the American College of Rheumatology Revised Criteria for the Classification of Systemic Lupus Erythematosus. *Arthritis Rheum.* **1997**, *40*, 1725. [CrossRef]
34. Petri, M.; Orbai, A.M.; Alarcón, G.S.; Gordon, C.; Merrill, J.T.; Fortin, P.R.; Bruce, I.N.; Isenberg, D.; Wallace, D.J.; Nived, O.; et al. Derivation and Validation of the Systemic Lupus International Collaborating Clinics Classification Criteria for Systemic Lupus Erythematosus. *Arthritis Rheum.* **2012**, *64*, 2677–2686. [CrossRef] [PubMed]
35. Available online: https://Elbusdelasalut.Cat/Professionals/Protocol-Estudi/ (accessed on 5 September 2023).
36. Shardlow, A.; McIntyre, N.J.; Kolhe, N.V.; Nellums, L.B.; Fluck, R.J.; McIntyre, C.W.; Taal, M.W. The Association of Skin Autofluorescence with Cardiovascular Events and All-Cause Mortality in Persons with Chronic Kidney Disease Stage 3: A Prospective Cohort Study. *PLoS Med.* **2020**, *17*, e1003163. [CrossRef]

Disclaimer/Publisher's Note: The statements, opinions and data contained in all publications are solely those of the individual author(s) and contributor(s) and not of MDPI and/or the editor(s). MDPI and/or the editor(s) disclaim responsibility for any injury to people or property resulting from any ideas, methods, instructions or products referred to in the content.

Article

Relationship between Disease Characteristics and Circulating Interleukin 6 in a Well-Characterized Cohort of Patients with Systemic Lupus Erythematosus

Julia Mercader-Salvans [1], María García-González [2], Fuensanta Gómez-Bernal [3], Juan C. Quevedo-Abeledo [4], Antonia de Vera-González [3], Alejandra González-Delgado [3], Raquel López-Mejías [5], Candelaria Martín-González [6,7], Miguel Á. González-Gay [8,9,*] and Iván Ferraz-Amaro [2,7,*]

1. Division of Dermatology, Hospital Universitario de Canarias, 38320 Tenerife, Spain; juliamercader96@gmail.com
2. Division of Rheumatology, Hospital Universitario de Canarias, 38320 Tenerife, Spain; margagon23@hotmail.com
3. Division of Central Laboratory, Hospital Universitario de Canarias, 38320 Tenerife, Spain; fuensanta95@gmail.com (F.G.-B.); adeverag@gmail.com (A.d.V.-G.); alejandra.gd88@gmail.com (A.G.-D.)
4. Division of Rheumatology, Hospital Doctor Negrín, 35010 Las Palmas de Gran Canaria, Spain; quevedojcarlos@yahoo.es
5. Epidemiology, Genetics and Atherosclerosis Research Group on Systemic Inflammatory Diseases, IDIVAL, 39011 Santander, Spain; rlopezmejias78@gmail.com
6. Division of Internal Medicine, Hospital Universitario de Canarias, 38320 Tenerife, Spain; mmartgon@ull.edu.es
7. Department of Internal Medicine, University of La Laguna (ULL), 38200 Tenerife, Spain
8. Division of Rheumatology, IIS-Fundación Jiménez Díaz, 28040 Madrid, Spain
9. Department of Medicine, University of Cantabria, 39005 Santander, Spain
* Correspondence: miguelaggay@hotmail.com (M.Á.G.-G.); iferrazamaro@hotmail.com (I.F.-A.)

Abstract: Interleukin-6 (IL-6) is a proinflammatory cytokine that mediates pleiotropic functions in immune responses and inflammatory diseases. The literature lacks studies, with a clinical perspective, on the relationship between IL-6 serum levels and the characteristics of the disease in patients with systemic lupus erythematosus (SLE). In the present work, we aimed to analyze the association between circulating IL-6 and disease manifestations in a well-characterized series of patients with SLE. Serum IL-6 levels and disease activity (SLEDAI-2K), severity (Katz) and damage index (SLICC-DI), complete lipid profile, and subclinical carotid atherosclerosis were evaluated in 284 patients with SLE. In addition, a complete characterization of the complement system was performed in samples from patients with SLE. A multivariate linear regression analysis was carried out to study the relationship between clinical and laboratory characteristics of the disease and IL-6 levels. Age (beta coef. 0.07 [95%CI 0.01–0.1] pg/mL, $p = 0.014$), C-reactive protein (beta coef. 0.21 [95%CI 0.16–0.25] pg/mL, $p < 0.01$), and male gender (beta coef. 2 [95%CI 0.3–0.5] pg/mL, $p = 0.024$), were positively associated with higher IL-6 levels in SLE patients. Most disease characteristics and damage and activity indices did not show significant relationships with IL-6. However, after multivariate analysis, IL-6 was associated with lower serum levels of HDL cholesterol (beta coef. -0.04 [95%CI -0.08–(-0.1)] pg/mL, $p = 0.011$), and apolipoprotein A1 (beta coef. -0.02 [95%CI -0.04–(-0.001)] pg/mL, $p = 0.035$). In contrast, the alternative complement cascade, C1inh, and C3a were all positively and independently associated with higher serum levels of IL-6. Moreover, stratification of the Systematic Coronary Risk Assessment 2 (SCORE2) results according to different categories of cardiovascular risk was associated with higher circulating serum IL-6 levels (beta coef. 0.2 [95%CI 0.02–0.4], pg/mL, $p = 0.028$). In conclusion, in a large series of SLE patients, IL-6 was not associated with disease-related features of SLE, including damage, severity, or activity indices. However, an association was found between serum IL-6 levels and circulating C3a and cardiovascular risk. Our study emphasizes the importance that IL-6 could have in cardiovascular disease and complement system disruption of SLE patients. Therapies targeting IL-6 could have a role in these two clinical manifestations of patients with SLE.

Keywords: interleukin-6; systemic lupus erythematosus; disease damage; complement system; SCORE2

1. Introduction

Systemic lupus erythematosus (SLE) is a chronic autoimmune disease characterized by various manifestations, frequent flare-ups, and the involvement of multiple organs. Patients display a wide range of clinical symptoms, ranging from mild joint and skin problems to severe complications involving the kidneys, blood, and central nervous system [1,2]. The etiology of SLE remains unknown but is clearly multifactorial, with many observations suggesting a role for genetic [3], hormonal [4], immunologic [5,6], and environmental factors [7]. Furthermore, SLE is primarily a disease with abnormalities in immune regulation, including the formation of autoantibodies and immune complexes [8]. Phagocytosis and clearance of immune complexes, apoptotic cells, and necrotic cell-derived material are defective in SLE, allowing the persistence of antigens and immune complexes. This leads to abnormal cell persistence, autophagy, and cytokine production [9]. Furthermore, accelerated atherosclerosis and increased risk of cardiovascular disease have been identified as major causes of morbidity and mortality in patients with SLE [10].

Interleukin-6 (IL-6) is a proinflammatory cytokine that plays a crucial role in various immunological processes associated with host infection, inflammatory disorders, hematopoiesis, and oncogenesis. IL-6 functions as a regulator of the immune response, influencing the proliferation and differentiation of T cells, as well as the final maturation of B cells [11]. Additionally, IL-6 activates macrophages and osteoclasts and is considered a key stimulator of acute phase reactants [12]. Working in conjunction with tumor necrosis factor-alpha and IL-1, IL-6 promotes the production of vascular endothelial growth factor and metalloproteinases. In addition, IL-6, together with transforming growth factor beta, also plays a key role in the generation of subsets of peripherally induced CD4+ and CD8+ cytokine-producing suppressor cells [13]. Furthermore, the role of IL-6 in autoimmunity has been suggested [14]. This has been attributed to the idea that the immune system tightly regulates Th17/Treg cell homeostasis through the IL-6 axis, and the disturbance of this balance causes autoimmunity [15]. However, the role of IL-6 in the pathogenesis of SLE is not fully understood.

The literature lacks studies with a large number of SLE patients in which the relationship between a complete characterization of disease features and serum levels of IL-6 has been studied. In the present work, we studied a considerable and well-characterized series of patients with SLE. In addition to the comprehensive evaluation of clinical and laboratory features, including lipid profile and assessment of insulin resistance, we also analyzed all three complement pathways. In addition, we estimated the cardiovascular risk using the Systematic Coronary Risk Assessment 2 (SCORE2) algorithm and carotid ultrasound to determine subclinical atherosclerosis. After this, we set out to study the relationship between all these characteristics and the serum levels of IL-6. If the expression of IL-6 was found to be associated with specific disease features, then the potential use of therapies targeting this interleukin in SLE could be suggested.

2. Results

2.1. Demographics and Disease-Related Data on Systemic Lupus Erythematosus Patients

The median (IQR) serum level of IL-6 in SLE patients was 3.5 (IQR 2.3–5.4) pg/mL. Table 1 provides an overview of the characteristics of the 284 patients included in this study. Most of the participants were women (92%), with a mean age $\pm$ SD of 50 $\pm$ 12 years. The average body mass index was 28 $\pm$ 6 kg/m^2, and the abdominal circumference was 92 $\pm$ 14 cm. Classic cardiovascular risk factors included current smoking in 24% of patients, hypertension in 39%, and obesity in 30%. Additionally, 25% of the patients were taking statins and 29% were taking aspirin (Table 1).

Table 1. Characteristics of patients with SLE included in this study.

	SLE Patients (n = 284)
Interleukin-6, pg/mL	3.5 (2.3–5.4)
Age, years	50 ± 12
Female, n (%)	261 (92)
Body mass index, kg/m^2	28 ± 6
Abdominal circumference, cm	93 ± 14
Hip circumference, cm	103 ± 12
Waist-to-hip ratio	0.90 ± 0.07
Systolic pressure, mmHg	127 ± 20
Diastolic pressure, mmHg	79 ± 11
Cardiovascular co-morbidity	
Smoking, n (%)	69 (24)
Diabetes, n (%)	18 (6)
Hypertension, n (%)	111 (39)
Obesity, n (%)	85 (30)
Statins, n (%)	72 (25)
Aspirin, n (%)	80 (29)
SLE related data	
Disease duration, years	16 (7–24)
CRP, mg/dl	2.0 (0.8–4.4)
SLICC-DI	1 (0–2)
SLICC-DI $\geq$ 1, n (%)	191 (68)
Katz Index	2 (1–4)
Katz $\geq$ 3, n (%)	126 (44)
SLEDAI-2K	2 (0–4)
SLEDAI-2k categories, n (%)	
No activity, n (%)	109 (40)
Mild, n (%)	107 (39)
Moderate, n (%)	41 (15)
High, n (%)	10 (4)
Very High, n (%)	4 (1)
Auto-antibody profile	
Anti-DNA positive, n (%)	151 (67)
Anti-ENA positive, n (%)	164 (69)
Anti-SSA, n (%)	55 (35)
Anti-SSB, n (%)	36 (21)
Anti-RNP, n (%)	64 (28)
Anti-Sm, n (%)	24 (10)
Anti-ribosome	13 (9)
Anti-nucleosome	32 (22)
Anti-histone	22 (15)
Antiphospholipid syndrome, n (%)	43 (16)
Antiphospholipid autoantibodies, n (%)	61 (32)
Lupus anticoagulant, n (%)	51 (28)
ACA IgM, n (%)	22 (11)
ACA IgG, n (%)	39 (20)
Anti beta2 glycoprotein IgM, n (%)	19 (10)
Anti beta2 glycoprotein IgG, n (%)	28 (15)
Current prednisone, n (%)	140 (50)
Prednisone, mg/day	5 (5–7.5)
Hydroxychloroquine, n (%)	194 (69)
Methotrexate, n (%)	31 (11)

Table 1. Cont.

	SLE Patients (n = 284)
Mycophenolate mofetil, n (%)	31 (11)
Azathioprine, n (%)	43 (15)
Rituximab, n (%)	8 (3)
Belimumab, n (%)	8 (3)

Data represent mean ± SD or median (interquartile range) when the data were not normally distributed. BMI: body mass index; C3 C4: complement; CRP: C reactive protein; LDL: low-density lipoprotein. DMARD: disease-modifying antirheumatic drug; ACA: anticardiolipin. HDL: high-density lipoprotein; ANA: antinuclear antibodies; Anti-ENA: extractable nuclear antibodies. SLEDAI: Systemic Lupus Erythematosus Disease Activity Index. SLEDAI categories were defined as 0, no activity; 1–5 mild; 6–10 moderate; >10 high; >20 very high activity. SLICC: Systemic Lupus International Collaborating Clinics/American College of Rheumatology Damage Index. IL-6: interleukin-6.

The median disease duration was 16 (IQR 7–24) years. The majority of SLE patients had no activity (40%) or mild to moderate activity (39%), as indicated by the SLEDAI-2K score. The SLICC-SDI and Katz indices were 1 (IQR 0–2) and 2 (IQR 1–4), respectively. A SLICC-SDI score of 1 or higher was found in 68% of the patients. Half of the patients (50%) were taking prednisone, with a median daily dose of 5 mg/day (IQR 5–7.5). At the time of recruitment, 67% of patients tested positive for anti-DNA antibodies, and 69% tested positive for anti-ENA antibodies, where anti-SSA was the most detected antibody (35%). Hydroxychloroquine was being used by 69% of the patients at the time of this study. Other less frequently used disease-modifying antirheumatic drugs included methotrexate (11%) and azathioprine (15%). Additional data on SLE-related information can be found in Table 1.

2.2. Demographic and Disease Characteristics in Relation to Serum IL-6 Levels

In the univariate analysis, age, waist-hip ratio, and serum CRP levels had a positive and significant relationship with IL-6. Furthermore, the female gender was associated with significantly lower circulating levels of IL-6 compared with male patients (beta coef. −2 [95%CI −5–(−0.03)] pg/mL, p = 0.024) (Table 2). Regarding disease-related data, the presence of lupus anticoagulant was the only disease feature that showed a significant association with IL-6 (beta coef. 2 [95%CI 0.3–3] pg/mL, p = 0.016). In contrast, the autoantibody profile, the use of various therapies, and the SLICC-DI, SLEDAI-2K, and Katz indices did not reveal any association with serum IL-6 levels.

Table 2. Relationship between demographics and disease characteristics with IL-6 serum levels.

	IL-6 pg/mL Beta Coef. (95%), p	
Age, years	0.07 (0.01–0.1)	0.014
Female	−2 (−5–(−0.03))	0.024
Body mass index, kg/m^2	0.07 (−0.04–0.2)	0.20
Abdominal circumference, cm	0.04 (−0.005–0.08)	0.078
Hip circumference, cm	0.02 (−0.03–0.08)	0.36
Waist-to-hip ratio	9 (0.04–17)	0.041
Systolic pressure, mmHg	0.03 (−0.004–0.06)	0.084
Diastolic pressure, mmHg	0.04 (−0.02–0.09)	0.19
Cardiovascular co-morbidity		
Smoking	0.5 (−0.9–2)	0.47
Diabetes	0.9 (−2–3)	0.47
Hypertension	0.8 (−0.4–2)	0.19
Obesity	0.1 (−1–1)	0.86
Statins	0.8 (−0.6–2)	0.26
Aspirin	0.6 (−0.7–2)	0.37
SLE-related data		

Table 2. Cont.

	IL-6 pg/mL Beta Coef. (95%), p	
Disease duration, years	0.06 (−0.004–0.1)	0.065
CRP, mg/dl	**0.2 (0.2–0.3)**	**<0.001**
SLICC-DI	0.2 (−0.2–0.5)	0.35
SLICC-DI ≥ 1, n (%)	1 (−0.3–2)	0.12
Katz Index	−0.2 (−0.5–0.2)	0.33
Katz ≥ 3	−0.6 (−2–0.6)	0.34
SLEDAI-2K	−0.01 (−0.2–0.1)	0.87
SLEDAI-2k categories		
No activity	-	-
Mild	−0.2 (−2–1)	0.83
Moderate to very high	−0.5 (−2–1)	0.60
Auto-antibody profile		
Anti-DNA positive	0.2 (−1–2)	0.75
Anti-ENA positive	0.3 (−1–2)	0.73
Anti-SSA	1 (−0.8–3)	0.23
Anti-SSB	0.6 (−3–5)	0.78
Anti-RNP	−0.6 (−2–0.9)	0.43
Anti-Sm	1 (−1–3)	0.42
Anti-ribosome	−0.6 (−4–3)	0.73
Anti-nucleosome	0.7 (−2–3)	0.56
Anti-histone	−0.7 (−3–2)	0.62
Antiphospholipid syndrome	−1 (−3–0.5)	0.17
Antiphospholipid autoantibodies		
Lupus anticoagulant	**2 (0.3–3)**	**0.016**
ACA IgM	2 (−1–4)	0.23
ACA IgG	−1 (−3–0.6)	0.18
Anti beta2 glycoprotein IgM	0.5 (−2–3)	0.71
Anti beta2 glycoprotein IgG	0.5 (−2–3)	0.65
Current prednisone	0.6 (−0.6–2)	0.32
Prednisone, mg/day	−0.05 (−0.3–0.2)	0.74
Hydroxychloroquine	−0.4 (−2–0.9)	0.56
Methotrexate	1 (−0.8–3)	0.26
Mycophenolate mofetil	−0.5 (−3–1)	0.60
Azathioprine	−0.8 (−3–1)	0.37
Rituximab	−1 (−4–4)	0.94
Belimumab	−2 (−6–2)	0.35

In this analysis, IL-6 was considered the dependent variable. ANA: antinuclear antibodies; Anti-ENA: extractable nuclear antibodies, ACA: anticardiolipin. SLEDAI-2k: Systemic Lupus Erythematosus Disease Activity Index. SLEDAI-2k categories were defined as 0, no activity; 1–5 mild; 6–10 moderate; >10 high activity, >20 very high activity. SLICC-DI: Systemic Lupus International Collaborating Clinics/American College of Rheumatology Damage Index. Significant p-values are depicted in bold.

Since the activity score and the damage and disease severity indices are a sum of different aspects of SLE, we analyzed the relationship between each item of these scores and IL-6 (Table 3). Regarding the Katz index, no associations were found between the items of this score and IL-6.

Table 3. Relationship between individual disease score items and serum IL-6 levels.

	n	%	IL-6, pg/mL Beta Coef. (95%)	p
Katz index				
History of cerebritis (seizure or organic brain syndrome)	12	6	−0.2 (−2–1)	0.77
History of pulmonary disease	10	5	0.4 (−1–2)	0.64
Biopsy proven diffuse proliferative glomerulonephritis	23	12	−1 (−2–0.1)	0.080
Four to six ARA criteria for SLE satisfied to date	139	73	0.3 (−1–2)	0.76
Seven or more ARA criteria for SLE satisfied to date	23	12	−0.88 (−2–0.4)	0.18
History of proteinuria (two or more)	62	32	−0.1 (−2–1)	0.87
Lowest recorded hematocrit to date = 30–37%	88	46	−0.1 (−2–1)	0.87
Lowest recorded hematocrit to date < 30%	47	25	−0.7 (−2–0.2)	0.12
Highest recorded creatinine to date = 1.3–3	28	15	0.7 (−1–3)	0.52
Highest recorded creatinine to date > 3	3	2	−1 (−5–2)	0.46
SLEDAI				
Seizures	1	0	1 (−9–11)	0.84
Psychosis	1	0	8 (−2–17)	0.12
Organic brain syndrome	0	0	-	
Visual disturbance	1	0	0.05 (−10–10)	0.99
Cranial nerve disorder	1	0	−3 (−12–7)	0.58
Lupus headache	1	0	-	
ACVA	0	0	-	
Vasculitis	1	0	6 (−4–15)	0.24
Arthritis	9	3	−2 (−5–2)	0.37
Myositis	0	0	-	
Urinary cylinders	7	3	3 (−1–8)	0.13
Hematuria	16	6	2 (−1–5)	0.23
Proteinuria	5	2	−2 (−7–4)	0.54
Pyuria	11	4	**4 (0.8–8)**	**0.017**
Rash	21	8	0.9 (−1–3)	0.46
Alopecia	11	4	−2 (−6–1)	0.18
Mucosal ulcers	14	5	−1 (−4–2)	0.37
Pleurisy	3	1	−2 (−11–8)	0.74
Pericarditis	1	0	−1 (−11–9)	0.84
Low complement	76	28	−0.6 (−2–0.8)	0.38
Elevated antiDNA	85	31	−0.6 (−2–0.7)	0.36
Fever	2	1	−0.2 (−7–7)	0.96
Thrombopenia	10	4	−1 (−4–2)	0.52
Leukopenia	19	7	−0.7 (−3–2)	0.58
SLICC domains				
Ocular	63	22	0.6 (−0.8–2)	0.40
Neuropsychiatric	40	14	−0.4 (−2–1)	0.69
Renal	28	10	−1 (−3–1)	0.30
Pulmonary	19	7	0.2 (−2–3)	0.86
Cardiovascular	23	8	1 (−1–3)	0.36
Peripheral vascular	34	12	−0.04 (−2–2)	0.97
Gastrointestinal	28	10	0.2 (−2–2)	0.85
Musculoskeletal	89	31	0.2 (−1–2)	0.81
Skin	39	14	1 (−0.3–3)	0.095
Premature gonadal failure	19	7	−0.2 (−3–2)	0.89
Diabetes (regardless of treatment)	18	6	0.9 (−1–3)	0.45
Malignancy (excluded dysplasia)	11	4	−0.5 (−3–2)	0.73

In this analysis, IL-6 was considered the dependent variable. Significant p-values are depicted in bold. History of pulmonary disease refers to the presence of lupus pneumonitis, pulmonary hemorrhage, or pulmonary hypertension. ARA: American Rheumatism Association; ACVA: acute cerebrovascular accident. SLEDAI: Systemic Lupus Erythematosus Disease Activity Index; SLE: systemic lupus erythematosus. SLICC: Systemic Lupus International Collaborating Clinics/American College of Rheumatology Damage Index. The presence of a SLICC domain involvement was shown if points in the domain were ≥1. See Table A1.

Similarly, SLEDAI-2K score items were generally not related to circulating IL-6. In this regard, only the presence of pyuria, which was present in 11 patients (4%), was the item that showed a significant relationship with higher levels of circulating IL-6. With respect to SLICC-SDI areas, only the cataract (n = 29, 11%), pleural fibrosis (n = 1, 0%), and skin ulceration (n = 4, 1%) items were significantly related to higher values of serum IL-6 (Tables 3 and A1).

2.3. Multivariate Analysis of the Relationship between Cardiovascular-Related Factors and IL-6

Values for lipid-related molecules, insulin resistance indices, cIMT, the presence of carotid plaque, and the SCORE2 in SLE patients are shown in Table 4.

Table 4. Association between factors related to the cardiovascular system and IL-6 in patients with SLE.

		IL-6 pg/mL			
		Beta Coef. (95%), p			
		Univariate		Multivariate	
Lipid profile					
Cholesterol, mg/dL	198 ± 36	−0.02 (−0.04−(−0.003))	0.024	−0.02 (−0.04−(−0.002))	0.026
Triglycerides, mg/dL	130 ± 78	0.007 (−0.002−0.02)	0.12	0.005 (−0.004−0.01)	0.32
LDL cholesterol, mg/dL	111 ± 29	−0.02 (−0.04−0.0008)	0.059	−0.02 (−0.04−0.003)	0.097
HDL cholesterol, mg/dL	61 ± 19	−0.05 (−0.08−(−0.01))	0.008	−0.04 (−0.08−(−0.01))	0.011
LDL:HDL cholesterol ratio	1.96 ± 0.75	0.4 (−0.5−1)	0.40		
Non-HDL cholesterol, mg/dL	137 ± 33	−0.01 (−0.03−0.009)	0.32		
Lipoprotein (a), mg/dL	39 (12–108)	0.005 (−0.002−0.01)	0.16	0.004 (−0.003−0.01)	0.25
Apolipoprotein A1, mg/dL	173 ± 35	−0.02 (−0.04−(−0.0008))	0.040	−0.02 (−0.04−(−0.001))	0.035
Apolipoprotein B, mg/dL	95 ± 23	−0.001 (−0.03−0.03)	0.92		
ApoB:Apo A ratio	0.57 ± 0.17	2 (−1−6)	0.19	3 (−1−6)	0.16
Atherogenic index	3.5 ± 1.1	0.4 (−0.1−1)	0.14	0.4 (−0.2−1)	0.21
Insulin resistance indices *					
Glucose, mg/dL	91 ± 9	0.02 (−0.05−0.08)	0.65		
Insulin, µU/mL	6.6 (4.4–9.8)	0.07 (−0.006−0.1)	0.073	0.05 (−0.02−0.1)	0.16
C-peptide, ng/mL	2.2 (1.5–3.3)	0.1 (−0.08−0.3)	0.22		
HOMA2-IR	0.86 (0.59–1.127)	0.5 (−0.04−1)	0.066	0.4 (−0.1−1)	0.14
HOMA2-S%	116 (79–172)	−0.005 (−0.01−0.0008)	0.091	−0.004 (−0.01−0.002)	0.16
HOMA2-B%-C-peptide	156 ± 89	0.006 (−0.0008−0.01)	0.085	0.004 (−0.003−0.01)	0.28
Carotid ultrasound					
cIMT, mm	0.628 ± 0.109	**6 (0.4–11)**	**0.035**	4 (−3−10)	0.26
Carotid plaque	99 (36)	**1 (0.05–3)**	**0.041**	1 (−0.4−2)	0.15
SCORE2 calculator					
SCORE 2	2.1 (0.9–3.9)	**0.2 (0.02–0.4)**	**0.028**		
SCORE2 categories, n (%)					
Low to moderate	224 (79)	ref.			
High	50 (18)	1 (−0.5−3)	0.17		
Very high	18 (4)	−0.7 (−4−3)	0.68		

In this analysis, IL-6 was considered the dependent variable. IL-6: interleukin-6. Significant p-values are depicted in bold. LDL: low-density lipoprotein, HDL: high-density lipoprotein, cIMT: carotid intima thickness. HOMA: homeostatic model assessment, SCORE: Systematic Coronary Risk Assessment. * In this analysis, the relationship between insulin resistance indices and IL-6 was only performed in non-diabetes patients and glucose < 110 mg/dL (n = 221). Multivariate analysis was adjusted for age, gender, abdominal circumference, and hypertension. The relationship between SCORE2 and IL-6 was not adjusted for covariables because this score was calculated using several composite variables.

Regarding lipid profile molecules, after the multivariate analysis, serum levels of total and HDL cholesterol (beta coef. −0.04 [95%CI −0.08−(−0.1)] pg/mL, p = 0.011) and apolipoprotein A1 (beta coef. −0.02 [95%CI −0.04−(−0.001)] pg/mL, p = 0.035) were significantly associated with lower IL-6 values. The presence of carotid plaque and cIMT and the insulin resistance indices were unrelated to IL-6 after multivariate adjustment.

However, SCORE2 results, considered as a continuous variable, were associated with significantly higher serum IL-6 levels (beta coef. 0.2 [95%CI 0.02–0.4], pg/mL, $p = 0.028$) (Table 4).

2.4. Multivariate Analysis of the Relationship between the Pathways and Components of the Complement System and IL-6

A full characterization of the complement system using an assessment of serum values for C1q, C2, C3, C3a, factors H and D, and C1-inhibitor, as well as functional assays of the three classical, alternative, and lectin pathways is listed in Table 5. After multivariate analysis, the alternative complement cascade and C1inh and C3a were found to be positively and independently associated with higher serum levels of IL-6 (Table 5).

Table 5. Multivariate analysis of the relationship between the pathways and components of the complement system and IL-6.

		IL-6, pg/mL Beta Coef. (95%CI), p			
		Univariate		Multivariate	
Classical pathway					
Functional assay, %	91 ± 38	0.01 (−0.006–0.03)	0.21		
C1q, mg/dL	34 ± 11	−0.03 (−0.09–0.03)	0.32		
Lectin pathway					
Functional assay, %	10 (1–41)	−0.0005 (−0.02–0.01)	0.95		
Common elements of the classic and lectin pathways					
C2, mg/dL	2.5 ± 1.2	−0.01 (−0.5–0.5)	0.96		
C4, mg/dL	21 ± 12	0.03 (−0.02–0.08)	0.27		
C1 inhibitor, mg/dL	32 ± 9	**0.07 (0.003–0.1)**	**0.040**	**0.07 (−0.0004–0.1)**	**0.049**
Alternative pathway					
Functional assay, %	41 (12–79)	0.01 (−0.001–0.03)	0.071	**0.02 (0.0002–0.03)**	**0.047**
Factor D, ng/mL	2593 ± 1836	0.0002 (−0.0002–0.0006)	0.41		
Common elements of the three pathways					
C3, mg/dL	130 ± 40	0.01 (−0.005–0.03)	0.20		
C3a, mg/dL	39 ± 10	**0.1 (0.05–0.2)**	**<0.001**	**0.1 (0.05–0.2)**	**<0.001**
Factor H, ng/mL × 10^{-3}	389 (281–564)	−0.0003 (−0.001–0.0005)	0.46		

Complement routes and elements are considered the independent variable. Significant *p*-values are depicted in bold. The multivariate analysis was adjusted for age, gender, abdominal circumference, and hypertension.

3. Discussion

To date, our work represents the most comprehensive characterization of IL-6 serum levels in patients with SLE. According to our findings, IL-6 levels do not show a relationship with most of the characteristics directly related to the disease when this association is studied cross-sectionally. However, other characteristics such as the lipid profile and the SCORE2 cardiovascular risk algorithm did show a relationship with IL-6. Of note, the alternative pathway of the complement system and C3a were also positively related to IL-6.

A recent meta-analysis reviewed the relationship between serum IL-6 levels and disease activity in SLE [16], which included 17 previous studies on this topic. According to the meta-analysis, IL-6 levels were significantly higher in SLE than in healthy controls. Furthermore, it showed a significant positive correlation between IL-6 levels and disease activity scores. In contrast, in our largest fully characterized series, we did not observe a relationship between various disease scores, including activity, damage, or severity, and IL-6.

A possible explanation for our findings could tight disease control since most of our patients were in the mild or no disease activity categories when SLEDAI-2k was applied. The literature is scarce regarding the relationship between IL-6 and specific manifestations of the disease. In this sense, urinary IL-6 levels in 29 patients with active class IV lupus nephritis were significantly higher than in patients with other classes of lupus nephritis [17]. After treatment, urinary levels of IL-6 decreased significantly. Furthermore, IL-6 was shown to be increased in the cerebrospinal fluid of patients with lupus psychosis [18,19] and to have an inverse correlation with hemoglobin levels in 171 patients with SLE [20]. However, the number of patients recruited in these studies was less than in our series, and none of the studies performed multivariate adjustments.

Remarkably, IL-6 and CRP highly correlated in our study. Hepatocytes are responsible for producing significant amounts of CRP, primarily triggered by IL-6 [21]. Due to this, this association is expected to occur. However, it is believed that autoimmune diseases where the type I interferon gene signature predominates, such as SLE, deviate from the usual pattern where CRP levels typically correlate with the degree of inflammation [22]. Two old previous reports, with a small number of patients, described the lack of association of CRP and IL-6 in patients with SLE [23,24]. This was not the case of our study. Moreover, CRP has been linked with cardiovascular disease in general population [25]. For this reason, the fact that there is a relationship between IL-6 and cardiovascular disease in our work could be mediated by the interrelation between both IL-6 and CRP.

Emerging research has provided substantial evidence indicating that IL-6 expression exhibits varying degrees of elevation in cardio-cerebrovascular conditions, such as atherosclerosis, myocardial infarction, heart failure, and ischemic stroke [26]. This cytokine actively contributes to the onset and progression of cardiovascular disease, particularly in response to triggers like ischemia, hypoxia, oxidative stress, inflammation, and vascular occlusion. This was supported by two large meta-analyses that confirmed the crucial role played by a variant allele of the *IL6R* gene encoding the IL-6 receptor in the generation of inflammation and the associated risk of coronary heart disease [27,28]. Furthermore, the hypothesis that IL6 is a potential target in cardiovascular disease is being currently tested in the ZEUS trial, which is being conducted to determine if ziltivekimab (a human anti-IL-6 monoclonal antibody) reduces the risk of cardiovascular events in people with cardiovascular disease, chronic kidney disease, and inflammation. In our study, we found a positive relationship between the SCORE2 cardiovascular risk calculation algorithm and IL-6. In addition, after adjusting for covariates, IL-6 was associated with lower levels of HDL cholesterol and apolipoprotein A1. Therefore, we believe that in patients with SLE, IL-6 may retain the deleterious role in cardiovascular disease that has been shown in the general population.

Our study is the first in the literature to evaluate the relationship between a complete characterization of the complement system and serum IL-6 levels. In this regard, after multivariate adjustment, we observed a relationship between IL-6 and the complement particles C3a and C1inh and the alternative complement pathway. Cytokines, such as IL-6, are typically released in sites of inflammation and then travel via circulation to the liver, where they increase the hepatic synthesis of complement proteins. C1inh is a known regulator of the complement system. It prevents excessive complement activation on a target as well as in plasma. This function is performed by binding to each C1r and C1s subcomponent of the C1 complex. Furthermore, the complement system promotes the inflammatory response primarily through the liberation of C3a anaphylatoxin. The positive association described in our work between IL-6 and these two complement elements matches with the pro-inflammatory role of IL-6 and its role in the stimulation of complement protein synthesis. The relationship with the alternative cascade, and not with the classic one, is notable. The alternative pathway is dominant over the classical pathway and the lectin pathway under normal physiological conditions. The continued activation of C3 by the alternative pathway is called "tick over", which generates low levels of C3a and is amplified if necessary [29]. It is possible that IL-6 could be more related to this production of complement and not to the activation/consumption that occurs in the disease.

4. Limitations

We acknowledge that we did not include healthy controls in our study. However, the comparison with controls was studied in previous work [13]. In addition, the design of our study was cross-sectional and, therefore, causality cannot be inferred from our results. Furthermore, because SLE is characterized by complexities in disease phases, flares, pathological states, treatment effects, etc., the cross-sectional design of our work did not allow us to identify how IL-6 varies during the disease progression.

5. Conclusions

In conclusion, IL-6 is not related to the damage, activity, or severity produced by SLE. However, certain abnormalities in complement system cascades are associated with IL-6. Furthermore, a positive relationship between cardiovascular risk and IL-6 exists. These findings are relevant since they could support the use of anti-IL-6 therapies for certain manifestations of the disease, such as complement system disruption, as well as the cardiovascular disease that frequently accompanies SLE.

6. Materials and Methods

6.1. Study Participants

Two hundred and eighty-four patients with SLE were assessed in a cross-sectional study. All patients were 18 years or older and met ≥ 4 American College of Rheumatology (ACR) classification criteria for SLE [30]. A diagnosis of SLE was performed by rheumatologists, and all the patients were regularly followed up in rheumatology outpatient clinics. Patients taking a prednisone dose equal to or lower than 10 mg/day were allowed to participate in this study since glucocorticoids are often used in the management of SLE. The research was conducted in accordance with the Declaration of Helsinki. The study protocol was approved by the Institutional Review Committee at Hospital Universitario de Canarias and at Hospital Universitario Doctor Negrín (both in Spain), and all patients provided informed written consent (Approval Number 2015_84).

6.2. Data Collection

The patients included in this study completed a questionnaire on cardiovascular risk factors and medication use and underwent a physical examination. Weight, height, body mass index, abdominal circumference, and systolic and diastolic blood pressure (measured with the participant in a supine position) were assessed under standardized conditions. Information regarding smoking status and hypertension treatment was obtained from the questionnaire. Medical records were reviewed to verify specific diagnoses and medications. SLE disease activity and damage were assessed using the Systemic Lupus Erythematosus Disease Activity Index—2000 (SLEDAI-2K) [31] and the Systemic Lupus International Collaborating Clinics/American College of Rheumatology (SLICC/ACR Damage Index -SDI-) [32], respectively. For the present study proposal, the SLEDAI-2k index was divided into none (0 points), mild (1–5 points), moderate (6–10 points), high (11–19), and very high activity (>20), as previously described [33]. The severity of the disease was measured using the Katz index [34]. In addition, carotid ultrasonography was performed to assess carotid intima-media wall thickness (cIMT) in the common carotid artery and to identify focal plaques in the extracranial carotid according to Mannheim consensus definitions [35]. In this study, HOMA2, the updated computer HOMA model, was utilized [36]. Also, the SCORE2 risk prediction algorithm, an updated model to estimate the 10-year risk of cardiovascular disease in Europe, was assessed in this cohort of patients [37]. Human IL-6 was measured using the electrochemiluminescence immunoassay method (Roche Diagnostics, Indianapolis, IN, USA).

6.3. Complement System Assessment

The SVAR functional complement assays under the Wieslab® brand (Sweden) were used to assess classical, alternative, and lectin pathways activity. These tests combine principles of the hemolytic assay for complement function with the use of labeled antibodies specific for the neoantigen produced as the result of C activation. The amount of neoantigen generated is proportional to the functional activity of C pathways. Microtiter strip wells are coated with classical, alternative, or lectin pathway-specific activators. The patient's serum is diluted in a diluent containing a specific blocker to ensure that only the studied pathway is activated. The specific coating activates C during the incubation of the diluted patient serum in the wells. The wells are then washed, and C5b-9 is detected with an alkaline phosphatase-labeled specific antibody against the neoantigen expressed during membrane attack complex (MAC) formation. After an additional washing step, the detection of specific antibodies is obtained using incubation with an alkaline phosphatase substrate solution. The amount of C activation correlates with the intensity of the color and is measured in terms of absorbance (optical density). The amount of formed MAC (neo-epitope) reflects the activity of the C cascade. The result is expressed semi-quantitatively using the optical density ratio between a positive control and the sample. The classical, alternative, and lectin cascade values should be interpreted as the lower the level, the greater the activation of the pathway. Wieslab® has validated these functional assays by studying their correlation and concordance with the classical CH50 and AH50 hemolytic tests (https://www.svarlifescience.com/ accessed on 15 April 2023). C2, C3, C3a, C4, and C1q were analyzed using turbidimetry (Roche), the C1-inhibitor was analyzed using nephelometry (Siemens), and factor D and factor H were assessed using an enzyme-linked immunosorbent assay (ELISA Duoset, R&D). Both the intra- and inter-coefficients of variability were <10% for these assays.

6.4. Statistical Analysis

Demographic and clinical characteristics in patients with SLE were described as mean ± standard deviation (SD) or percentages for categorical variables. For non-normally distributed continuous variables, data were expressed as the median and interquartile range (IQR). The relationship between disease characteristics and circulating IL-6 was evaluated using multivariate linear regression analysis. Univariate relations with a *p*-value less than 0.20 were adjusted for covariates. In the analysis of the association between the complement system, cardiovascular risk factors, and IL-6, confounders were selected from demographics if they had a relationship with both the independent and dependent variables and a *p*-value less than 0.20. All the analyses used a 5% two-sided significance level and were performed using Stata software, version 17/SE (StataCorp, College Station, TX, USA). p-values < 0.05 were considered statistically significant.

Author Contributions: Conception, design, and interpretation of the data: I.F.-A. and M.Á.G.-G.; acquisition of the data: J.M.-S., F.G.-B., M.G.-G., J.C.Q.-A., A.d.V.-G., A.G.-D., C.M.-G. and R.L.-M. All authors have agreed to be personally accountable for the author's own contributions and to ensure that questions related to the accuracy or integrity of any part of the work, even ones in which the author was not personally involved, are appropriately investigated, resolved, and the resolution documented in the literature. All authors have read and agreed to the published version of the manuscript.

Funding: This work was supported by a grant to I.F.-A. from the Spanish Ministry of Health, Instituto de Salud Carlos III (Fondo de Investigaciones Sanitarias, PI20/00084).

Institutional Review Board Statement: This research was carried out in accordance with the Declaration of Helsinki. The study protocol was approved by the Institutional Ethics Committees of the Hospital Universitario de Canarias and the Hospital Universitario Doctor Negrín (both in Spain), and all subjects provided informed written consent (approval number 2015_84).

Informed Consent Statement: Informed consent was obtained from all subjects involved in this study.

Data Availability Statement: The data sets used and/or analyzed in the present study are available from the corresponding author upon request.

Conflicts of Interest: The authors declare no conflict of interest. Nevertheless, Iván Ferraz-Amaro would like to acknowledge that he received grants/research support from Abbott, MSD, Jansen and Roche, as well as consultation fees from company-sponsored speakers' bureaus associated with Abbott, Pfizer, Roche, Sanofi, Celgene, and MSD. M.A. González-Gay has received grants/research support from AbbVie, MSD, Jansen, and Roche, as well as consultation.

Appendix A

Table A1. Relationship between SLICC score items and, IL-6.

	n	%	IL-6, pg/mL Beta Coef. (95%)	p
Ocular				
Any cataract ever	29	11	**2 (0.02–4)**	**0.048**
Retinal change or optic atrophy	33	12	−0.2 (−2–2)	0.84
Points ≥ 1 in the domain	63	22	0.6 (−0.8–2)	0.40
Neuropsychiatric				
Cognitive impairment	7	3	−0.6 (−5–3)	0.78
Seizures requiring therapy for 6 months	15	5	−1 (−4–2)	0.41
Cerebrovascular accident ever	13	5	−0.8 (−3–2)	0.57
Cranial or peripheral neuropathy	5	2	4 (−1–9)	0.12
Transverse myelitis	1	0	−1 (−11–9)	0.82
Points ≥ 1 in the domain	40	14	−0.4 (−2–1)	0.69
Renal				
Estimated or measured glomerular filtration rate < 50%	13	5	−0.7 (−4–3)	0.68
Proteinuria 3.5 gm/24 h	7	3	−2 (−7–3)	0.34
End-stage renal disease	4	1	−0.4 (−2–1)	0.67
Points ≥ 1 in the domain	28	10	−1 (−3–1)	0.30
Pulmonary				
Pulmonary hypertension	4	1	3 (−1–8)	0.21
Pulmonary fibrosis	4	1	−1 (−6–4)	0.70
Shrinking lung	2	1	−3 (−12–7)	0.61
Pleural fibrosis	1	0	**10 (0.9–20)**	**0.033**
Pulmonary infarction	1	0	−3 (−12–7)	0.57
Points ≥ 1 in the domain	19	7	0.2 (−2–3)	0.86
Cardiovascular				
Angina or coronary artery bypass	4	1	1 (−4–6)	0.60
Myocardial infarction ever	2	1	−0.2 (−7–7)	0.96
Cardiomyopathy	2	1	7 (−3–16)	0.17
Valvular disease	9	3	2 (−0.8–6)	0.14
Pericarditis for 6 months, or pericardiectomy	2	1	0.06 (−10–10)	0.99
Points ≥ 1 in the domain	23	8	1 (−1–3)	0.36
Peripheral vascular				
Claudication for 6 months	3	1	−0.2 (−6–5)	0.95
Minor tissue loss (pulp space)	5	2	−0.5 (−6–5)	0.85
Significant tissue loss ever	0	0	-	
Venous thrombosis	14	5	0.8 (−2–4)	0.55
Points ≥ 1 in the domain	34	12	−0.04 (−2–2)	0.97
Gastrointestinal				
Infarction or resection of bowel	22	8	0.5 (−2–3)	0.66
Mesenteric insufficiency	1	0	−3 (−13–6)	0.49
Infarction or resection of bowel below duodenum, spleen, liver, or chronic peritonitis	1	0	−3 (−13–7)	0.55
Stricture or upper gastrointestinal tract surgery ever	0	0	-	
Pancreatic insufficiency	0	0	-	
Points ≥ 1 in the domain	28	10	0.2 (−2–2)	0.85
Musculoskeletal				

Table A1. Cont.

	n	%	IL-6, pg/mL Beta Coef. (95%)	p
Muscle atrophy or weakness	3	1	−2 (−9–5)	0.60
Deforming or erosive arthritis	40	15	−0.5 (−2–1)	0.62
Osteoporosis with fracture or vertebral collapse	23	9	2 (−0.6–4)	0.14
Avascular necrosis	7	3	−0.5 (−5–4)	0.82
Osteomyelitis	1	0	0.06 (−10–10)	0.99
Tendon rupture	4	2	3 (−2–8)	0.19
Points ≥ 1 in the domain	89	31	0.2 (−1–2)	0.81
Skin				
Scarring chronic alopecia	16	6	0.7 (−2–3)	0.63
Extensive scarring or panniculum	10	4	−0.06 (−3–3)	0.97
Skin ulceration	4	1	**11 (6–16)**	**<0.001**
Points ≥ 1 in the domain	39	14	1 (−0.3–3)	0.095
Premature gonadal failure	19	7	−0.2 (−3–2)	0.89
Diabetes (regardless of treatment)	18	6	0.9 (−1–3)	0.45
Malignancy (exclude dysplasia)	11	4	−0.5 (−3–2)	0.73

SLICC items and domains represent the independent variable. SLICC: Systemic Lupus International Collaborating Clinics/American College of Rheumatology Damage Index. Significant *p*-values are depicted in bold.

References

1. Szeto, C.-C.; So, H.; Poon, P.Y.-K.; Luk, C.C.-W.; Ng, J.K.-C.; Fung, W.W.-S.; Chan, G.C.-K.; Chow, K.-M.; Lai, F.M.-M.; Tam, L.-S. Urinary Long Non-Coding RNA Levels as Biomarkers of Lupus Nephritis. *Int. J. Mol. Sci.* **2023**, *24*, 11813. [CrossRef]
2. Ruaro, B.; Casabella, A.; Paolino, S.; Alessandri, E.; Patané, M.; Gotelli, E.; Sulli, A.; Cutolo, M. Trabecular Bone Score and Bone Quality in Systemic Lupus Erythematosus Patients. *Front. Med.* **2020**, *7*, 574842. [CrossRef]
3. Boackle, S.A. Advances in lupus genetics. *Curr. Opin. Rheumatol.* **2013**, *25*, 561–568. [CrossRef]
4. McMurray, R.W.; May, W. Sex hormones and systemic lupus erythematosus: Review and meta-analysis. *Arthritis Rheum. Off. J. Am. Coll. Rheumatol.* **2003**, *48*, 2100–2110. [CrossRef]
5. Hahn, B.H.; Ebling, F.; Singh, R.R.; Singh, R.P.; Karpouzas, G.; La Cava, A. Cellular and molecular mechanisms of regulation of autoantibody production in lupus. *Ann. N. Y. Acad. Sci.* **2005**, *1051*, 433–441. [CrossRef] [PubMed]
6. Ahmad, A.; Brylid, A.; Dahle, C.; Saleh, M.; Dahlström, Ö.; Enocsson, H.; Sjöwall, C. Doubtful Clinical Value of Subtyping Anti-U1-RNP Antibodies Regarding the RNP-70 kDa Antigen in Sera of Patients with Systemic Lupus Erythematosus. *Int. J. Mol. Sci.* **2023**, *24*, 10398. [CrossRef]
7. Parks, C.G.; Santos, A.D.S.E.; Barbhaiya, M.; Costenbader, K.H. Understanding the role of environmental factors in the development of systemic lupus erythematosus. *Best Pract. Res. Clin. Rheumatol.* **2017**, *31*, 306–320. [CrossRef] [PubMed]
8. Arbuckle, M.R.; McClain, M.T.; Rubertone, M.V.; Scofield, R.H.; Dennis, G.J.; James, J.A.; Harley, J.B. Development of autoantibodies before the clinical onset of systemic lupus erythematosus. *N. Engl. J. Med.* **2003**, *349*, 1526–1533. [CrossRef] [PubMed]
9. Katsuyama, T.; Tsokos, G.C.; Moulton, V.R. Aberrant T Cell Signaling and Subsets in Systemic Lupus Erythematosus. *Front. Immunol.* **2018**, *9*, 1088. [CrossRef]
10. Restivo, V.; Candiloro, S.; Daidone, M.; Norrito, R.; Cataldi, M.; Minutolo, G.; Caracci, F.; Fasano, S.; Ciccia, F.; Casuccio, A.; et al. Systematic review and meta-analysis of cardiovascular risk in rheumatological disease: Symptomatic and non-symptomatic events in rheumatoid arthritis and systemic lupus erythematosus. *Autoimmun. Rev.* **2022**, *21*, 102925. [CrossRef]
11. Choy, E.H.; De Benedetti, F.; Takeuchi, T.; Hashizume, M.; John, M.R.; Kishimoto, T. Translating IL-6 biology into effective treatments. *Nat. Rev. Rheumatol.* **2020**, *16*, 335–345. [CrossRef] [PubMed]
12. Gauldie, J.; Richards, C.; Harnish, D.; Lansdorp, P.; Baumann, H. Interferon beta 2/B-cell stimulatory factor type 2 shares identity with monocyte-derived hepatocyte-stimulating factor and regulates the major acute phase protein response in liver cells. *Proc. Natl. Acad. Sci. USA* **1987**, *84*, 7251–7255. [CrossRef] [PubMed]
13. Okuda, Y. Review of tocilizumab in the treatment of rheumatoid arthritis. *Biologics* **2008**, *2*, 75–82. [CrossRef]
14. Hirano, T. IL-6 in inflammation, autoimmunity and cancer. *Int. Immunol.* **2021**, *33*, 127–148. [CrossRef]
15. Knochelmann, H.M.; Dwyer, C.J.; Bailey, S.R.; Amaya, S.M.; Elston, D.M.; Mazza-McCrann, J.M.; Paulos, C.M. When worlds collide: Th17 and Treg cells in cancer and autoimmunity. *Cell. Mol. Immunol.* **2018**, *15*, 458–469. [CrossRef]
16. Pattanaik, S.S.; Panda, A.K.; Pati, A.; Padhi, S.; Tripathy, R.; Tripathy, S.R.; Parida, M.K.; Das, B.K. Role of interleukin-6 and interferon-α in systemic lupus erythematosus: A case–control study and meta-analysis. *Lupus* **2022**, *31*, 1094–1103. [CrossRef]
17. Iwano, M.; Dohi, K.; Hirata, E.; Kurumatani, N.; Horii, Y.; Shiiki, H. Urinary levels of IL-6 in patients with active lupus nephritis. *Clin. Nephrol.* **1993**, *40*, 16–21.

18. Hirohata, S.; Kanai, Y.; Mitsuo, A.; Tokano, Y.; Hashimoto, H. Accuracy of cerebrospinal fluid IL-6 testing for diagnosis of lupus psychosis. A multicenter retrospective study. *Clin. Rheumatol.* **2009**, *28*, 1319–1323. [CrossRef]
19. Hirohata, S.; Kikuchi, H. Role of Serum IL-6 in Neuropsychiatric Systemic lupus Erythematosus. *ACR Open Rheumatol.* **2021**, *3*, 42–49. [CrossRef] [PubMed]
20. Ripley, B.J.M.; Goncalves, B.; Isenberg, D.A.; Latchman, D.S.; Rahman, A. Raised levels of interleukin 6 in systemic lupus erythematosus correlate with anaemia. *Ann. Rheum. Dis.* **2005**, *64*, 849–853. [CrossRef]
21. Black, S.; Kushner, I.; Samols, D. C-reactive Protein. *J. Biol. Chem.* **2004**, *279*, 48487–48490. [CrossRef] [PubMed]
22. Enocsson, H.; Karlsson, J.; Li, H.Y.; Wu, Y.; Kushner, I.; Wetterö, J.; Sjöwall, C. The Complex Role of C-Reactive Protein in Systemic Lupus Erythematosus. *J. Clin. Med.* **2021**, *10*, 5837. [CrossRef] [PubMed]
23. Meijer, C.; Huysen, V.; Smeenk, R.T.; Swaak, A.J. Profiles of cytokines (TNF alpha and IL-6) and acute phase proteins (CRP and alpha 1AG) related to the disease course in patients with systemic lupus erythematosus. *Lupus* **1993**, *2*, 359–365. [CrossRef] [PubMed]
24. Gabay, C.; Roux-Lombard, P.; De Moerloose, P.; Dayer, J.M.; Vischer, T.; Guerne, P.A. Absence of correlation between interleukin 6 and C-reactive protein blood levels in systemic lupus erythematosus compared with rheumatoid arthritis. *J. Rheumatol.* **1993**, *20*, 815–821. [PubMed]
25. C-Reactive Protein, Fibrinogen, and Cardiovascular Disease Prediction. *N. Engl. J. Med.* **2012**, *367*, 1310–1320. [CrossRef] [PubMed]
26. Su, J.H.; Luo, M.Y.; Liang, N.; Gong, S.X.; Chen, W.; Huang, W.Q.; Ying, T.; Wang, T. Interleukin-6: A Novel Target for Cardio-Cerebrovascular Diseases. *Front. Pharmacol.* **2021**, *12*, 745061. [CrossRef]
27. Swerdlow, D.I.; Holmes, M.V.; Kuchenbaecker, K.B.; Engmann, J.E.L.; Shah, T.; Sofat, R.; Guo, Y.; Chung, C.; Peasey, A.; Pfister, R.; et al. The interleukin-6 receptor as a target for prevention of coronary heart disease: A mendelian randomisation analysis. *Lancet* **2012**, *379*, 1214–1224.
28. Sarwar, N.; Butterworth, A.S.; Freitag, D.F.; Gregson, J.; Willeit, P.; Gorman, D.N.; Gao, P.; Saleheen, D.; Rendon, A.; Nelsom, C.P.; et al. Interleukin-6 receptor pathways in coronary heart disease: A collaborative meta-analysis of 82 studies. *Lancet* **2012**, *379*, 1205–1213.
29. García-González, M.; Gómez-Bernal, F.; Quevedo-Abeledo, J.C.; Fernández-Cladera, Y.; González-Rivero, A.F.; de Vera-González, A.; de la Rua-Figueroa, I.; López-Mejias, R.; Diaz-Gonzalez, F.; González-Gay, Á.M.; et al. Full characterization of the three pathways of the complement system in patients with systemic lupus erythematosus. *Front. Immunol.* **2023**, *14*, 1167055. [CrossRef]
30. Hochberg, M.C. Updating the American College of Rheumatology revised criteria for the classification of systemic lupus erythematosus. *Arthritis Rheum.* **1997**, *40*, 1725. [CrossRef]
31. Gladman, D.D.; Ibañez, D.; Urowltz, M.B. Systemic lupus erythematosus disease activity index 2000. *J. Rheumatol.* **2002**, *29*, 288–291. [PubMed]
32. Gladman, D.; Ginzler, E.; Goldsmith, C.; Fortin, P.; Liang, M.; Urowitz, M.; Bacon, P.; Bombardieri, S.; Hanly, J.; Isenberg, D.; et al. The development and initial validation of the Systemic Lupus International Collaborating Clinics/American College of Rheumatology damage index for systemic lupus erythematosus. *Arthritis Rheum. Off. J. Am. Coll. Rheumatol.* **1996**, *39*, 363–369. [CrossRef] [PubMed]
33. Mosca, M.; Bombardieri, S. Assessing remission in systemic lupus erythematosus. *Clin. Exp. Rheumatol.* **2006**, *24* (Suppl. 43), S99–S104.
34. Katz, J.D.; Senegal, J.L.; Rivest, C.; Goulet, J.R.; Rothfield, N. A Simple Severity of Disease Index for Systemic Lupus Erythematosus. *Lupus* **1993**, *2*, 119–123. [CrossRef]
35. Touboul, P.J.; Hennerici, M.G.; Meairs, S.; Adams, H.; Amarenco, P.; Bornstein, N.; Csiba, L.; Desvarieux, M.; Ebrahim, S.; Fatar, M.; et al. Mannheim carotid intima-media thickness consensus (2004–2006). An update on behalf of the Advisory Board of the 3rd and 4th Watching the Risk Symposium, 13th and 15th European Stroke Conferences, Mannheim, Germany, 2004, and Brussels, Belgium, 2006. *Cerebrovasc. Dis.* **2007**, *23*, 75–80. [CrossRef] [PubMed]
36. Wallace, T.M.; Levy, J.C.; Matthews, D.R. Use and abuse of HOMA modeling. *Diabetes Care* **2004**, *27*, 1487–1495. [CrossRef]
37. ESC Cardiovasc Risk Collaboration; SCORE2 Working Group. SCORE2 risk prediction algorithms: New models to estimate 10-year risk of cardiovascular disease in Europe. *Eur. Heart J.* **2021**, *42*, 2439–2454. [CrossRef]

Disclaimer/Publisher's Note: The statements, opinions and data contained in all publications are solely those of the individual author(s) and contributor(s) and not of MDPI and/or the editor(s). MDPI and/or the editor(s) disclaim responsibility for any injury to people or property resulting from any ideas, methods, instructions or products referred to in the content.

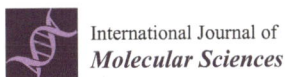

Article

Elevated Serum Levels of Soluble Transferrin Receptor Are Associated with an Increased Risk of Cardiovascular, Pulmonary, and Hematological Manifestations and a Decreased Risk of Neuropsychiatric Manifestations in Systemic Lupus Erythematosus Patients

Agnieszka Winikajtis-Burzyńska [1], Marek Brzosko [2] and Hanna Przepiera-Będzak [2,*]

[1] Individual Laboratory for Rheumatologic Diagnostics, Pomeranian Medical University in Szczecin, Unii Lubelskiej 1, 71-252 Szczecin, Poland; agawb@o2.pl
[2] Department of Rheumatology, Internal Medicine, Geriatrics and Clinical Immunology, Pomeranian Medical University in Szczecin, Unii Lubelskiej 1, 71-252 Szczecin, Poland; marek.brzosko@pum.edu.pl
* Correspondence: hanna.przepiera.bedzak@pum.edu.pl; Tel.: +48-91-4253321; Fax: +48-91-4253344

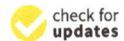

Citation: Winikajtis-Burzyńska, A.; Brzosko, M.; Przepiera-Będzak, H. Elevated Serum Levels of Soluble Transferrin Receptor Are Associated with an Increased Risk of Cardiovascular, Pulmonary, and Hematological Manifestations and a Decreased Risk of Neuropsychiatric Manifestations in Systemic Lupus Erythematosus Patients. *Int. J. Mol. Sci.* **2023**, *24*, 17340. https://doi.org/10.3390/ijms242417340

Academic Editor: Ludmilla A. Morozova-Roche

Received: 3 November 2023
Revised: 4 December 2023
Accepted: 8 December 2023
Published: 11 December 2023

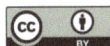

Copyright: © 2023 by the authors. Licensee MDPI, Basel, Switzerland. This article is an open access article distributed under the terms and conditions of the Creative Commons Attribution (CC BY) license (https:// creativecommons.org/licenses/by/ 4.0/).

Abstract: The aim of this study was to analyze the relationship between the serum levels of soluble transferrin receptor (sTfR) and interleukin 4 (IL-4), and the disease activity and organ manifestations in SLE patients. We studied 200 SLE patients and 50 controls. We analyzed disease activity, organ involvement, serum sTfR, IL-4 and interleukin-6 (IL-6) levels, and antinuclear and antiphospholipid antibody profiles. The median serum levels of sTfR ($p > 0.000001$) and IL-4 ($p < 0.00001$) were higher in the study group than in the controls. SLE patients, compared to the controls, had significantly lower HGB levels ($p < 0.0001$), a lower iron concentration ($p = 0.008$), a lower value of total iron-binding capacity (TIBC) ($p = 0.03$), and lower counts of RBC ($p = 0.004$), HCT ($p = 0.0004$), PLT ($p = 0.04$), neutrophil ($p = 0.04$), and lymphocyte ($p < 0.0001$). Serum sTfR levels were negatively correlated with lymphocyte ($p = 0.0005$), HGB ($p = 0.0001$) and HCT ($p = 0.008$), and positively correlated with IL-4 ($p = 0.01$). Elevated serum sTfR > 2.14 mg/dL was associated with an increased risk of myocardial infarction (OR: 10.6 95 CI 2.71–464.78; $p = 0.001$), ischemic heart disease (OR: 3.25 95 CI 1.02–10.40; $p = 0.04$), lung manifestations (OR: 4.48 95 CI 1.44–13.94; $p = 0.01$), and hematological manifestations (OR: 2.07 95 CI 1.13–3.79; $p = 0.01$), and with a reduced risk of neuropsychiatric manifestations (OR: 0.42 95 CI 0.22–0.80; $p = 0.008$). Serum IL-4 was negatively correlated with CRP ($p = 0.003$), and elevated serum IL-4 levels > 0.17 mg/L were associated with a reduced risk of mucocutaneous manifestations (OR: 0.48 95 CI 0.26–0.90; $p = 0.02$). In SLE patients, elevated serum levels of sTfR were associated with an increased risk of cardiovascular, pulmonary, and hematological manifestations, and with a decreased risk of neuropsychiatric manifestations. In contrast, elevated serum IL-4 levels were associated with a decreased risk of mucocutaneous manifestations.

Keywords: systemic lupus erythematosus; serum soluble transferrin receptor; interleukin 4; organ manifestations

1. Introduction

Systemic lupus erythematosus (SLE) is a chronic autoimmune disease. The clinical picture of the disease varies from a mild course to a life-threatening disease [1]. In the course of the disease, skin, mucosal, hematological, musculoskeletal, cardiovascular, neurological, gastrointestinal, pulmonary, and renal organ manifestations may develop. In addition, SLE patients have an increased risk of accelerated atherosclerosis and cardiovascular complications, the development of which may be influenced by both the disease itself and the treatment used [1,2].

Hematologic disorders associated with abnormal iron metabolism are common in SLE. A lack of normal regulation in iron homeostasis can cause anemia of chronic disease (ACD) or iron deficiency anemia (IDA) [3]. Anemia in the course of SLE occurs in approximately 50% of patients [3,4]. The incidence of anemia is influenced by many factors such as inflammation, renal failure, gastrointestinal complications, and hemolysis. Numerous studies in SLE patients have reported that the prevalence of ACD ranges from 30% to 80% [4,5]. In many SLE patients, the differentiation of ACD and IDA is difficult. The determination of soluble transferrin receptor (sTfR), which is the plasma-soluble form of the transferrin receptor and an indicator of tissue iron deficiency, is helpful in differentiating between ACD and IDA. Elevated sTfR concentrations are indicative of an existing iron body deficiency or IDA. In ACD, sTfR concentrations are unchanged [6].

The dysregulation of iron homeostasis has been associated with several diseases including cardiovascular, neurodegenerative, depression, epilepsy, and respiratory tract diseases [7–11].

Interleukin 4 (IL-4) is an anti-inflammatory cytokine with a broad spectrum of effects. IL-4 stimulates the proliferation and differentiation of B lymphocytes and Th2 lymphocytes, inactivates the differentiation of Th1 lymphocytes and regulatory T cells (Treg), affects the production of IgE and IgG4, and is involved in granulopoiesis and erythropoiesis [12,13]. The role of IL-4 in SLE patients is ambiguous [13,14]. The available literature lacks a comprehensive analysis of the serum concentrations among sTfR and IL-4 and iron metabolism parameters, as well as organ manifestations in SLE patients.

The aim of this study was to analyze the relationship among serum sTfR and IL-4 levels, disease activity, and organ manifestations in SLE patients.

2. Results

The characteristics of the study group are shown in Table 1.

The median concentration of sTfR was higher in the study group than in the control group ($p > 0.000001$). The median serum IL-4 concentration was higher in the study group than in the control group ($p < 0.00001$) (Table 2).

The analysis of the hematological parameters showed that SLE patients, compared to the control group, had a significantly lower count of red blood cells (RBC) ($p = 0.004$), hematocrit (HCT) ($p = 0.0004$), platelets (PLT) ($p = 0.04$), neutrophil ($p = 0.04$), and lymphocytes ($p < 0.0001$), a lower HGB concentration ($p < 0.0001$), and significantly lower values of indices including the mean corpuscular hemoglobin (MCH) ($p = 0.03$) and mean corpuscular hemoglobin concentration (MCHC) ($p < 0.0001$). There was no significant difference between the study group and the control group regarding the white blood cell (WBC) count, the mean corpuscular volume (MCV) index value, and the number of reticulocytes (Ret) (all $p > 0.05$) (Table 2).

The analysis of the iron metabolism parameters showed that SLE patients, compared to the control group, had significantly lower iron (Fe) concentrations ($p = 0.008$) and lower total iron-binding capacity (TIBC) values ($p = 0.03$). There was no significant difference regarding the unsaturated iron-binding capacity (UIBC) value, nor in the ferritin, transferrin (Tf), and transferrin saturation (TfS) concentrations between the study and the control group (all $p > 0.05$) (Table 2).

The SLE patients showed a positive correlation between serum sTfR and IL-4 levels ($p = 0.01$). There was no significant correlation between sTfR levels and the patients' age, disease duration, and IL-6 levels (all $p > 0.05$).

In SLE patients, a negative correlation was found between serum sTfR levels and HGB levels ($p = 0.0001$), HCT ($p = 0.008$), MCV ($p = 0.0001$), MCH ($p < 0.00001$), and MCHC indexes ($p < 0.00001$), and the lymphocyte count ($p = 0.0005$). A positive correlation was found between the sTfR and WBC count ($p = 0.03$), Ret count ($p = 0.001$), and neutrophil count ($p = 0.002$). There was no significant correlation between the serum sTfR and RBC, PLT, monocytes, and eosinophils levels (all $p > 0.05$) (Table 3).

Table 1. Clinical characteristics of systemic lupus erythematosus patients and healthy controls.

Assessed Parameters		Study Group n = 200 Mean ± SD Number (%)	Control Group n = 50 Mean ± SD Number (%)	p
Sex		F: 181 (90.5); M: 19 (9.5)	F: 44 (88.0); M: 6 (12.0)	0.6
Age (years)		46.97 ± 13.73	42.72 ± 12.48	0.5
Disease duration (years)		10.40 ± 9.10	-	-
SLEDAI		10.07 (5.81)	-	-
Constitutional		52 (26.50)	-	-
Mucocutaneous			-	-
	Any change	135 (68.90)		
	Malar rash	115 (57.50)		
	Discoid rash	12 (6.00)		
	Oral ulcerations	44 (22.00)		
Arthritis		155 (77.50)	-	-
Heart		80 (40.4)	-	-
Myocardial infarction		10 (5.0)		
Ischemic heart disease		17 (9.6)	-	-
Hypertension		65 (32.5)	-	-
Lung			-	-
	Any change	12 (10.0)		
	Interstitial changes	6 (3.0)		
	Nodular lesions	4 (2.0)		
	Pleural effusion	2 (1.0)		
Haematologic involement				
	Any change	139 (69.50)	-	-
	Hemolytic anemia	10 (8.50)		
	Deficiency anemia	82 (43.40)		
	Leucopenia	75 (37.69)		
	Lymphopenia	87 (43.50)		
	Trombocytopenia	42 (21.11)		
Vascular system		29 (14.8)	-	-
Neuropsychiatric		68 (34.34)	-	-
Renal lupus		43 (21.50)	-	-
Treatment				
Antimalarials		154 (77)	-	-
Cs		162 (81)	-	-
Azathioprine		30 (15)	-	-
Cyclophosphamide		43 (21.5)	-	-
MMF		10 (5)	-	-
Methotrexate		7 (3.5)	-	-
Cyclosporin A		4 (2)	-	-
Immunoglobulins		12 (6)	-	-
Epratuzumab		2 (1)	-	-

n: number; F: female; M: men; SLEDAI: Systemic Lupus Erythematosus Activity Index; Cs: corticosteroids, MMF: mycophenolate mofetil.

Table 2. Laboratory characteristics of systemic lupus erythematosus patients and healthy controls.

Assessed Parameters	Study Group n = 200 Mean ± SD Median (Q1, Q3) Number (%)	Control Group n = 50 Mean ± SD Median (Q1, Q3) Number (%)	p
Sex	F: 181 (90.5); M: 19 (9.5)	F: 44 (88.0); M: 6 (12.0)	0.6
IL-4 (pg/mL)	0.00 (0.00, 1.58)	0.00 (0.00, 0.00)	<0.00001
sTfR [mg/L]	2.15 (1.6, 2.83)	1.51 (1.22, 2.04)	<0.00001
IL-6 (pg/mL)	2.50 (0.89, 5.40)	0.84 (0.30, 1.26)	<0.00001
ESR (mm/h)	16.00 (8.00, 30.00)	6.00 (4.00, 10.00)	<0.0001
CRP (mg/L)	1.89 (1.00, 5.83)	-	-
Complement factor C3 (mg/dL)	97.45 ± 25.2	-	-
Complement factor C4 (mg/dL)	16.86 ± 7.52	-	-
Fibrinogen (mg/dL)	349.5 ± 108.4	280.0 ± 65.5	0.0001
Positive direct Coombs test	25 (27.17)	-	-
False positive syphilis test (VDRL)	2 (1.90)	-	-
Hematological parameters			
WBCs ($10^3/\mu L$)	5.71 (4.36, 7.46)	5.97 (4.73, 6.65)	0.7
Lymphocytes ($10^3/\mu L$)	1.36 (0.99, 1.82)	1.81 (1.57, 2.17)	<0.0001
Neutrofils ($10^3/\mu L$)	3.65 (2.55, 5.31)	3.33 (1.32)	0.04
HGB (g/dl)	12.67 ± 1.70	13.85 ± 1.08	<0.0001
RBCs (mln/μL)	4.39 ± 0.53	4.65 ± 0.40	0.004
HGB (g/dL)	12.67 ± 1.70	13.85 ± 1.08	<0.0001
HCT (%)	38.05 ± 4.51	40.49 ± 3.03	0.0004
MCV (fl)	86.93 ± 6.55	87.32 ± 4.24	0.7
MCH (pg)	28.97 ± 2.74	29.87 ± 1.67	0.03
MCHC (g/dL)	33.26 ± 1.32	34.21 ± 0.89	<0.0001
PLTs ($10^3/\mu L$)	227.4 ± 78.2	251.2 ± 55.6	0.04
Ret (‰)	10.00 (7.00, 14.00)	10.99 ± 5.07	0.5
Iron metabolism parameters			
Ferritin (ng/mL)	55.3 (23.6, 133.6)	43.1 (20.4, 109.6)	0.2
Tf (mg/dL)	260.0 ± 53.3	275.8 ± 54.6	0.06
Fe ug/dL	81.5 ± 46.2	100.7 ± 43.4	0.008
TIBC (ug/dL)	309.8 ± 64.6	331.0 ± 51.4	0.03
UIBC ug/dL	227.4 ± 84.0	230.3 ± 67.6	0.8
TfS (%)	27.40 ± 16.45	31.15 ± 13.01	0.14
Immunological assessment			
ANA IgG	198 (99.00)	1 (2)	-
Anti-dsDNA IgG	86 (45.70)	-	-
Anti-NuA IgG	57 (32.90)	-	-
Anti-Sm IgG	9 (5.10)	-	-
Anti-SS-A/Ro IgG	68 (39.10)	-	-
Anti-SS-B/La IgG	25 (14.90)	-	-
Anti-SS-A/Ro IgG	68 (39.10)	-	-
Anti-SS-B/La IgG	25 (14.90)	-	-
Anti-ARPA IgG	6 (3.50)	-	-
Anti-histones IgG	24 (14.00)	-	-
Anti-U1-snRNP IgG	22 (12.60)	-	-
Anti-CL IgG	49 (28.00)	-	-
Anti-CL IgM	66 (37.70)	-	-
Anti-ß2-GPI screen IgA, IgG, IgM	61 (35.30)	-	-

IL-4: interleukin 4; IL-6: interleukin 6; sTfR: soluble transferrin receptor; ESR: erythrocyte sedimentation rate; CRP: C-reactive protein; WBCs: white blood cells; HGB: hemoglobin; RBCs: red blood cells; PLT: blood platelets; HCT: hematocrit; MCV: mean corpuscular volume; MCH: mean corpuscular hemoglobin; MCHC: mean corpuscular hemoglobin concentration; PLTs: platelets; Ret: reticulocytes; Tf: transferrin; Fe: iron; TIBC: total iron-binding capacity; UIBC: unsaturated iron-binding capacity; TfS: transferrin saturation; VDRL: Venereal Diseases Research Laboratory; ANA: anti-nuclear antibodies; Anti-dsDNA: anti-double-stranded DNA antibodies; Anti-NuA: anti-nucleosome antibodies; Anti-Sm: anti-Smith antibodies; Anti-SS-A/Ro: anti-Rose antibodies; Anti: ARPA: anti-ribosomal P protein antibodies; Anti-CL: anticardiolipin antibodies; Anti-B2GP-I: β2-glycoprotein I antibodies; Ig A: immunoglobulin A; Ig G: immunoglobulin G; Ig M: immunoglobulin M.

Table 3. The results of correlation analysis between sTfR and IL-4 levels and hematological, and iron metabolism parameters in patients with systemic lupus erythematosus.

Assessed Parameters	Levels of sTfR [mg/L]		Levels of IL-4 [pg/mL]	
	Spearman's Rank Correlation Coefficient, R	p	Spearman's Rank Correlation Coefficient, R	p
WBCs (tys/μL)	0.15	0.03	−0.11	0.1
RBCs (mln/μL)	0.00	1.0	−0.07	0.3
HGB (g/dL)	−0.28	0.0001	−0.04	0.6
HCT (%)	−0.19	0.008	−0.04	0.5
MCV (fl)	−0.28	0.0001	0.01	0.9
MCH (pg)	−0.36	<0.00001	−0.01	0.9
MCHC (g/dL)	−0.40	<0.00001	0.00	1.0
Ret (‰)	0.23	0.001	0.01	0.8
PLTs (tys/μL)	0.04	0.6	−0.06	0.4
Neutrofils (10^3/μL)	0.21	0.002	−0.03	0.6
Lymphocytes (10^3/μL)	−0.24	0.0005	−0.06	0.4
Monocytes (10^3/μL)	0.02	0.8	0.04	0.6
Basophils (10^3/μL)	−0.15	0.04	−0.01	0.9
Eosinophils (10^3/μL)	−0.07	0.3	0.08	0.3
Ferritin (ng/mL)	−0.29	<0.00001	−0.04	0.5
Tf (mg/dL)	0.24	0.001	−0.09	0.2
TIBC (μg/dL)	0.24	0.0007	−0.09	0.2
Fe (μg/dL)	−0.39	<0.00001	−0.03	0.7
TfS (%)	−0.42	<0.00001	0.00	1.0
UIBC (μg/dL)	0.38	<0.00001	−0.05	0.5
sTfR (nmol/L)			0.17	0.01
Folic acid (ng/mL)	−0.02	0.8	−0.08	0.3
Vitamin B12 (pg/mL)	−0.07	0.3	0.00	1.0
CRP (mg/L)	0.08	0.3	−0.22	0.003
ESR (mm/h)	0.09	0.2	−0.07	0.3
SLEDAI	−0.02	0.7	−0.12	0.1

IL-4: interleukin 4; sTfR: soluble transferrin receptor; WBCs: white blood cells; RBCs: red blood cells; HGB: hemoglobin; HCT: hematocrit; MCV: mean corpuscular volume; MCH: mean corpuscular hemoglobin; MCHC: mean corpuscular hemoglobin concentration; Ret: reticulocytes; PLTs: blood platelets; Tf: transferrin; TIBC: total iron-binding capacity; Fe: iron; TfS: transferrin saturation; UIBC: unsaturated iron-binding capacity; CRP: C-reactive protein; ESR: erythrocyte sedimentation rate; SLEDAI: Systemic Lupus Erythematosus Activity Index.

The study group showed a negative correlation between the serum sTfR and ferritin concentration ($p < 0.00001$), Fe concentration ($p < 0.00001$), and TfS index ($p < 0.00001$). In SLE patients, there was a positive correlation between the serum sTfR and Tf concentration ($p = 0.001$), TIBC ($p = 0.007$), and UIBC ($p < 0.00001$). There was no significant correlation between serum sTfR levels and CRP levels, fibrinogen levels, ESR values, and folic acid and vitamin B12 levels (all $p > 0.05$) (Table 3).

The comparison of SLE patients with and without different organ involvement, and with different severities of organ manifestations, showed elevated serum sTfR levels in SLE patients with myocardial infarction ($p = 0.003$), ischemic heart disease ($p = 0.03$), lung involvement ($p = 0.02$), and hematological manifestations ($p = 0.002$). SLE patients with heart lesions ($p = 0.01$), myocardial infarction ($p < 0.00001$), pericardial effusion ($p = 0.01$), and ischemic heart disease ($p < 0.00001$) were older compared to SLE patients without these lesions (Table 4). However, there was no correlation between the age of the SLE patients and the serum concentration of sTfR ($R = -0.06$, $p = 0.3$). Only one SLE patient had the coexistence of pericardial effusion with myocardial infarction and heart failure.

Table 4. Comparison of serum sTfR and IL-4 levels in SLE patients with and without different organ involvement.

Organ Manifestations		Number of Patients	Age (Years)	p	Levels sTfR [mg/L] Median (Q1, Q3)	p	Levels of IL-4 pg/mL Median (Q1, Q3)	p
Mucocutaneous	-	61	46.43	0.5	30.34		0.34	
	+	135	47.36		28.34	0.12	0.00	0.01
	Malar rash	115	47.76	0.2	29.13	0.33	0.00	0.34
	Oral ulcerations	44	47.93	0.5	23.54	0.04	0.00	0.45
Heart	-	120	45.16	0.01	28.66	0.87	0.00	0.64
	+	80	49.98		29.45		0.00	
Myocardial infarction	-	173	45.96	<0.00001	28.62	0.0003	0.00	0.28
	+	10	67.20		43.02		0.00	
Number of myocardial infarctions	1	7	66.29	0.0002	51.29	0.0008	0.00	0.28
	>2	3	69.33		39.93		0.00	
Pericardial effusion	-	120	45.16	0.01	28.52	0.90	0.00	0.81
	+	73	49.98		29.45		0.00	
Ischemic heart disease	-	160	44.80	<0.00001	28.83	0.03	0.00	0.04
	+	17	66.82		38.04		0.00	
Lung	-	155	46.06	0.02	28.13	0.002	0.00	0.86
	+	12	56.92		36.82		0.00	
Type of lung lesions	Interstinal changes	6	46.43	0.08	33.44	0.46	0.00	0.75
	Other	6	52.75		34.01		0.00	
Haematological	-	107	47.48	0.09	23.71	0.002	0.00	0.66
	+	92	42.15		31.29		0.00	
Anemia	Haemolytic	10	37.50	0.05	32.40	0.003	0.00	0.84
	deficiency	82	47.33		18.27		0.00	
Thrombocytopenia	-	157	46.72	0.8	28.00	0.09	0.00	0.34
	+	42	47.64		32.02		0.00	
PLT (tys/μL)	<100	30	49.77	0.5	27.77	<0.00001	0.00	0.89
	≥100 <400	163	46.45		32.04		0.00	
	>400	7	47.14		61.13		0.00	
Leucopenia	-	124	48.02	0.1	28.67	0.37	0.00	0.54
	+	75	45.17		29.61		0.00	
Neuropsychiatric	-	131	46.66	0.5	30.27	0.27	0.00	0.56
	+	68	47.99		27.39		0.00	
Number of TIA or strokes	0	136	46.73	0.7	30.25	0.16	0.00	0.22
	1	51	48.22		23.71		0.00	
	>2	13	44.62		28.34		0.00	
Renal lupus	-	157	47.84	0.09	28.72	0.96	0.00	0.87
	+	43	43.79		30.29		0.00	

IL-4: interleukin 4; sTfR: soluble transferrin receptor; -: absence of organ involvement; +: presence of organ involvement; PLT: blood platelets; TIA: transient ischemic attack.

A multivariate logistic regression analysis and stepwise analysis showed that in SLE patients, elevated serum sTfR > 2.14 mg/dL was associated with an increased risk of myocardial infarction (OR: 10.6 95 CI 2.71–464.78; p = 0.001), ischemic heart disease (OR: 3.25 95 CI 1.02–10.40; p = 0.04), lung involvement (OR: 4.48 95 CI 1.44–13.94; p = 0.01), and hematological manifestations (OR: 2.07 95 CI 1.13–3.79; p = 0.01), and with a reduced risk of neuropsychiatric manifestations (OR: 0.42 95 CI 0.22–0.80; p = 0.008) (Table 5). In SLE patients, there was no significant correlation between serum IL-4 levels and IL-6 levels (all p > 0.05). In the study group, there was no significant correlation between serum IL-4 levels and the patients' age, disease duration, and the blood count parameters WBCs, neutrophils, lymphocytes, RBCs, HGB, HCT, MCV, MCH, MCHC, PLTs, and Ret (all p > 0.05) (Table 3). There were no significant correlations between serum IL-4 levels and other indicators of iron metabolism (all p > 0.05) (Table 3). No significant correlation was found between serum IL-4 levels and vitamin B12 or folic acid levels (all p > 0.05) (Table 3). In SLE patients, there was a negative correlation between serum IL-4 and CRP levels (p = 0.003) (Table 3). There was no significant correlation between serum IL-4 and fibrinogen levels or ESR values (all p > 0.05) (Table 3).

Table 5. A logistic regression model of the OR of the increased serum sTfR and IL-4 levels, and organ involvement in patients with systemic lupus erythematosus.

Organ Manifestations	Levels sTfR > 2.14 mg/L			Levels of IL-4 > 0.17 pg/mL		
	OR	95% CI	p	OR	95% CI	p
Constitutional	0.79	0.42–1.49	0.4	0.78	0.41–1.52	0.4
Mucocutaneous	0.74	0.40–1.35	0.3	0.48	0.26–0.90	0.02
Arthritis	0.74	0.38–1.42	0.3	0.76	0.39–1.47	0.4
Heart	1.14	0.65–2.02	0.6	1.04	0.58–1.86	0.8
Myocardial infarction	10.60	2.71–464.78	0.001	0.36	0.07–1.74	0.2
Ischemic heart disease	3.25	1.02–10.40	0.04	0.29	0.08–1.05	0.05
Hypertension	0.93	0.51–1.71	0.8	0.59	0.31–1.10	0.09
Lung	4.48	1.44–13.94	0.01	1.06	0.41–2.72	0.9
Haematological	2.07	1.13–3.79	0.01	0.96	0.53–1.77	0.9
Vascular system	1.47	0.66–3.26	0.3	1.34	0.61–2.97	0.4
Neuropsychiatric	0.42	0.22–0.80	0.008	0.59	0.31–1.13	0.1
Renal lupus	1.16	0.59–2.29	0.6	1.00	0.50–2.00	0.9

OR: Odds ratio, adjusted for gender and age; 95% CI: confidence interval; IL-4: interleukin 4; sTfR: soluble transferrin receptor.

In a multivariate logistic regression analysis model and stepwise analysis, elevated serum IL-4 and elevated serum sTfR were not associated with the presence of antibodies in SLE patients (all p > 0.05).

The comparison of SLE patients with and without different organ involvement, and with different severities of organ manifestations, showed elevated serum IL-4 levels in SLE patients with mucocutaneous manifestations (p = 0.01) (Table 4).

In a multivariate logistic regression analysis model and stepwise analysis, elevated serum IL-4 levels > 0.17 mg/L in SLE patients were associated with a reduced risk of mucocutaneous manifestations (OR: 0.48 95 CI 0.26–0.90; p = 0.02) (Table 5).

3. Discussion

Based on our knowledge, our work represents the first comprehensive study of SLE patients, and we revealed that elevated serum sTfR levels are associated with an increased risk of cardiovascular, pulmonary, and haematological manifestations, and a decreased risk of neuropsychiatric manifestations. Additionally, elevated serum IL-4 levels showed an association with a reduced risk of skin and mucosal lesions.

Systemic lupus erythematosus is an autoimmune disease, during the course of which the occurrence of hematological and other organ manifestations is a significant clinical problem, and a variety of cytokines, such as IL-4, IL-6, and interleukin 10 (IL-10), can have a significant impact on this.

We conducted a study of SLE patients in whom serum levels of sTfR and IL-4 were evaluated in association with selected markers of disease activity, namely, hematological and other organ manifestations, iron metabolism parameters, and antibodies.

SLE patients have hematologic abnormalities which can either appear as an independent symptom or accompany other clinical manifestations [3]. Tomczyk-Socha et al. [15] compared the prevalence of hematologic manifestations in 71 SLE patients with short and long disease duration in a Caucasian population. They found the presence of hematological disorders in 53.5% of SLE patients at the time of diagnosis. In SLE patients with short and long disease duration, they found anemia in 33.8% and 42.3%, respectively, leukopenia in 32.4% and 33.8%, respectively, and thrombocytopenia in 18.3% and 12.7%, respectively. In another study of SLE patients from Turkey, the presence of hematologic symptoms was found in 67.3% of the subjects, of which AIHA was present in 6.5% and thrombocytopenia in 18.0% of the patients [16]. In SLE patients from Morocco, Zian et al. [17] found hematologic disorders in 46.0% of patients, including AIHA in 16.0%, lymphopenia in 30.0%, leukopenia in 8.0%, and thrombocytopenia in 8.0%. In our study, hematological symptoms were present in 69.5% of SLE patients, including AIHA in 8.5%, anemia of other types (ACD, IDA and ACD with IDA) in 43.4%, lymphopenia in 43.5%, leukopenia in 37.7%, and thrombocytopenia in 21.1%. These results are in agreement with data presented by other investigators [15–17]. This confirms the influence of iron metabolism disturbances on the development of hematological changes in SLE patients.

Soluble transferrin receptor is the plasma-soluble form of the transferrin receptor and is an indicator of tissue iron deficiency. Elevated sTfR concentrations are indicative of an existing iron deficiency or IDA. In ACD, the concentration of sTfR is unchanged [6]. In our study, we found significantly higher serum sTfR concentrations in the study group compared to the control group. Elevated serum sTfR levels in SLE patients may be indicative of impaired iron metabolism, suggesting an iron deficiency or increased erythropoiesis. In SLE patients, elevated serum sTfR levels may suggest the presence of IDA [18–20]. In our study, we demonstrated a positive correlation between serum sTfR levels and IL-4 levels in SLE patients. In the available literature, we did not find any studies showing a direct association between sTfR levels and IL-4 levels in SLE patients. In Kuvibidila et al.'s [21] study conducted on an animal model, it was found that serum IL-4 was positively correlated with Fe, the HGB concentration, and the HCT value. The hemoglobin level is an anemia marker with low-sensitivity and low-specificity, and it is unable to distinguish the type of anemia. HCT is an unreliable indicator in the diagnosis of anemia [19]. Reduced serum Fe levels stimulate sTfR synthesis. Our results suggest that IL-4 may have a stimulatory effect on the development of iron deficiency anemia in SLE patients.

IL-4 is a monomeric glycoprotein produced by Th2 lymphocytes, NK cells, mast cells, and basophils [22,23]. Interleukin 4 is an anti-inflammatory cytokine that inhibits the production of pro-inflammatory cytokines and acute-phase proteins such as haptoglobin, CRP, and albumin [20]. Observations of the results of IL-4 concentrations in SLE patients obtained by different investigators are divergent [13,24–26]. Zhou et al. [25] obtained comparable results regarding serum IL-4 concentrations in SLE patients and controls. On the other hand, Guimarães et al. [24] showed significantly reduced serum IL-4 concentrations in SLE patients compared to healthy subjects. In contrast, other researchers showed that IL-4 serum levels in SLE patients were significantly higher compared to the controls, which is in agreement with our results [15]. The discrepancy in these studies indicates that further research into the role of IL-4 in the pathogenesis of SLE is required.

Arora et al. [26] found a negative correlation between serum IL-4 levels and disease activity, as measured using the SLEDAI scale, and linked this to the anti-inflammatory and immunosuppressive effects of IL-4. In our study, we found no significant correlation between serum IL-4 levels and patient age, disease duration, and disease activity, as measured using the SLEDAI scale, but we demonstrated a negative correlation between serum IL-4 and CRP levels, confirming the anti-inflammatory effect of this cytokine in SLE patients. This confirms the inhibitory effect of IL-4 on disease activity in SLE patients.

In a study by Zhou et al. [25], it was shown that patients with positive anti-double-stranded DNA antibodies (anti-dsDNA) had lower IL-4 levels compared to patients with negative results regarding anti-dsDNA antibodies. Thus, serum IL-4 is likely to have an inhibitory effect on anti-dsDNA antibodies formation. In our study, no such relationship was confirmed.

The determination of blood count and Iron metabolism parameters is crucial in diagnosing the type of anemia. Determining the type of anemia in SLE patients using conventional laboratory parameters is often difficult. The analysis of iron metabolism parameters in our study showed that SLE patients had significantly lower Fe and TIBC levels compared to the controls, which is in line with previous findings [4,27]. The results of a study conducted by Kunireddy et al. [4] in SLE patients showed significantly lower Fe, TIBC, and Tf levels compared to the controls, as well as elevated ferritin and hepcidin levels. In another study of SLE patients, elevated ferritin and reduced Tf and TIBC levels were observed compared to the controls [28]. In our study, there was no significant difference in the UIBC, Tf, or ferritin levels, nor in the TfS index between the study group and the control group. However, we showed that reduced ferritin levels were correlated with the risk of IDA, which is consistent with previous studies [4].

In the course of SLE, patients may develop lesions in multiple organs, but we do not have markers to predict that.

Iron disturbance is associated with abnormal cardiomyocyte function. Myocardial manifestations are most often accompanied by iron deficiency and/or anemia, which appear to be important factors contributing to a patient's deterioration. Recently, sTfR levels were proposed as a potential new marker of iron metabolism in cardiovascular diseases. In the AtheroGene study, increased serum sTfR levels were strongly associated with future myocardial infarction and cardiovascular death [7]. In our study, when comparing SLE patients with and without different organ involvement, as well as varying severities of organ manifestations, we found that SLE patients with myocardial infarction and ischemic heart disease exhibited elevated serum sTfR levels. Additionally, we showed that elevated serum sTfR levels (>2.14 mg/dL) were associated with an increased risk of cardiovascular manifestations, such as myocardial infarction and ischemic heart disease, in patients with SLE. This confirms the influence of iron metabolism disturbances on the development of cardiovascular changes in SLE patients.

The mechanisms causing alterations in iron metabolism in the development of lung disorders are incompletely understood [8]. An increased accumulation of pulmonary iron is considered to play a key role in the pathogenesis of idiopathic pulmonary fibrosis and lung function decline [8,10]. In the available literature, we found no data on iron homeostasis dysregulation in SLE patients with pulmonary involvement. In our study, the comparison of SLE patients with and without different organ involvement, and with different severities of organ manifestations, showed elevated serum sTfR levels in SLE patients with lung lesions. Additionally, we demonstrated that elevated serum sTfR levels (>2.14 mg/dL) were associated with an increased risk of pulmonary manifestations in SLE. Therefore, we can conclude that in SLE patients, iron deficiency in conjunction with the autoimmune process may influence the occurrence of pulmonary lesions. Conducting further studies to identify the role of iron metabolism in the development of lung changes in SLE would be necessary.

Abnormal iron metabolism is associated with several neurological disorders. Iron deficiency anemia is associated with severe neurological impairments such as mental, neurophysiological, and emotional dysfunctions [11]. On the other hand, iron overload is one of the common causes of refractory epilepsy in patients with hemorrhagic stroke. However, the correlation between epilepsy and iron metabolism is not yet clarified and needs further exploration [10]. In our study, elevated serum sTfR levels (>2.14 mg/dL) were associated with a decreased risk of neuropsychiatric manifestations in SLE. However, we did not observe a significant difference in serum sTfR levels in the comparison of patients with and without neurological changes. In our opinion, these results confirm the ambiguous role of iron metabolism in the pathogenesis of neuropsychiatric changes in SLE patients. Further research on this problem is needed.

The results of Kalkan et al.'s [29] study suggested that there is a possible association between the functional IL4 VNTR genetic polymorphism and oral mucosal diseases of Turkish SLE patients. In our study, we showed that elevated serum IL-4 levels (>0.17 pg/mL) are associated with a reduced risk of skin and mucosal lesions in SLE patients. This confirmed the influence of IL-4 on the development of mucocutaneous changes in SLE patients.

Conducting further studies to identify the cytokines involved in organ manifestation may be helpful in personalized immunotherapy for SLE patients.

The fact that we found an association between sTfR levels and the occurrence of organ changes in SLE patients, without a correlation of this parameter with disease activity as measured by SLEDAI, may allow us to consider sTfR determination as a potential prognostic marker for the occurrence of selected organ changes in SLE patients.

Our study's strength lies in it highlighting the association of iron metabolism disturbances with the occurrence of organ manifestations in SLE patients. The control of iron metabolism markers, such as serum sTfR, may be helpful in assessing organ involvement and predicting disease progression. Additionally, this suggests the necessity to address iron metabolism disturbances as another treatment goal for SLE patients. The results of our study were not always in agreement with data from the literature, indicating that the mechanism of this relationship must be complex and requires further research. Therefore, a further analysis of these correlations will be the subject of our further research.

Limitations

We acknowledge the limitations in our study due to the majority of patients having low SLEDAI scores. Consequently, we could not evaluate changes in the serum sTfR and IL-4 levels in patients with very low and very high disease activity, due to the small size of these groups. The majority of the patients were women, which is obvious because SLE occurs mainly in women. However, the limited number of male participants prohibits us from generalizing the obtained results to male SLE patients.

4. Materials and Methods

4.1. Patients and Controls

We studied 200 Caucasian patients with confirmed diagnoses of SLE and recorded data concerning their age, sex, disease duration, organ involvement, disease activity, and treatment. Recruitment of patients for the study took place during their routine visits to the outpatient clinic or at our rheumatology clinic. The control group consisted of 50 healthy individuals (44 females, 6 males), matched for age and sex with the study group and without data indicating organ changes. The ethics committee of the Pomeranian Medical University in Szczecin approved this study (KB-0012/11/13), and all participants provided informed consent.

The diagnosis of SLE was established according to the American College of Rheumatology (ACR) criteria of 1982 (modified in 1997) and the classifications developed by the Systemic Lupus International Collaborating Clinics (SLICC) of 2012 [30].

We assessed organ changes based on the SLIIC criteria, incorporating clinical, laboratory, and imaging data. Mucocutaneus manifestations encompassed the medical history of acute cutaneous lupus (malar rash and others), chronic cutaneous lupus (discoid rash and others), oral ulcerations, and nonscarring alopecia. Lung involvement was identified based on the presence of pleural effusions or pleural rub diagnosed using routine X-ray or computed tomography (CT). In addition, we documented data on nodular or interstitial lung lesions. Heart involvement was diagnosed based on the presence of typical pericardial pain lasting more than one day, pericardial effusion (confirmed through a two-dimensional echocardiography examination using a Philips Epiq 5 ultrasound machine), pericardial rub, or pericarditis observed in an electrocardiogram (ECG) (in the absence of other causes). Furthermore, we collected data on medical history related to hypertension, ischemic heart disease, and the number of myocardial infarctions. Renal lesions were diagnosed based on a 24 h urine protein output of 500 mg protein/24 h, or the presence of red blood cell casts. Neuropsychiatric involvement was considered based on clinical data of seizures, psychosis, mononeuritis multiplex (in the absence of other known causes such as primary vasculitis), myelitis, peripheral or cranial neuropathy (in the absence of other known causes such as primary vasculitis, infection, and diabetes mellitus), and acute confusional state (in the absence of other causes, including toxic/metabolic, uremia, drugs). Moreover, we collected data on medical history related to transient ischemic attacks and the number of strokes. Hematologic abnormalities were diagnosed based on assessments of blood morphology parameters, Coombs test results, and parameters of iron metabolism [30].

The disease activity of SLE was assessed according to the Systemic Lupus Erythematosus Disease Activity Index (SLEDAI) scale in a modified version: SLEDAI-2000 (SLEDAI-2K) [31].

4.2. Laboratory and Serological Diagnostics

For the estimation of sTfR, IL-4, and IL-6 levels, serum was stored at −80 °C until analysis using a sensitive sandwich enzyme-linked immunosorbent assay (ELISA) method using the Human sTfR Immunoassay Quantikine® ELISA kit, Human IL-4 Immunoassay Quantikine® ELISA kit, and the Human IL-6 Immunoassay Quantikine® ELISA kit (R&D Systems, Minneapolis, MN, USA).

IgG antinuclear antibodies (ANA) were assessed in a HEp-2 cell line contaminated with CVCL-0030 cervical adenocarcinoma human HeLa using indirect immunofluorescence assay (IIFA). Monospecific tests were also performed using the ELISA method to detect anti-double-stranded DNA (anti-dsDNA), anti-Sm, anti-SS-A/Ro, anti-SS-B/La, anti-nucleosome (anti-NuA), anti-ribosomal P protein, anti-histone, and anti-U1-RNP antibodies (EUROIMMUN AG Medizinische Labordiagnostika tests, Lűbeck, Germany). The reference values of ANA were established as absent when the titer was <1:160 and present when the titer was ≥1:160. The titers were divided into three groups: low titers from 1:160 to 1:320, medium titers from 1:640 to 1:1280, and high titers > 1:1280.

The profiles of anti-phospholipid antibodies (aPL), including anticardiolipin (aCL) and anti-beta 2 glycoprotein I (aβ2-GPI), were determined using the ELISA method (EUROIMMUN AG Medizinische Labordiagnstika tests, Lűbeck, Germany). The lupus anticoagulant (LA) was tested using coagulological methods according to the criteria of the International Society of Thrombosis and Hemostasis [32].

Additionally, blood was taken for the assessment of ESR (Westergren method), C-reactive protein (CRP) (turbidimetric nephelometry), fibrinogen (Clauss method), and complement factors C3 and C4 (nephelometry) levels.

Blood count examination was performed using an automated method with XN-2000 and XN-550 hematology instruments from Sysmex (Kobe, Japan), using fluorescence flow cytometry (FFC).

The following blood morphology parameters were determined: hemoglobin (HGB), hematocrit (HCT), red blood cells (RBCs), white blood cells (WBCs), and blood platelets (PLT). The following blood cell indices were determined: mean corpuscular volume (MCV), mean corpuscular hemoglobin (MCH), mean corpuscular hemoglobin concentration (MCHC).

The following parameters of iron metabolism were determined: iron (Fe), ferritin, (Tf), transferrin saturation (TfS), total iron-binding capacity (TIBC), and unsaturated iron-binding capacity (UIBC), using COBAS 8000 (Roche Diagnostics, Mannheim, Germany).

The vitamin B12 concentration and folic acid concentration were determined using the ECLIA method with COBAS 8000 (Roche Diagnostics, Mannheim, Germany).

4.3. Statistical Analysis

Data distributions were evaluated using the Kolmogorov–Smirnov test. Data are presented as means (SD) and medians (Q1, Q3). The R values of correlations were also determined. The groups were compared using a Student's t-test, Mann–Whitney U test, and Kruskal–Wallis test. The parameters were evaluated using a Pearson's chi-squared test (χ^2), logistic regression analysis, and stepwise analysis, and $p < 0.05$ was considered statistically significant. All statistical data were analyzed using STATA 11: license number 30110532736 (StatSoft Inc., Tulsa, OK, USA).

5. Conclusions

In SLE patients, elevated serum levels of sTfR were associated with an increased risk of cardiovascular, hematological, and pulmonary manifestations, and a decreased risk of neuropsychiatric manifestations. In contrast, elevated IL-4 levels were associated with a decreased risk of mucocutaneous lesions.

Author Contributions: A.W.-B. participated in the design and coordination of the study, carried out the immunoassays, performed the statistical analysis, and drafted the manuscript. M.B. participated in the design and coordination of the study, and helped draft the manuscript. H.P.-B. participated in the design and coordination of the study and drafted the manuscript. All authors have read and agreed to the published version of the manuscript.

Funding: This research received no external funding.

Institutional Review Board Statement: The study was conducted in accordance with the Declaration of Helsinki, and approved by the ethics committee of the Pomeranian Medical University in Szczecin (KB-0012/11/13).

Informed Consent Statement: Informed consent was obtained from all subjects involved in the study.

Data Availability Statement: The data used to support the findings of this study are available from the corresponding author upon request.

Conflicts of Interest: The authors declare no conflict of interest.

References

1. Kuhn, A.; Bonsmann, G.; Anders, H.J.; Herzer, P.; Tenbrock, K.; Schneider, M. The Diagnosis and Treatment of Systemic Lupus Erythematosus. *Dtsch. Arztebl. Int.* **2015**, *112*, 423–432. [CrossRef] [PubMed]
2. Stojan, G.; Petri, M. Epidemiology of systemic lupus erythematosus: An update. *Curr. Opin. Rheumatol.* **2018**, *30*, 144–150. [CrossRef] [PubMed]
3. Velo-García, A.; Castro, S.G.; Isenberg, D.A. The diagnosis and management of the haematologic manifestations of lupus. *J. Autoimmun.* **2016**, *74*, 139–160. [CrossRef]
4. Kunireddy, N.; Jacob, R.; Khan, S.A.; Yadagiri, B.; Sai Baba, K.S.S.; Rajendra Vara Prasad, I.; Mohan, I.K. Hepcidin and Ferritin: Important Mediators in Inflammation Associated Anemia in Systemic Lupus Erythematosus Patients. *Indian J. Clin. Biochem.* **2018**, *33*, 406–413. [CrossRef] [PubMed]
5. El-Shafey, A.M.; Kamel, L.M.; Fikry, A.A.; Nasr, M.M.; Galil, S.M.A. Serum hepcidin and interleukin-6 in systemic lupus erythematosus patients: Crucial factors for correction of anemia. *Egypt Rheumatol. Rehabil.* **2020**, *47*, 14. [CrossRef]
6. Braga, F.; Infusino, I.; Dolci, A.; Panteghini, M. Soluble transferrin receptor in complicated anemia. *Clin. Chim. Acta* **2014**, *431*, 143–147. [CrossRef] [PubMed]

7. Weidmann, H.; Bannasch, J.H.; Waldeyer, C.; Shrivastava, A.; Appelbaum, S.; Ojeda-Echevarria, F.M.; Schnabel, R.; Lackner, K.J.; Blankenberg, S.; Zeller, T.; et al. Iron Metabolism Contributes to Prognosis in Coronary Artery Disease: Prognostic Value of the Soluble Transferrin Receptor Within the AtheroGene Study. *J. Am. Heart Assoc.* **2020**, *9*, 015480. [CrossRef]
8. Ali, M.K.; Kim, R.Y.; Karim, R.; Mayall, J.R.; Martin, K.L.; Shahandeh, A.; Abbasian, F.; Starkey, M.R.; Loustaud-Ratti, V.; Johnstone, D.; et al. Role of iron in the pathogenesis of respiratory disease. *Int. J. Biochem. Cell Biol.* **2017**, *88*, 181–195. [CrossRef]
9. Berthou, C.; Iliou, J.P.; Barba, D. Iron, neuro-bioavailability and depression. *EJHaem* **2021**, *3*, 263–275. [CrossRef]
10. Chen, S.; Chen, Y.; Zhang, Y.; Kuang, X.; Liu, Y.; Guo, M.; Ma, L.; Zhang, D.; Li, Q. Iron Metabolism and Ferroptosis in Epilepsy. *Front. Neurosci.* **2020**, *14*, 601193. [CrossRef]
11. Shah, H.E.; Bhawnani, N.; Ethirajulu, A.; Alkasabera, A.; Onyali, C.B.; Anim-Koranteng, C.; Mostafa, J.A. Iron Deficiency-Induced Changes in the Hippocampus, Corpus Striatum, and Monoamines Levels That Lead to Anxiety, Depression, Sleep Disorders, and Psychotic Disorders. *Cureus* **2021**, *13*, e18138. [CrossRef] [PubMed]
12. Mohammadoo-Khorasani, M.; Salimi, S.; Tabatabai, E.; Sandoughi, M.; Zakeri, Z.; Farajian-Mashhadi, F. Interleukin-1β (IL-1β) & IL-4 gene polymorphisms in patients with systemic lupus erythematosus (SLE) & their association with susceptibility to SLE. *Indian J. Med. Res.* **2016**, *143*, 591–596. [PubMed]
13. Ul-Haq, Z.; Naz, S.; Mesaik, M.A. Interleukin-4 receptor signaling and its binding mechanism: A therapeutic insight from inhibitors tool box. *Cytokine Growth Factor Rev.* **2016**, *32*, 3–15. [CrossRef] [PubMed]
14. Sugimoto, K.; Morimoto, S.; Kaneko, H.; Nozawa, K.; Tokano, Y.; Takasaki, Y.; Hashimoto, H. Decreased IL-4 producing CD4+ T cells in patients with active systemic lupus erythematosus-relation to IL-12R expression. *Autoimmunity* **2002**, *35*, 381–387. [CrossRef] [PubMed]
15. Tomczyk-Socha, M.; Sikorska-Szaflik, H.; Frankowski, M.; Andrzejewska, K.; Odziomek, A.; Szmyrka, M. Clinical and immunological characteristics of Polish patients with systemic lupus erythematosus. *Adv. Clin. Exp. Med.* **2018**, *27*, 57–61. [CrossRef] [PubMed]
16. Pamuk, O.N.; Akbay, F.G.; Dönmez, S.; Yilmaz, N.; Calayir, G.B.; Yavuz, S. The clinical manifestations and survival of systemic lupus erythematosus patients in Turkey: Report from two centers. *Lupus* **2013**, *22*, 1416–1424. [CrossRef] [PubMed]
17. Zian, Z.; Maamar, M.; Aouni, M.E.; Barakat, A.; Nourouti, N.G.; El Aouad, R.; Arji, N.; Bennani Mechita, M. Immunological and Clinical Characteristics of Systemic Lupus Erythematosus: A Series from Morocco. *Biomed. Res. Int.* **2018**, *2018*, 3139404. [CrossRef] [PubMed]
18. Jain, S.; Narayan, S.; Chandra, J.; Sharma, S.; Jain, S.; Malhan, P. Evaluation of serum transferrin receptor and sTfR ferritin indices in diagnosing and differentiating iron deficiency anemia from anemia of chronic disease. *Indian J. Pediatr.* **2010**, *77*, 179–183. [CrossRef]
19. Mittal, S.; Agarwal, P.; Wakhlu, A.; Kumar, A.; Mehrotra, R.; Mittal, S. Anaemia in Systemic Lupus Erythematosus Based on Iron Studies and Soluble Transferrin Receptor Levels. *J. Clin. Diagn. Res.* **2016**, *10*, EC08–EC11.
20. Shin, D.H.; Kim, H.S.; Park, M.J.; Suh, I.B.; Shin, K.S. Utility of Access Soluble Transferrin Receptor (sTfR) and sTfR/log Ferritin Index in Diagnosing Iron Deficiency Anemia. *Ann. Clin. Lab. Sci.* **2015**, *45*, 396–402.
21. Kuvibidila, S.R.; Velez, M.; Gardner, R.; Penugonda, K.; Chandra, L.C.; Yu, L. Iron deficiency reduces serum and in vitro secretion of interleukin-4 in mice independent of altered spleen cell proliferation. *Nutr. Res.* **2012**, *32*, 107–115. [CrossRef] [PubMed]
22. Paul, W.E. History of interleukin-4. *Cytokine* **2015**, *75*, 3–7. [CrossRef] [PubMed]
23. Silva-Filho, J.L.; Caruso-Neves, C.; Pinheiro, A.A.S. IL-4: An important cytokine in determining the fate of T cells. *Biophys. Rev.* **2014**, *6*, 111–118. [CrossRef] [PubMed]
24. Guimarães, P.M.; Scavuzzi, B.M.; Stadtlober, N.P.; Franchi Santos, L.F.D.R.; Lozovoy, M.A.B.; Iriyoda, T.M.V.; Costa, N.T.; Reiche, E.M.V.; Maes, M.; Dichi, I.; et al. Cytokines in systemic lupus erythematosus: Far beyond Th1/Th2 dualism lupus: Cytokine profiles. *Immunol. Cell Biol.* **2017**, *95*, 824–831. [CrossRef] [PubMed]
25. Zhou, H.; Li, B.; Li, J.; Wu, T.; Jin, X.; Yuan, R.; Shi, P.; Zhou, Y.; Li, L.; Yu, F. Dysregulated T Cell Activation and Aberrant Cytokine Expression Profile in Systemic Lupus Erythematosus. *Mediat. Inflamm.* **2019**, *2019*, 8450947. [CrossRef]
26. Arora, V.; Verma, J.; Marwah, V.; Kumar, A.; Anand, D.; Das, N. Cytokine imbalance in systemic lupus erythematosus: A study on northern Indian subjects. *Lupus* **2012**, *21*, 596–603. [CrossRef] [PubMed]
27. El-Hady, A.; Sennara, S.; Mosaad, Y.; Mahmoud, N. Serum ferritin, transferrin and metabolic syndrome are risk factors for subclinical atherosclerosis in Egyptian women with systemic lupus erythematosus (SLE). *Egypt. Rheumatologist* **2019**, *41*, 35–40. [CrossRef]
28. Ripley, B.J.M.; Goncalves, B.; Isenberg, D.A.; Latchman, D.S.; Rahman, A. Raised levels of interleukin 6 in systemic lupus erythematosus correlate with anaemia. *Ann. Rheum. Dis.* **2005**, *64*, 849–853. [CrossRef]
29. Kalkan, G.; Yigit, S.; Karakus, N.; Baş, Y.; Seçkin, H.Y. Association between interleukin 4 gene intron 3 VNTR polymorphism and recurrent aphthous stomatitis in a cohort of Turkish patients. *Gene* **2013**, *527*, 207–210. [CrossRef]
30. Petri, M.; Orbai, A.M.; Alarcón, G.S.; Gordon, C.; Merrill, J.T.; Fortin, P.R.; Bruce, I.N.; Isenberg, D.; Wallace, D.J.; Nived, O.; et al. Derivation and validation of the Systemic Lupus International Collaborating Clinics classification criteria for systemic lupus erythematosus. *Arthritis Rheum.* **2012**, *64*, 2677–2686. [CrossRef]

31. Mikdashi, J.; Nived, O. Measuring disease activity in adults with systemic lupus erythematosus: The challenges of administrative burden and responsiveness to patient concerns in clinical research. *Arthritis Res. Ther.* **2015**, *17*, 183. [CrossRef] [PubMed]
32. Miyakis, S.; Lockshin, M.D.; Atsumi, T.; Branch, D.W.; Brey, R.L.; Cervera, R.; Derksen, R.H.; De Groot, P.G.; Koike, T.; Meroni, P.L.; et al. International consensus statement on an update of the classification criteria for definite antiphospholipid syndrome (APS). *J. Thromb. Haemost.* **2006**, *4*, 295–306. [CrossRef] [PubMed]

Disclaimer/Publisher's Note: The statements, opinions and data contained in all publications are solely those of the individual author(s) and contributor(s) and not of MDPI and/or the editor(s). MDPI and/or the editor(s) disclaim responsibility for any injury to people or property resulting from any ideas, methods, instructions or products referred to in the content.

MDPI AG
Grosspeteranlage 5
4052 Basel
Switzerland
Tel.: +41 61 683 77 34

International Journal of Molecular Sciences Editorial Office
E-mail: ijms@mdpi.com
www.mdpi.com/journal/ijms

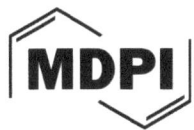

Disclaimer/Publisher's Note: The title and front matter of this reprint are at the discretion of the Guest Editors. The publisher is not responsible for their content or any associated concerns. The statements, opinions and data contained in all individual articles are solely those of the individual Editors and contributors and not of MDPI. MDPI disclaims responsibility for any injury to people or property resulting from any ideas, methods, instructions or products referred to in the content.